Gender and Psychopathology

Gender and Psychopathology

Edited by

Mary V. Seeman, M.D., C.M., F.R.C.P.C.
Vice-Chair, Department of Psychiatry
University of Toronto
Clarke Institute of Psychiatry
Toronto, Ontario, Canada

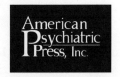

Washington, DC
London, England

Copyright © 1995 American Psychiatric Press, Inc.
ALL RIGHTS RESERVED
Manufactured in the United States of America on acid-free paper
98 97 96 95   4 3 2 1
First Edition

American Psychiatric Press, Inc.
1400 K Street, N.W., Washington, DC   20005

Library of Congress Cataloging-in-Publication Data
Gender and psychopathology / edited by Mary V. Seeman. — 1st ed.
      p.   cm.
   Includes bibliographical references and index.
   ISBN 0-88048-564-7 (casebound : alk. paper)
   1. Mental illness—Sex factors.   2. Sex differences (Psychology)
   I. Seeman, M. V. (Mary Violette), 1935-   .
   [DNLM: 1. Mental Disorders.   2. Sex Factors.   WM 140 G325
1995]
   RC455.4.S45G475   1995
   616.89′071—dc20
   DNLM/DLC
   for Library of Congress   95-4161
                                                                        CIP

British Library Cataloguing in Publication Data
A CIP record is available from the British Library.

To the memory of my father, Oles,
who was clearsighted and foresighted when it mattered,
but blind to frailty.

Contents

Contributors

William C. Friend, M.Sc., M.D., C.M., F.R.C.P.C.
Assistant Professor, Department of Psychiatry, McGill University;
and Director, Psychogeriatric Program, Douglas Hospital, Verdun,
Quebec

Jill M. Goldstein, Ph.D.
Assistant Professor, Department of Psychiatry, Harvard Medical
School, Consolidated Department of Psychiatry at Massachusetts
Mental Health Center, Boston, Massachusetts

Edith S. Lisansky Gomberg, Ph.D.
Professor of Psychology, Department of Psychiatry, School of
Medicine, University of Michigan, Alcohol Research Center, Ann
Arbor, Michigan

George Gurguis, M.D.
Assistant Professor, Department of Psychiatry, University of Texas
Southwestern Medical Center, Dallas, Texas

Ian Hacking, Ph.D., F.R.S.C.
University Professor of Philosophy, Institute for the History and
Philosophy of Science and Technology, Victoria College,
University of Toronto, Toronto, Ontario

Russell T. Joffe, M.D.
Professor and Chair, Department of Psychiatry, McMaster
University, Hamilton, Ontario

Sidney H. Kennedy, M.D., F.R.C.P.C.
Head, Mood & Anxiety Division, Clarke Institute of Psychiatry;
and Professor and Head, Mood Disorders Program, University of
Toronto, Toronto, Ontario

Richard R. J. Lewine, Ph.D.
Director, Schizophrenic Disorders Program; and Professor,
Department of Psychiatry and Behavioural Sciences, Emory
University, School of Medicine, Atlanta, Georgia

Barbara W. Lex, Ph.D., M.P.H.
Associate Professor of Psychiatry (Anthropology), Department of
Psychiatry, Harvard Medical School, Alcohol and Drug Abuse
Research Center, McLean Hospital, Belmont, Massachusetts

Carol C. Nadelson, M.D.
Clinical Professor of Psychiatry, Harvard Medical School; and
Editor-in-Chief, American Psychiatric Press; The Cambridge
Hospital, Cambridge, Massachusetts

Susan Nolen-Hoeksema, Ph.D.
Associate Professor, Department of Psychology, Stanford
University, Stanford, California

Malkah T. Notman, M.D.
Acting Chair and Clinical Professor of Psychiatry, Harvard
Medical School, The Cambridge Hospital and Harvard University,
Cambridge, Massachusetts

Mary V. Seeman, M.D., C.M., F.R.C.P.C.
Professor and Vice-Chair, Department of Psychiatry, University of
Toronto, Clarke Institute of Psychiatry, Toronto, Ontario

Colin M. Shapiro, M.B., Ph.D., M.R.C.Psych., F.R.C.P.C.
Professor, Department of Psychiatry, University of Toronto,
The Toronto Hospital—Western Division, Toronto, Ontario

Jennifer Shaw, M.D.
Formerly Staff Psychiatrist, Sunnybrook Hospital, University of
Toronto, Toronto, Ontario

Eileen P. Sloan, Ph.D.
Assistant Professor and Research Fellow, Department of
Psychiatry, The Toronto Hospital—Western Division,
Toronto, Ontario

Brenda B. Toner, Ph.D.
Associate Professor and Head, Women's Mental Health Research
Program, Clarke Institute of Psychiatry, Toronto, Ontario

D. Blake Woodside, M.D., M.Sc., F.R.C.P.C.
Assistant Professor and Director, Eating Disorder Inpatient
Program, The Toronto Hospital, Toronto, Ontario

Kimberly A. Yonkers, M.D.
Assistant Professor, Departments of Psychiatry and Obstetrics &
Gynecology, University of Texas Southwestern Medical Center,
Dallas, Texas

Preface

The proposed chapters in the original table of contents for this book, in its planning stages, were to constitute a perspective and commentary on current psychiatric nosology, highlighting the metamorphic role of gender. The undertaking was to involve working systematically through each diagnostic entity and critically examining gender effects on epidemiology, expression of symptoms, age at onset, sequelae, differential treatment, and treatment response. The original project proved to be unrealistic. Much was known about some categories of illness; little was known about others. The ideal was abandoned for the feasible, and, serendipitously, a many-splendored text arose out of the ashes of the initial plan.

The organization of the book is flexible. It allows the interested reader to start at any chapter and be cross-referred to analogous or opposing constructs in other chapters.

I have chosen to begin with an update on psychodynamic views on female and male development because differences in later psychopathology may owe their origins to divergences in early childhood. A historical chapter follows. Here, the author traces the concept of multiple personality disorder and shows how historical forces shape illness expression. Psychopathology is also shaped by mutant genes, and various non-Mendelian mechanisms are reviewed in the next chapter, although none seem, at present, to be able to explain such gender differences as are known to exist. Depression and anxiety disorders are traditionally associated with women. Two chapters on depression and one on the various forms that anxiety takes examine competing biopsychosocial theories of gender difference.

There is a disproportionate number of chapters on schizophrenia because a large amount of literature exists on the relatively subtle gender differences in this disorder and because there is some "hard" evidence (i.e., reproducible measurement differences) on brain scans and in postmortem studies.

Eating disorders, somatoform disorders, and sleep disorders further illustrate the complex ways in which gender effects can influence symptom expression. Finally, two chapters focus on addictions—addiction to alcohol and illegal substances, both more prevalent in men, and dependence on prescribed drugs, a disorder more common to women. The last chapter weaves the many themes together and points to fertile avenues of exploration.

I thank the American Psychiatric Association Press, particularly Dr. Carol Nadelson, for encouragement of this project. I would not have started this without Carol's continuing insistence. I am grateful to the contributors who worked diligently and kept their tempers through several rewrites. I thank Blanche Stuart, who ran the department while I worked on this volume, and I thank Tammy LePage for patience, industry, and found time. I am especially grateful to Jackie Ralph, who put it all together in the end.

I am indebted to my father and my mother who first taught me about gender. I am grateful to the women and men in my life, in particular my life's partner, Philip, and our sons, Marc, Bob, and Neil. Sex differences could not escape my attention in their company. As much as (so he says) my clinical fascination with schizophrenia shaped Phil's scientific discoveries, so, and much more, Phil's intense, unswerving pursuit of researchable questions led me to try to examine this most interesting question of all, why psychopathology differs in women and men.

CHAPTER 1

Gender, Development, and Psychopathology

A Revised Psychodynamic View

Malkah T. Notman, M.D.
Carol C. Nadelson, M.D.

Knowledge about personality development and the interrelationships between personality and psychopathology has increased substantially in the past few decades. Emerging views of development have incorporated psychoanalytic constructs and findings from developmental psychology and other fields. Although many areas of controversy remain, there appears to be agreement about the interacting and reciprocal influences of nature and nurture and the role of genetic endowment, cultural context, gender, relationships with family and others, and specific developmental experiences in shaping personality.

In this chapter, we provide an overview of gender differences in psychological development, emphasizing areas that appear to be related to differences in psychopathology. The framework is psychodynamic, integrating recent thinking as it has modified classical psychoanalytic theory.

1

Early Influences on Development

Early influences, both biological and psychosocial, help to shape personality. The presence or absence of continued, stable care; styles of child rearing; the richness, responsiveness, and nurturance of people and the environment; the presence or absence of physical illness, loss, and trauma; and biological endowment are all integral to the ultimate configuration of personality and to the evolution of a cohesive sense of self. Early developmental milestones, many of which are genetically influenced, such as motor and speech abilities, are also important; these milestones, in turn, influence the experience of the child. Complex integrative tasks, such as the capacity to conceptualize and learn language and social skills, derive from both biological and psychosocial influences and are determined very early in life.

The role of particular cultural practices, including gender differences in child rearing, are manifest from infancy. Differences in parental behavior, especially those related to concepts of male and female roles, are powerful forces contributing to differences in male and female development.

Emerging and expanding views of development have incorporated psychoanalytic constructs and findings from developmental biology, psychology, and other fields to evolve an increasingly cohesive framework for understanding. From the biological perspective, it has become clear that circulating prenatal hormones influence genital development, but they also influence gender development in a more complex way. The relational environment within the family and in the particular cultural group to which the child is exposed also affects the child's self-concept. Early in the history of psychoanalysis, the role of anatomy, particularly the genitals and the difference between the male genitals and the female genitals in determining gender development, was considered critical. Concepts have shifted away from the classical view that accorded the presence or absence of a penis and the child's interpretation of this reality with major significance in gender development. This classical view held that, after an initial period of development essentially similar in the two sexes, children notice their genital differences, and their perception of their body image is thereafter affected.

For the boy, fear of bodily injury, sometimes accompanied by the thought that this might be deserved punishment for forbidden impulses or wishes, may take the form of castration anxiety. Boys can be made anxious at the sight of girls' genitals, interpreting their anatomy as representing "loss" of the penis. Girls can be envious of boys' visible genitals and of their seemingly masterful functions. However, this is not inevitable or universal, and the envy can be aroused by the boys' perceived favored status in society rather than by the sight of the penis.

The little girl perceives that there are special advantages to being a little boy, and the genitals are symbolic of this. In classical psychoanalytic theory, the concept of penis envy is derived from the male perspective in which internal genitals are perceived as absent rather than as situated within the body. Thinking that female genitals are "absent," rather than present but hidden, is not consistent with the adult realization that other organs besides the genitals are internal and not visible, but present (e.g., the heart or the stomach). This thinking reflects a child's view that what is not seen does not exist in the same sense as that which is seen.

By the second and third year of life, the challenges of developing independence and learning to explore one's world while maintaining a consistent, predictable, and close relationship with parents are reflected in the process of separation-individuation (Mahler et al. 1975). Important aspects of this phase are the capacity to retain an internalized image of the parent that remains real even when the parent is physically absent and the ability to sustain a sense of closeness in the face of conflicting feelings. A disruption, such as illness, major loss, trauma, or family dysfunction, leads to increased vulnerability to later psychopathology, particularly depression and specific personality disorders (Adler 1985; Zanarini et al. 1989). For example, the connection between early trauma and the development of borderline personality disorder has been widely discussed in the literature (Gunderson and Sabo 1993; Herman 1992; Herman et al. 1989; Perry and Herman 1993).

Some characteristics of borderline personality disorder, which is more common in women than in men, are consistent with a hypothesis that developmental disruptions occur when an individual is traumatized early in life. These individuals characteristically have unstable relationships in which they swing between extremes of affect or behavior. They cannot tolerate being alone and are intensely fearful of abandonment. They appear to be unable to form reliable, integrated inner representations even of those close to them or to achieve object constancy (Clarkin and Kernberg 1993; Gunderson 1984). Why some people can apparently withstand early trauma with greater resilience than others is not well understood (Gunderson and Sabo 1993).

Gender Identity and Gender Role

The concepts of gender identity and gender role have become important in considerations of male and female development (Money and Ehrhardt 1972; Stoller 1976). Gender identity, that is, the sense of one's gender and what it means, is crucial in the development of a sense of self. Gender identity refers to the internalized sense of maleness or femaleness and the knowledge of one's biological sex, including the associated psychological attributes. Core gender identity is the earliest experience of gender identity. It evolves in early childhood as a developmental phenomenon; it is not entirely based on the resolution of the oedipal phase, as early analysts held (Stoller 1976). As the child gets older, gender identity continues to evolve.

Gender identity appears to be established by approximately age 1½ years, arising from many influences, including identifications with parents and their attitudes, expectations, and behaviors. Once established, gender identity does not appear to be reversible (Kleeman 1976; Money and Ehrhardt 1972). Evidence supports some hormonal basis for the development of core gender identity (Hines and Green 1991), although other determinants, including culture, are major contributors. As we indicated above, recent theoreticians have suggested that there are separate lines of male and female development from very early in childhood (Stoller 1976; Tyson 1984). That is, boys and girls have different experiences, and their gender impacts on many aspects of their relationships. Parents and others relate to even very young children in gender-specific ways (Block 1982). Note, however, that many aspects of male and female development are similar and overlapping.

Gender role is a culturally constructed concept referring to the expectations, attitudes, and behaviors that are considered to be appropriate for each gender in that particular culture. It is possible to have a clear sense of gender identity, as a male or female, and at the same time not be comfortable with this identity. It is also possible to feel some conflict about particular role behavior. One can behave in a traditional gender-stereotyped "masculine" or "feminine" manner, yet not be consciously pleased with or accepting of this behavior. One can also behave in ways that are departures from parental or societal expectations and, despite a conscious decision to adopt these particular behaviors, one can feel some conflict about them. For example, a man may decide to be an "involved" father and participate actively in child care, yet be uncomfortable, consciously or unconsciously, with the perceived societal disapproval of this "feminine" role. Similarly, a woman may choose to take an active, aggressive stance in her career or in politics, yet feel guilty about being successful and living a life that is not the same as her mother's.

Many factors influence the evolution of gender role. Kohlberg (1966) speaks of the cognitive task of self-categorization as a critical organizer of gender role, in association with cognitive maturation and adaptation to physical and social realities.

As we suggested above, there is some degree of gender polarization of roles in almost every society, although there are enormous cultural variations in the roles and expectations of men and women. Some societies dictate more rigid and fixed roles than others. Not all cultures value the same traits or see traits as gender specific in the same ways. The range of roles assigned to men and women in the world's subcultures is considerable. For example, despite their smaller size and lesser physical strength, in some cultures women are assigned the heavy work. The one consistent role assigned to women cross-culturally is child rearing (LeVine 1991), but the role and expectations of men with regard to child rearing vary.

In Western cultures, despite recent changes, fathers continue to take less active roles in early child rearing. This remains true despite the dramatic increase in the numbers of mothers of young children employed outside of the home (Kahne 1991). This gender role expectation has important implications that go beyond statements of conviction about equality and sharing between the sexes; it has an effect on the personality development of young children.

Because the mother is the primary caretaker, the first physical and emotional bond is likely to be made with her. She becomes the primary identification figure in early childhood, for both boys and girls. The father often continues to be a more distant figure. Thus, for girls, the first identification is with the parent of the same sex. For boys, the first identification is with the parent of the opposite sex and, consequently, with a parent who is different from him.

As the girl grows up, this same-sex identification does not have to change in order for her feminine gender identity to consolidate. That is, she learns, consciously and unconsciously, about being female via her identification with her mother. In order for the boy to consolidate his masculine identity, however, he must shift his primary identification away from his mother and develop an identification with a male figure. During this process, he moves away from his early attachment. This may leave some unresolved conflicts, particularly regarding dependency.

Many of these developmental experiences have been thought to lead to the personality differences that have been observed between men and women (Chodorow 1978). For men, a regressive pull toward their early attachments may bring about a struggle to reinforce the distance and separation they managed to achieve from their early ties to their mothers. Any pressure toward closeness and intimacy can seem threatening, as if leading inevitably to regression. For men, this often leads to a persistent need to define and maintain boundaries (Chodorow 1978). Consequently, qualitative distinctions in intimacy, "dependency," and attachment often exist between men and women.

It is interesting to note that gender identity disorders are more common in males than in females (American Psychiatric Association 1987). Perhaps this is related to the complex process of establishing a male identity and to the separation from early attachments that seems necessary to the process of the development of a masculine identity.

In the early years beyond toddlerhood, the child begins to relate to each parent differently. The period of growth up until age 5–6 years is accompanied by tangible development milestones, as well as emotional, cognitive, and social growth. In most cultures, formal education begins at about this time, when cognitive processes have become organized for formal learning and there appears to be a capacity for logical organization, with an ability to control activity and fantasy. This increases until puberty begins.

Gender segregation and gender role definition appear to be fairly well established by midchildhood. During this period, the child's functioning and interests extend beyond the family into the larger world. Friends, peers, teachers, and others add to the range of resources and models available to the developing child.

Although girls usually function better as students in the primary grades and present fewer behavior problems than boys, these characteristics reinforce social stereotypes. Thus, girls are expected to be more compliant and conforming, and this can inhibit the activity and ambition that lead to a sense of competence and self-esteem (Wellesley College Center for Research on Women 1992).

The relationship between mother and child changes in various ways as the child grows older. In many cultures, puberty rites function to demarcate the passing from childhood to adulthood, especially for boys. They also reinforce the separateness of male and female roles. A wide range of rituals generally remove boys from the society of women and place them into the world of men. In some cultures, boys are abruptly taken from the maternal environment, whereas in others, increasing a boy's involvement with the men of the group is a more gradual process, without physical separation from mothers.

Erikson (1964) described a model of development with stages from infancy to old age. He contrasted the boy's evolution toward independence and identity consolidation, later followed by the development of the capacity for intimacy, with the girl's maturational process in which the sequence is somewhat different. The girl, according to Erikson's original formulation, waits for completion of her own identity consolidation until later in her life, when she develops a relationship with a man. Erikson was criticized for not conceptualizing the development of the girl's identity in her own right, rather than in connection with the man in her life. He was, however, describing a prevailing pattern that has now been recognized as representing a real difference between girls and boys.

Because girls do not have to struggle against regressive pulls in their identification process in the same way that boys do, they appear to have a capacity for moving back and forth between the closeness and attachment to primary figures and the outside world (Blos 1980).

The girl has greater difficulty establishing her autonomy and independence while retaining important relationships. Aggression and anger may be difficult to manage because they threaten these relationships and generate anxiety about the possible loss of love and societal disapproval. It is particularly difficult for the girl to express herself and, at the same time, to remain close, especially when she experiences anger and aggression.

The primary and ongoing identification of the girl with her mother has been recognized as potent throughout development, even when it is negatively or ambivalently experienced. Normal female development builds on the ongoing importance of attachments and relationships (Gilligan 1982; Jordan 1991; Jordan et al. 1982). The normal sense of self in women evolves in the context of relationships in a way that appears to be different from that for men (Notman et al. 1991). Developing autonomy while negotiating aggression, anger, and competitiveness and sustaining attachments can thus present conflicts for the girl. The balance is difficult to achieve and may be seen later in life in women's conflict with anger and aggression, manifested in difficulty in being appropriately assertive and in inhibited risk-taking behavior (Nadelson et al. 1982). Qualities such as independence, initiative, and competitiveness have been considered positive characteristics for males in our culture but not for females.

Because of the primacy of relational ties, women also may be more vulnerable to loss throughout their lives. One of the syndromes that has been seen as related to the conflict about autonomy and independence and the sense of vulnerability to loss is agoraphobia, which is more commonly diagnosed in women than in men (Bourdon et al. 1988; Symmonds 1971). It represents anxiety about moving out into the world and feeling alone.

At times, women may fail to act in their own best interest because of their desire to preserve relationships, even those that are abusive. For some women, this can result in behavior that may continue to put them at risk for victimization. The threat of loss and women's conflict about aggression may motivate behavior that can be interpreted as masochistic, which diminishes self-esteem. Culturally supported passivity and inactivity, with consequent feelings of helplessness, can be risk factors for depression.

Problems in the development of self-esteem, for girls, appear to be intensified in adolescence (Gilligan 1987). The direction of women toward doing for others can also be one of sacrifice and service, with conflict about achievement, mastery, and pursuing one's own goals, in order to gain approval and not risk loss of love (Miller et al. 1981). When the mother is depressed, her child is at greater risk for developmental difficulties. Some children become stimulus seekers in an effort to generate responses and interest. Others identify with the depressed mother. Because women have often been devalued in society and even in their families, identification with a devalued mother has implications for self-esteem and may increase the potential for depression.

Gilligan (1987) found gender differences in her studies of self-concept and identity in adolescence. Males defined themselves in terms of individual achievement and work, and females saw themselves in relational terms. Gilligan found that girls in midadolescence experienced a "crisis of connection," with conflicts between "selfish" or individual solutions to relational problems and "selflessness and self-sacrifice."

Classic psychoanalytic theory viewed superego development as different in males and females. The idea that women's superegos were less advanced was proposed by Freud (1925/1961): "I cannot evade the notion . . . that for women the level of what is ethically sound is different from what it is in men. Their superego is never so inexorable, so impersonal, so independent of its emotional origins as we require it to be in men . . . [women] are more often influenced in their judgments by feelings of affection or hostility" (pp. 257–258).

More recent thinking has emphasized that men's and women's superegos are in some ways distinct, rather than that one is less advanced than the other. Gilligan (1982) described women's moral development as anchored in responsiveness to others. She viewed the self as developing toward connection and interdependence and suggested that male experience has a different emphasis. She contrasted the "justice voice" that predominates in men with the "care voice" of women. Her studies of adolescents reveal that although both voices are found in both sexes, the care voice is more frequently found in adolescent girls than in boys. Gilligan (1982) suggested that women's moral development occurs along a different line, in which concern about harming others is a more compelling criterion of justice than abstract ideals. This is consistent with the theory that women's development takes place within a relational context.

Body Image and Reproduction

Although we focus on puberty as the time for major changes in the body and in the body image, earlier experiences related to the body are very important. Sexual maturation does not occur all at once. Hormonal changes begin at age 8 or 9, or even earlier, and genital exploration and masturbation are part of normal development. For a time, the extent and importance of masturbation in girls were not acknowledged (Clower 1976). The girl's confusion about her genitals, because they were not as visible as the boy's, was accentuated by parental mislabeling or failure to name (Lerner 1976). This is part of our cultural taboo about female sexuality and its expression.

As puberty approaches, the girl's maturing body brings her reproductive potential into the foreground. Menarche signals a capacity for pregnancy, but this change also brings a potential vulnerability that is not part of the male experience. Girls are often told that the main reason for menarche is the potential for pregnancy. It is both a positive concept and a source of risk and anxiety. The girl also develops a new "organ," the breasts, which have no parallel in the boy. This transforms her body. It is both sexual and nurturant.

The effects of puberty, menarche, and the further elaboration of gender identity at this life stage continue to be important developmental organizers. The changing body and its representation as part of the self-concept contribute to the maturational process, which, in turn, contributes to the reorganization of the body image and the further differentiation of gender identity and role. Menarche organizes the girl's sense of sexual identity. It is also an undeniable physical experience, and it can be a source of conflict about growing up and about femininity. Many girls feel embarrassed, self-conscious, dirty, and messy but also feel pleased at the visible indication of their maturity.

The adolescent girl is constantly bombarded with media images of thin, glamorous women who are loved because of the way they look. A specific model of physical attractiveness continues to be more important for women than for men, for whom strength and performance are more valued. For both, self-esteem and self-confidence rest heavily on physical attributes and body image, especially during adolescence. As a girl enters adolescence, her mother is less likely to be seen by her as the authority on looks or acceptability, as peer influences become more important.

Conflicts about control and ownership of her body become more prominent during adolescence. Discomfort with body image and fear and ambivalence about mastery, independence, separation from family, and facing adulthood, including sexuality, are difficult issues that are thought to contribute to the dramatic incidence of eating disorders in adolescent girls, who may literally attempt to starve themselves back into childhood.

The acknowledgment of a women's reproductive capacity is an important component of her sense of identity and femininity, regardless of whether she actually bears children. The knowledge that there is a finite time for reproduction also influences her concept of time and her own life cycle. She must make decisions about career and family in a way that is different from that for men.

There has been a great deal of debate about the male and female sexual response. Stoller (1985) described the recognition of a greater intensity of the drive for genital sexual expression for the adolescent boy. The girl is described as being more invested in the relational aspect of the sexual experience than in genitally focused sexual responses. The importance of sexual performance to the maintenance of a sense of masculinity has been contrasted with the more relational sexuality of the female (Person 1980; Stoller 1985). For women, intimacy, affection, and pleasing their partner can be of greater importance than performance. Although sexual norms change, and women have become more concerned with orgasm and sexual satisfaction, the relational aspects have remained important (Notman et al. 1991; Person 1980). It is interesting that, until recently, sexual dysfunction was primarily a complaint of men. More recently, women have presented with sexual problems.

Adolescence can be a time of experimentation with sexual orientation, and both heterosexual and homosexual experimentation is frequent. For some, homosexual exploration is part of a developmental process leading to heterosexuality; for others, it marks the beginning of a homosexual identity.

Gender and Psychopathology: Some Examples

The appearance of depression and the effects of early life trauma can be understood as examples of prior problems and distortions of development. Depression is significantly more common in women than in men (see Chapters 4 and 5). In contrast, disturbances involving violent, aggressive behavior and problems with impulsiveness are more common in men (Weissman 1991). Conflicts about intimacy and socialization toward aggression and action are consistent with this.

Early trauma, especially sexual abuse (which is more common in women), the impact of the trauma itself, and the betrayal by parental figures or those in authority, can result in the failure to achieve a cohesive self-image and can have profound implications for future development and vulnerability. It can be understood as an etiological factor in the observation that survivors of childhood abuse are more likely to be victimized as adults (Herman 1992).

It has been suggested that the child needs to retain a good impression of the parent in order to blot out the distress and anguish that result from the abuse (Reiker and Carmen 1986). This distress can lead to anger against the self or others throughout life. Several studies report profoundly self-destructive behaviors emerging after victimization (Lystad 1986). Green (1978) concluded that "the abused child's sense of worthlessness, badness and self-hatred as a consequence of parental assault, rejection and scapegoating form the nucleus of self-destructive behavior" (p. 581).

The aftermath of abuse, particularly if the abuse is repeated, is often a residual sense of helplessness and a loss of autonomy (Nadelson and Notman 1979; Notman and Nadelson 1976). This may intensify conflicts about dependency and stimulate self-criticism, shame, and guilt in many areas of life. Difficulty handling anger and aggression and persistent feelings of vulnerability are also common repercussions.

The long-term responses to abuse appear to be different for women and men. Some data suggest that abused men tend to identify with the aggressor and are more likely to victimize others later, whereas women are more likely to establish relationships with abusive men in which they and their children are victimized (Jaffe et al. 1986; van Der Kolk 1989). This is consistent with the meaning of relationships for men and women and the importance of relationships for the development and maintenance of self-esteem, as well as the differences between men and women in the perception and expression of aggression and dependency (Chodorow 1978; Gilligan 1982; Miller 1981).

Conclusion

It is clear that gender-related developmental differences exist, although it is not possible to be definitive about their etiology. The nature versus nurture debate can only be resolved, we believe, by acknowledging the complex interaction of forces that shape an individual's life, rather than by oversimplified attribution of causality. Even if men and women live in the same cultures and families, they have unique biological and psychological environments. Their relationships differ from early infancy as do societal expectations, prohibitions, and reinforcements. They grow up with specific vulnerabilities deriving from their biology and their experience. Thus, their developmental experience is divergent and may lead directly or indirectly to some of the gender variations we find in psychopathology.

References

Adler G: Borderline Psychopathology and Its Treatment. New York, Jason Aronson, 1985

American Psychiatric Association: Diagnostic and Statistical Manual of Mental Disorders, 3rd Edition, Revised. Washington, DC, American Psychiatric Association, 1987

Block JH: Psychological development of female children and adolescents, in Women: A Developmental Perspective (NIH Publ No 82-2298). Edited by Berman P, Rainey E. Washington, DC, U.S. Department of Health and Human Services, Public Health Services, National Institutes of Health, 1982

Blos P: Modifications in the traditional psychoanalytic theory of female adolescent development, in Adolescent Psychiatry. Edited by Feinstein S. Chicago, IL, University of Chicago Press, 1980, pp 8–24

Bourdon K, Bloyd J, Rae D, et al: Gender differences in phobias: results of the ECA community survey. Journal of Anxiety Disorders 2:227–241, 1988

Chodorow N: The Reproduction of Mothering: Psychoanalysis and the Sociology of Gender. Berkeley, University of California Press, 1978

Clarkin JF, Kernberg OF: Developmental factors in borderline personality disorder and borderline personality organization, in Borderline Personality Disorder: Etiology and Treatment. Edited by Paris J. Washington, DC, American Psychiatric Press, 1993, pp 161–184

Clower V: Theoretical implications on current views of masturbation in latency girls. J Am Psychoanal Assoc 24:109–125, 1976

Erikson E: Inner and outer space: reflections on womanhood. Daedalus 93:582–608, 1964

Freud S: Some psychical consequences of the anatomic differences between the sexes (1925), in The Standard Edition of the Complete Psychological Works of Sigmund Freud, Vol 19. Translated and edited by Strachey J. London, Hogarth Press, 1961, pp 243–258

Gilligan C: In a Different Voice. Cambridge, MA, Harvard University Press, 1982

Gilligan C: Adolescent development reconsidered, in Adolescent Social Behavior and Health (New Directions for Child Development No 37). Edited by Irwin C. San Francisco, CA, Jossey-Bass, 1987, pp 63–92

Green A: Self-destructive behavior in battered children. Am J Psychiatry 135:579–582, 1978

Gunderson JG: Borderline Personality Disorder. Washington, DC, American Psychiatric Press, 1984

Gunderson JG, Sabo AN: The phenomenological and conceptual interface between borderline personality disorder and PTSD. Am J Psychiatry 150:19–27, 1993

Herman JL: Trauma and Recovery. New York, Basic Books, 1992

Herman JL, Perry JC, van Der Kolk BA: Childhood trauma in borderline personality disorder. Am J Psychiatry 146:490–500, 1989

Hines M, Green R: Human hormonal and neural correlates of sex-typed behaviors, in American Psychiatric Press Review of Psychiatry, Vol 10. Edited by Tasman A, Goldfinger SM. Washington, DC, American Psychiatric Press, 1991, pp 536–555

Jaffe P, Wolfe D, Wilson S, et al: Family violence and child adjustment: a comparative analysis of girls' and boys' behavioral symptoms. Am J Psychiatry 143:74–77, 1986

Jordan JV: Empathy and the mother-daughter relationship, in Women's Growth in Connection. Edited by Jordan JV, Kaplan AG, Miller JB, et al. New York, Guilford, 1991, pp 28–34

Jordan JV, Surrey J, Kaplan A: Women and Empathy. Wellesley, MA, Stone Center for Developmental Studies, 1982

Kahne H: Economic perspectives on work and family issues, in Women and Men: New Perspectives on Gender Differences. Edited by Notman MT, Nadelson CC. Washington, DC, American Psychiatric Press, 1991, pp 9–22

Kleeman J: Freud's views on early female sexuality in the light of direct child observation. J Am Psychoanal Assoc 24:3–27, 1976

Kohlberg L: A cognitive-developmental analysis of children's sex-role concepts and attitudes, in The Development of Sex Differences. Edited by Maccoby E. Stanford, CA, Stanford University Press, 1966, pp 82–172

Lerner H: Parental mislabelling of female genitals as a determinant of penis envy and learning inhibitions in women. J Am Psychoanal Assoc 24:269–283, 1976

LeVine RA: Gender differences: interpreting anthropological data, in Women and Men: New Perspectives on Gender Differences. Edited by Notman MT, Nadelson CC. Washington, DC, American Psychiatric Press, 1991, pp 1–8

Lystad M (ed): Violence in the Home: Interdisciplinary Perspectives. New York, Brunner/Mazel, 1986

Mahler M, Pine F, Bergman A: The Psychological Birth of the Human Infant. New York, Basic Books, 1975

Miller JB, Notman MT, Nadelson CC, et al: Some considerations of self-esteem and aggression in women, in Changing Concepts in Psychoanalysis. Edited by Klebanow S. New York, Gardner Press, 1981, pp 157–167

Money J, Ehrhardt AA: Man and Woman, Boy and Girl: The Differentiation and Dimorphism of Gender Identity From Concept to Maturity. Baltimore, MD, Johns Hopkins University Press, 1972

Nadelson CC, Notman MT: Psychoanalytic considerations of the response to rape. International Review of Psychoanalysis (NIM) 6:97–103, 1979

Nadelson CC, Notman MT, Miller JB, et al: Aggression in women: conceptual issues and clinical impressions, in The Woman Patient, Vol 3. Edited by Notman MT, Nadelson CC. New York, Plenum, 1982, pp 17–28

Notman MT, Nadelson CC: The rape victim: psychodynamic considerations. Am J Psychiatry 133:408–413, 1976

Notman MT, Klein R, Jordan JV, et al: Women's unique developmental issues across the life cycle, in American Psychiatric Press Review of Psychiatry, Vol 10. Edited by Tasman A, Goldfinger SM. Washington, DC, American Psychiatric Press, 1991, pp 556–577

Perry JC, Herman JL: Trauma and defense in the etiology of borderline personality disorder, in Borderline Personality Disorder: Etiology and Treatment. Edited by Paris J. Washington, DC, American Psychiatric Press, 1993, pp 123–140

Person E: Sexuality as the mainstay of identity: psychoanalytic perspectives. Signs 5:605–630, 1980

Reiker P, Carmen E: The victim-to-patient process: the disconfirmation and transformation of abuse. Am J Orthopsychiatry 56:360–370, 1986

Stoller RJ: Primary femininity. J Am Psychoanal Assoc 24:59–78, 1976

Stoller RJ: Observing the Erotic Imagination. New Haven, CT, Yale University Press, 1985

Symmonds A: Phobias after marriage—women's declaration of dependence. Am J Psychoanal 31:144–152, 1971

Tyson P: A developmental line of gender identity, gender role, and choice of love object. J Am Psychoanal Assoc 30:61–86, 1984

van Der Kolk BA: The compulsion to repeat the trauma: re-enactment, revictimization, and masochism. Psychiatr Clin North Am 12:389–411, 1989

Weissman MM: Gender differences in the rates of mental disorders, in Assessing Future Research Needs: Mental and Addictive Disorders in Women. Washington, DC, Institute of Medicine, 1991, pp 8–13

Wellesley College Center for Research on Women: How Schools Shortchange Girls. Washington, DC, American Association of University Women, 1992

Zanarini M, Gunderson JM, Frankenburg F, et al: Childhood experiences of borderline patients. Compr Psychiatry 30:18–25, 1989

CHAPTER 2

Multiple Personality and Gender

A Historical Approach

Ian Hacking, Ph.D., F.R.S.C.

lmost all historical cases, known from the literature, that appear to satisfy the criteria for dissociative identity disorder in DSM-IV (American Psychiatric Association 1994) have been women. The ratio of women to men is 9:1. In addition, it is now common for these patients to develop a large number of alter personalities or personality fragments, some of which are of the opposite sex. Are these instabilities in sexuality a superficial phenomenon, or is sexual ambivalence integral to the disorder and its causes?

Multiple personality disorder (MPD) was recognized in DSM-III (American Psychiatric Association 1980) and relabeled dissociative identity disorder (DID) in DSM-IV. It is not acknowledged in ICD-10 (World Health Organization 1992). For criticism of this omission, see Coons (1990), Garcia (1990), Spiegel (1990), and Young (1990). The DSM-IV criteria are listed in Table 2–1.

In all nineteenth-century cases, alter personalities had at least one-way amnesia; for example, the less lively alter personality would have no memory of the actions of the more lively one. Sometimes the personalities were mutually amnesic. Various types of partial amnesia

Table 2–1. DSM-IV diagnostic criteria for dissociative identity disorder

A. The presence of two or more distinct identities or personality states (each with its own relatively enduring pattern of perceiving, relating to, and thinking about the environment and self).
B. At least two of these identities or personality states recurrently take control of the person's behavior.
C. Inability to recall important personal information that is too extensive to be explained by ordinary forgetfulness.
D. The disturbance is not due to the direct physiological effects of a substance (e.g., blackouts or chaotic behavior during alcohol intoxication) or a general medical condition (e.g., complex partial seizures).

Source. Reprinted from American Psychiatric Association: *Diagnostic and Statistical Manual of Mental Disorders, 4th Edition.* Washington, DC, American Psychiatric Association, 1994, p. 487. Used with permission.

remain the rule among DID patients. DSM-IV has included inability to recall as a third necessary condition for the diagnosis, a requirement that was absent in DSM-III-R (American Psychiatric Association 1987) but present in DSM-III. The most obvious difference between cases reported in the early literature and the present is that, formerly, there were seldom more than two or three alter personalities. In the most recent large questionnaire survey, the average number of personalities at the time of reporting was 15.7 ($N = 236$) (Ross et al. 1989). Patients with approximately 100 alter personalities or personality fragments are mentioned (Kluft 1988).

Multiple personality was rarely reported before 1970. Only in the past decade has MPD become widely diagnosed, and then only in North America. This increased awareness is reflected in the growth of the International Society for the Study of Multiple Personality Disorder and Dissociation. Its scientific journal, *Dissociation,* is now in its fifth year of publication. There is now a widely recognized textbook on diagnosis and treatment of MPD (Putnam 1989). The question of why far more women are diagnosed with this condition than are men is beginning to be studied.

In one extreme view, well represented by Ross and colleagues (1989), MPD is one of the most readily identifiable of dissociative disorders. Ross and colleagues have found definitive examples in records from ancient Egypt. They argue that, in many cultures, dissociation and even multiple personality are manifested in the diverse states that Western anthropologists have varyingly called possession, trance, shamanism, and so forth. Thus, in Ross' and his colleagues' view, the prevalence of the syndrome is relatively insensitive to cultural surroundings, although its expression will be culture specific. Ross and his co-workers (1990) have developed a diagnostic tool—Dissociative Disorders Interview Schedule (DDIS)—that may be used in conjunction with an older screening instrument, the Dissociative Experiences Scale (DES; Bernstein and Putnam 1986). A midscore on the DDIS correlates strongly with the diagnosis. Ross and associates (1992) conjectured that the incidence of DID in North America may be as high as 2% and even higher among college students.

Others doubt not only the incidence but the diagnosis itself. Of 73 inpatient admissions seen by Ross in 1987, 8 were given the diagnosis of MPD; no other doctor at his hospital diagnosed MPD in any patients (Ross 1987). It must be pointed out, too, that the average age of the sample of 385 "college students" was 27, suggesting an atypical sample (Ross et al. 1992). Merskey (1992) maintains that MPD has become a culturally reinforced mode of manifesting distress, buttressed not only in clinics but also in the popular media. He believes the diagnosis is never warranted. He does not believe that the behavior is feigned but rather that mental health professionals provide an environment in which fragmenting into a number of antagonistic and even mutually amnesic personalities can flourish. In his opinion, these patients could be more effectively helped by actively discouraging, rather than encouraging, the florid development of a number of alter personalities.

Two other attitudes about this condition should be noted. One is that MPD (or DID) is a real and extremely rare condition, with a fairly constant incidence in Western industrialized societies for over two centuries. The psychiatrists who treated the famous case of Eve (Thigpen and Cleckly 1957) forcefully stated that opinion and held that almost all recent diagnoses are unfounded (Thigpen and Cleckly 1984). A quite different attitude is that dissociation and multiplicity form a continuum of which MPD is only one extreme. Multiplicity is the human condition, as stated by Crabtree (1985). From a philosophical perspective, DID is perhaps even to be expected (Dennett

1991). From a more clinical point of view, we all have subpersonalities, which, in times of trouble, benefit from developing in a therapeutic setting (Rowan 1990).

The two opposed extremes—complete skepticism and commitment to the diagnosis—are stated and defended, not only in medical circles but also by distinguished psychiatrists writing in semipopular journals (see, e.g., Putnam 1992 and McHugh 1992).

Beliefs about DID touch on larger issues. It has been firmly established—for clinicians who believe in the diagnosis—that the disorder is primarily a consequence of childhood trauma, usually early and repeated child abuse, and especially sexual abuse within the child's family network. According to Kluft's four-factor model, MPD (DID) begins in childhood and occurs when 1) a child able to dissociate is exposed to overwhelming stimuli; 2) these stimuli cannot be managed by less drastic defenses; 3) dissociated contents become linked to underlying substrates for personality organization; and 4) there are no restorative influences, or there are too many "double-binds" (Kluft 1984). Putnam and associates' (1986) questionnaire showed that of 100 patients with MPD, 96 reported early childhood trauma, usually including sexual abuse. All data subsequently published are consistent with an etiology of early and repeated child sexual abuse. The correlation has become so well accepted that, in relatively informal public presentations, clinicians often speak as if early sexual abuse were part of the very definition of DID.

Hence, this disorder transcends medical territory. The question of the prevalence of child abuse, especially incest, has become political, moral, and ideological. It has become a controversial issue in practical and theoretical feminism. Let us recall some recent history (Hacking 1991a). Child abuse, in the form of battered baby syndrome, was drawn to public and medical attention in 1961 (Kempe et al. 1962). Incest came to be regarded as a form of child abuse only in the late 1970s, as a consequence of the work of feminist activists, such as Rush (1980) and Herman (1981). Herman (1992, p. 9) states that "the systematic study of psychological trauma therefore depends upon the support of a political movement."

The diagnosis of DID is therefore seen to be connected with different possible stances about the family and about the relationships between men and women in industrialized Western societies. One active clinician believes that child abuse and associated DID are symptomatic of the socialization of women into subservient roles (Rivera 1991). These concerns extend in other directions as well. Herman (1992) addresses one current approach to forgotten trauma—the concept of posttraumatic stress disorder (PTSD). This concept is applied to battered women, combat veterans, terrorist hostages, concentration camp survivors, and adults who were abused during childhood. DID is seen as a type of dissociation closely allied to, and perhaps a variant of, PTSD. In one view, MPD (DID) is simply the most extreme form of PTSD (Spiegel 1984). Conversely, PTSD has been described as an "adult-onset analogue" to MPD (Branscomb 1992).

Most authorities who work with DID patients expect that significant traumata have been forgotten. Appropriate therapy involves recollection and abreaction of traumatic events, followed by a maturing ability to live with the recollections. This type of therapy has been standard for two decades and goes back at least as far as Prince (1905), who was deeply influenced by Janet (1889). Prior to any attempt at integration or resolution, patients are now encouraged to become aware of a large number of alter personalities, each of which is a reaction to a specific trauma. The alter personalities themselves provide a window through which to recall forgotten incidents of abuse. Because these recollections commonly involve allegations about living family members, they are not easily contained in the clinical setting. Relatives who deny the recollected incidents propose that the memories are delusions that have been cultivated by the patient and therapist. At the time of this writing, this issue is provoking increasingly sharp confrontations.

Other matters are also contested. Even if we consider only the pathologies discussed in other chapters of this book, we have disputes over territory. It is urged, for example, that although MPD had been a viable diagnosis in the United States until the end of the first quarter of the twentieth century, it was replaced by the diagnosis of schizophrenia (Rosenbaum 1980). It is argued that patients wrongly diagnosed with schizophrenia must be rediagnosed with DID.

Woodside and Kennedy (see Chapter 11) provide a classic account of eating disorders. They do not even consider dissociation, although they do mention child abuse. An alternative view, associated with an increasingly widely practiced therapy, holds that eating disorders are often consequences of child abuse and that many patients with eating disorders have latent multiple personalities (Torem 1990). Indeed, the resistance of many anorexic patients to therapy is explained by the fact that one alter personality is telling the host personality not to eat, while another is telling it to binge eat.

It is not common, in survey chapters such as this one, to state political, ideological, and territorial disputes at the outset. In the case of DID, however, it would have been irresponsible not to do so.

Incidence

At present, it is not possible to determine the epidemiology of DID. The best predictor of DID diagnosis is a practitioner, clinic, or center that specializes in the disorder. This in no way implies that the disorder is iatrogenic, a proposition that has been firmly refuted (Kluft 1989). It is universally agreed that many DID patients initially fit other diagnoses and may also have concurrent disorders. Diagnosis may require special sensitivity or training. There is, moreover, a strong element of patient-therapist selection: in many communities in North America, a well-established network of information enables patients who suspect such symptoms to reject earlier diagnoses and to gravitate to sympathetic clinicians. One may thus state, without taking any position on the nature of the disorder, that there is no terrain-neutral DID epidemiology.

Before 1970

Writers on MPD (DID) commonly allude to a canonical list of early cases, all of which involved women patients. The cases have been well summarized by Ellenberger (1970). They begin with the once much discussed case of Gmelin (1791). Most famous is the American, Mary Reynolds (Mitchill 1817). There is Estelle (Despine 1844), Félida X (Azam 1876), Léonie (Janet 1889), Miss Beauchamp (Prince 1905) and another patient of Prince (Bean 1908), Norma (Goddard 1926), Mrs. X (Wholey 1933), and Eve (Thigpen and Cleckly 1957).

After 1887, there was, interestingly, a population in French clinical practice that matched MPD (DID), but in which males predominated. The disorder was known as fugue (Tissié 1887) or *automatisme ambulatoire* (Charcot 1888, 1889). In a survey of 94 published French cases of fugue in 1850–1910 (excluding 3 prima facie cases of DID) there were 74 males and 20 females (Beaune 1987). Historical analysis has determined that similar figures exist in Italy (1890–1914), Germany (1895–1914), and Russia (1902–1914) (with fugue having become a clinical entity in those countries only during the periods indicated). In America, where the diagnosis of fugue was not in use, many males described as having double consciousness or multiple personality would now be said to have had amnesia or fugue episodes—for example, Ansel Bourne (Hodgson 1891), Henry Rowlands (Angell 1910), and Charles Poulting (Franz 1933), who also had organic brain disease (Lewis 1953).

After 1970

Cornelia Wilbur's patient Sybil (Schreiber 1973) ushered in a new era in three distinct ways. First, her analysis established a close connection between Sybil's multiple personalities and her sexual abuse as a child. Second, Sybil had 17 personalities, far more than reported for any previous patient. Third, she had two alter personalities of the opposite sex. The emphasis on all three features was relatively novel, but it has been characteristic of DID since that time. What Boor (1982) called a "multiple personality epidemic" followed. With a far larger series of patients on which to draw, gender prevalence could be determined. As can be seen in the gender ratios of seven series presented in Table 2–2, most patients are women.

Explanations

Most people who have received the diagnosis of MPD (DID) have been women. Why? Many explanations have been proposed, and all are heavily influenced by background opinions. The following explanations are by no means mutually exclusive and the order of presentation is random:

Table 2–2. Female prevalence of multiple personality disorder (dissociative identity disorder)

Practitioners	Total number of cases reported	Number of females
Bliss (1980)	14	14
Bliss (1984)	32	20
Stern (1984)	8	7
Horevitz and Braun (1984)	33	24
Kluft (1984)	33	25
Putnam et al. (1986)	100	92
Ross et al. (1989)	236	207

Note. The first five entries are series observed by a single practitioner or clinic; the last two are based on responses to questionnaires.

++ *Choice in a cultural milieu.* At any time, people who experience severe psychological distress that is not of biological origin "choose" culturally available and clinically reinforced ways to express this distress. Women prefer various types of dissociative behavior (Berman 1974). Men choose other ways of expressing distress. During the nineteenth and twentieth centuries, for example, men often expressed their distress through alcoholism; in the late nineteenth century, women often expressed their distress through hysteria; however, now, in the late twentieth century, women often express their distress through dissociative symptoms. There may be a parallel diagnostic mutation, also associated with social factors, from neurasthenia to chronic fatigue syndrome (Wessley 1990). It is further suggested that current stereotypes of male and female behavior determine the expression of psychological distress.

++ *Migration to the criminal justice system in DID males* (Wilbur 1985). This thesis (DID male violence brings them to jail) is accompanied by the observation that the anger of female DID patients tends to be self-directed, with self-mutilation being quite common. One report focuses on men with DID who have never been arrested or behaved violently (Loewenstein 1990). These 22 cases do, however, confirm the pattern of men's not seeking help from within the mental health system, except in connection with related difficulties such as alcohol abuse or marital discord.

↔ *Etiology.* DID is strongly associated with early and repeated child abuse, especially sexual abuse. Far more girls are thought to be subject to this type of abuse than boys. Traditionally, the ratio has been stated to be about 9:1. This provides a standard explanation of the 9:1 sex ratio among diagnosed DID patients. Ross and co-workers (1989, p. 97), however, suggest that "the clinical ratio will probably drop over the next decade as MPD is diagnosed in prisons and other settings." They note that hypnotizability is strongly correlated with MPD and with scores on the DES (Bernstein and Putnam 1986). They argue: "Given that men and women are equally hypnotizable and do not appear to differ in dissociative experiences in the general population, the sex ratio of MPD ought to be about the same as the ratio for abuse (somewhere between 1:1 and 9:1)" (Ross et al. 1989, p. 97).

↔ *Suggestion.* Even though DID is not strictly iatrogenic, critics attend to statements by clinicians like, "MPD patients rarely come for treatment with obvious or overt multiplicity" (Ross et al. 1989, p. 93). Skeptics suppose that there is a strong element of suggestion (a concept not rigorously defined) in the patient-therapist relationship. Why then do more women than men have DID? Perhaps women request help for a variety of inner-directed problems that respond readily to suggestion. There may also be the implication that troubled North American women in a therapeutic or clinical setting, even one that rigorously tries to avoid a stereotypical power structure, may cooperate more readily with therapeutic expectations than men experiencing comparable distress.

Discussion

A Changing Ratio of Females to Males?

Ample evidence suggests that, in the short run, an increasing proportion of the symptoms in males will be diagnosed as DID. Ross, quoted above, has mentioned an interest in prison populations, which are primarily male. There are also mostly male patients treated in United States Veterans Administration hospitals where PTSD has become a common diagnosis. An increasing proportion of PTSD diagnoses are being supplemented by a diagnosis of DID. In another direction, there is a growing interest in DID in children and adolescents. In a short series of adolescents with DID, 7 of 11 were male (Dell and Eisenhower 1990). In a series of children with multiple personalities, 4 of 6 were male (Tyson 1992). Abuse of male children by their mothers may also become an increasingly pertinent factor as this concept is applied to the treatment of men in unsatisfactory marriages who become alcoholic patients and womanizers (Brodie 1992).

Historical Perspectives

Hacking (1992) distinguishes four "waves" of multiple personality, of which the present one is the most striking. There is 1) double consciousness in the nineteenth century; 2) France after Azam's Félida X (1875–1900); 3) America in the era of Morton Prince (1900–1926); and 4) 1970 to the present. Hacking asserts that, in each case, at least one feature in society at large made dissociative behavior acceptable and, at the same time, rendered it subject to medical diagnosis. Can any aspects of these four waves be associated with the long-standing ratio for DID of about nine females to one male?

The first wave occurred during the nineteenth century in an era of social restraint. Alter personalities were, in every case, more lively than the personality taken to be the normal self. Words such as "merry," "gay," and "vivacious" were among those used to describe the alter personality. Double consciousness may have provided a way for American Protestant women, whose social options were severely curtailed, to adopt a freer pattern of life. There is inadequate information about the social and religious background of the women in a survey of British cases (Hacking 1991b), but there are some consistent findings. These women were either confined to middle-class social obligations, which were limiting, or were employed as serving girls in authoritarian households. Thus, double consciousness can be viewed as a way of legitimately transgressing social propriety. This "unconscious choice" was influenced by the cultural milieu, although other explanatory possibilities are not excluded.

Note that the second wave, in France after 1875, coincides with the dominance of Charcot and his diagnosis of *grande hystérie*. All people with multiple personalities were described as having hysterical conditions, including quite florid conversion symptoms. They were all drawn from a "pool" of hysterical patients. Although male hysteria was known and much discussed (Ellenberger 1970), the vast majority of the pool of patients with hysterical symptoms were female. Hence, a special explanation of the preponderance of women with DID is not necessary; one should instead explain the preponderance of women called "hysterics." The etiological explanation, namely that female hysterics had been the victims of family violence, could fit the entire class of hysterical patients. That is the thesis of Herman (1992). In fact, child abuse, although amply reported (Tardieu 1860), was not regularly mentioned in connection with hysteria, and Charcot himself had a hereditary theory about the disease. Trauma and sexual violence were, nevertheless, regularly connected with hysteria, even when it was denied that hysteria was essentially a psychosexual disorder (Briquet 1859). Although familial violence in connection with hysteria was not emphasized by Charcot, it was very explicitly mentioned in the survey of *grande hystérie* by his associate, Richer (1881).

We have little information about men during this period. The most intensely studied man with MPD was Louis Vivé (Camuset 1882). He had epilepsy, and, in the diagnostic terminology of the day was a "hysteric." He had served repeated prison terms for minor crimes, perhaps illustrating the force of type II explanations, namely, that men with DID can be found in the justice system. As noted earlier, after 1887–1888, many men with symptoms that matched those of MPD were diagnosed as exhibiting fugue. Here, there were several complicating factors. First, Charcot insisted that the patients he saw with *automatisme ambulatoire* actually had latent epilepsy and that fugue episodes were analogous to epileptic seizures. Thus, along the main line of division, Charcot saw two distinct subpopulations: 1) DID and hysteria, almost all females; and 2) fugue and epilepsy, mostly males. Second, today's practitioner may well suspect that head injuries played a larger role in late nineteenth-century fugue than appears in the literature. Finally, fugue was closely associated with vagrancy (*vagabondage*), which in France was believed to be a critical social problem. It has been argued that vagrants' symptoms were diagnosed as fugue in order to bring them under medical care and take them off the streets without jailing them (Beaune 1987). Once again, we are on strongly political territory to the extent that vagrancy, psychogenic fugue, and the 1890s wave of French anti-Semitism are closely connected (Goldstein 1985).

The above observations only indirectly address gender and DID in France in 1875–1900. They connect gender and hysteria and admit a possible association with family violence according to an etiological connection between child abuse and DID. Migration to the criminal system for DID males makes child abuse an unnecessary explanation for male DID patients. However, these observations do not address the specific syndrome of DID. In 1875, it appears to have been seized upon for reasons having nothing to do with gender, except that the DID patients were drawn from the pool of those with hysterical symptoms who were highly hypnotizable. Specific interest in dissociation was closely connected, as Janet (1906) was later to state explicitly, with a positivist view of human consciousness as defined by memory and experience rather than any transcendental or religious "ego" or soul. That, in turn, was standard ideology of republican intellectuals during the political strife following the Franco-Prussian war. We are reminded once again of Herman's (1992) assertion that these psychiatric issues are closely connected to political ones.

The third wave—that of Americans with multiple personalities—was strongly associated with Morton Prince (1905). The group of patients was somewhat different from what it had been in France and was strongly influenced by the spiritist movement. Most mediums were women, and aside from *The Journal for Abnormal Psychology,* founded by Prince in 1905, most American cases of DID were reported in the *Proceedings of the Society for Psychical Research* or its American counterpart. Prince himself formally rejected any suggestion that Sally, an alter personality of his most famous patient, Miss Beauchamp, was a spirit. But William McDougall, perhaps America's leading academic psychologist of the day, explicitly stated that the alter personality was a spirit (McDougall 1907). When Prince was out of town or otherwise occupied, he consigned Beauchamp to the care of Richard Hodgson, Boston's most famous psychic investigator. It is not surprising, in this milieu, that Sally stated "I am a spirit" (Prince 1905, p. 377).

The pool of patients with multiple personalities in this period included spiritists and spiritualists, with a high proportion of women, and particular mediums, almost all of whom were women. This is in every way consistent with an abuse etiology—for example, mediums may in fact have had serious traumatic experiences, and multiple personalities may have been their way of working out their trauma in a socially accepted manner. Beauchamp herself certainly had had a severe shock, associated with sex; she was also, in her word, "terrified" of her violent father (Prince 1905, pp. 375, 427). The skeptic will urge that the multiple personalities of that day should be given no more credence than mediums. Braude (1991) examines the opposite case, that mediumship is a type of dissociation.

Finally, in the fourth and present wave of multiple personalities, child abuse is central. That is one thing on which DID advocates and critics can agree, although they may interpret the fact differently. Child abuse activists began with battering, cruelty, and neglect in the 1960s and turned their attention to sexual abuse and incest in the 1970s. Were it not for greatly heightened awareness of these problems, and the freedom to discuss them, the diagnosis and treatment of MPD would not have been able to flourish as it did. Until very recently, the focus has been on the abuse of girls and women, which might in itself be sufficient to explain the sex ratio among those with symptoms meeting the diagnostic criteria for DID.

Feminist Analyses

An unduly brief summary of one feminist analysis is as follows. DID is a possible response to child abuse. Although the distress of individual DID patients must be resolved immediately, and in personal terms, far larger issues exist in the background. Child abuse is not an isolated aspect of present North American society that can be removed by economic and psychological palliatives, preventatives, and controls. Just as DID is one indicator of child abuse, child abuse is only an expression of the violence inherent in our present patriarchal power structure (Rush 1980). The sexually abusive male may be condemned, but his behavior is only an extreme form of aggression toward women and children that is condoned and even encouraged, both in popular media and within the economic power structure.

The most detailed analysis of this type, specifically worked out in the context of DID, is by Rivera (1991). She takes trauma and violence against women as a basis from which to start but may regard DID more metaphorically than most other clinicians. Traumas, she writes "are sequestered in desegregated self-states called alters" (Rivera 1991, p. 79). Her approach to therapy, nevertheless, has much in common with standard practices as described by Putnam (1989) and in the work of other clinicians. Its aim is "the strategic reworking of the history of experiences of trauma" leading to nondissociative coping skills. Her approach to therapy may differ in encouraging patients to gain a larger and more political awareness of their plight.

The majority feminist perspective is straightforward. It is well represented by Herman (1992) and, in more general terms, for example, by MacKinnon (1987). Women are abused. Children are abused. Females are far more often abused than males. Repeated early abuse is the primary cause of DID. Hence, far more women than men have DID.

A minority feminist view is represented by Leys (1992), drawing on the work of Rose (1986). This type of analysis urges a rethinking of the role and meaning of violence. Leys writes that Rose poses a challenge to

> Catherine MacKinnon, Jeffrey Masson and others who, rejecting the notion of unconscious conflict, embrace instead a rigid dichotomy between the internal and the external such that violence is imagined as coming to the subject entirely from the outside—a point of view that inevitably reinforces a politically retrograde stereotype of the female as a purely passive victim. (Leys 1992, p. 168)

She holds that discourse like that of MacKinnon "in effect denies the female subject of all possibility of agency" (Leys 1992, p. 204). This opinion, although strongly differing in intention from the skeptical view about clinical suggestion, implies that the preponderance of women with a diagnosis of DID is a result of a covert alliance between clinicians and patients, intended to be supportive of women, but which, in fact, merely continues the old system of disempowerment.

Unlike the skeptical positions previously mentioned, this is a genuinely radical critique of current theories and practices connected with DID. It does not dispute the prevalence of family violence or question its societal foundations. It does not deny that past abuse can, in a cultural and clinical milieu, lead to DID symptomatology of a florid sort. It does question the complacence of a theory that purports to take the part of the patient; it conjectures that the theory, practice, and underlying assumptions reinforce the patient's self-image as a passive victim. One possible conclusion of this type of analysis might suggest that current theories of abuse, trauma, and DID are part of another cycle of oppression of women, all the more dangerous because they represent themselves as being so entirely on the side of the "victim," whom they thereby construct as a helpless pawn rather than as an autonomous human being.

Expression of Gender

Only three features of DID phenomenology have been constant from 1791 to the present. One feature is that most patients are women. The second feature is that it is very common for one alter personality to be younger than the host, often a child. The third feature is ambivalence about sexuality. Virtually every female patient for whom much has been reported is said to have a second personality that is more lively than the personality regarded as the host. Words used to describe this second personality include "vivacious," "mischievous," "naughty," and "promiscuous." As early as Dewar (1823), a woman had sex with a man who had "taken advantage" of her second state. Félida X conceived and gave birth in her second state, while denying pregnancy in her first state; variations on this sequence of events are well known for many patients (Van der Hart et al. 1991). In the early twentieth century, ample evidence suggests that the main alter of Prince's Miss Beauchamp behaved in a way that would now be described as bisexual (Leys 1992). Indeed, Rosenzweig (1987) suggested that not only was Miss Beauchamp bisexual but that Breuer's Anna O. (Breuer and Freud 1893–1895/1955), described by many as having DID, was similar in many respects to Prince's patient, including her bisexuality. The alter reported by

Dewey (1907) was lesbian. Male personality fragments appear in Wholey's (1933) study. The 67 patients with a diagnosis of multiple personality in the report by Taylor and Martin (1944) include some whose symptoms do not closely match the DSM-IV criteria; however, note that there were nine instances of gender ambivalence, namely, either a homosexual alter or a male alter for a female host. Nevertheless, there is much truth in the following statement about Wilbur's patient Sybil:

> The uniqueness which, before, was based on Sybil's having developed more alternating selves than had any other known multiple personality, was now founded as well on her being the only multiple personality to have crossed the borders of sexual difference to develop personalities of the opposite sex. (Schreiber 1973, p. 214)

Alters of the opposite sex multiplied after the publication of *Sybil*. There is a close correlation between the emergence of theoretical perspectives and the emergence of different types of cross-sex alter personalities. Thus, in the late 1970s, "imaginary playmates" were widely canvassed as an origin of DID—many children have imaginary playmates, and it was thought that, in some, the imagined figure coalesces and develops into a personality that uses the body of the host. One such male alter of a female patient is described in Bliss (1980). A second source of the male alters is found in male self-fantasies of the growing female child herself—Sybil's two male alters are prepubertal boys who never quite grew up. Also around 1980, there was a notable stylization of the range of alter personalities so that one would find one or more persecutor alters and one or more protector alters. Females developed male protector alters who were strong, heavyset, and reliable (e.g., cowboys or truckers). Throughout this period, the sexuality of cross-sex alters was not discussed in published reports.

As the number of reported alters increased from a typical 3 or 4 to the present average of about 17, the number of patients with disclosed opposite-sex alters radically increased, as did the numbers of patients with alters of more obviously stereotypical contrasts with the host, such as alters of different race or ethnicity. The questionnaire by Ross and co-workers (1990) showed that 62% of reported MPD patients had alters of the opposite sex.

Current reports of sexuality play an increased role in the characteristics of the alters. The resulting options for combinations and permutations of gender identity are thereby greatly enhanced. The contrast between inhibited and outgoing personalities is commonplace, but the choices of alters have been augmented. Each alter personality can now be characterized by choices made from each of the following categories: same sex/opposite sex, inhibited/outgoing, heterosexual/bisexual/homosexual, and infantile/prepubertal/adolescent/mature. Therefore, a patient can assume 48 alter states; in the United States, these states are doubled for white patients who opt for a number of black alters.

What are the relationships between alters chosen from the possible combinations of gender roles? Rivera (1987) observed that

> in my experience of working with women who experience multiple personalities, it is very common for their vulnerable child personalities and their seductive and/or compliant personalities to be female and their aggressive protector personalities to be male, and other therapists with a wider range of experience than I have confirmed my clinical impression (Kluft 1987), though there has not been any research done so far that would document it. The experience of these alter personalities as they fight with each other for status, power and influence over the individual is powerfully illustrative of the social construction of masculinity and femininity in our society. (p. 43)

Conclusion

This chapter has been a self-consciously neutral inspection of territory that is intensely contested. It has been tempting to back away from the question, What is *my* explanation of the fact that most people with symptoms diagnosed as multiple personality are women? Is this a fact about women, for example, about the way that they respond to cruel treatment? Is this a fact about clinicians and the way in which they perceive and interact with their patients? Or are we to understand multiple personality as a primarily social phenomenon in which patients and diagnosticians act out contemporary roles for which women are more easily selected?

These questions are misleading, as is the overarching and overly popular query, "Is DID *real* or not?" If one answers "yes" to one of the questions, it does not imply answering "no" to the other three. Examine an extreme phenomenon, the *grande hystérie* elucidated in Jean-Martin Charcot's public lectures during the 1880s. It is amply described in many sources, such as Ellenberger (1970), but it is most vividly captured in the illustrations of the day (e.g., in the textbook by Charcot's pupil, Paul Richer [1881]). With respect to gender, the example seems especially pertinent, for most patients with hysteria were women; but Charcot himself made current the awareness that many male patients also had hysteria. A former student of Charcot studied 31 men in a series of 100 cases, and the photographs and engravings in this text (Pitres 1891) are almost as striking as Richer's plates. All historians of medicine agree that the stigmata of *grande hystérie* disappeared after Charcot's death in 1893. Of course, the behavior had much to do with Charcot's clinic and the way in which Charcot and his students interacted with their patients. One can fully assent to that theory but also agree with Herman (1992) that *fin-de-siècle* hysteria was a consequence of the condition of women and their responses to repressive or brutal familial life. In addition, every historian will insist that it was essential to both patient and helper that hysteria (and also neurasthenia) was socially acceptable both as a mode of behavior and as a type of diagnosis. I do not mean that it was "socially acceptable" to have hysteria, although there was sometimes something in that too, but that this was a type of description, with ample implications for action and interaction, that was intelligible and accepted without question. It was in the framework of that style of description and understanding that female *grande hystérie* flourished. Likewise, I am not prepared to single out the patient, the clinician, or the cultural milieu as "the" explanation of the sex ratio among diagnoses of DID. My emphasis, if there must be one, is nevertheless on the cultural and anthropological vector to the extent of saying that patient and clinician act and interact within a set of social norms that makes intelligible what they are doing. Only within that set of meanings could DID exist, and that set of meanings must be investigated to understand why more women than men have this disorder.

I conclude with a further warning about any search for "the" explanation. I have mentioned several earlier waves of multiple personality (or "double consciousness") preceding the present epidemic of DID. It is far from obvious that we are speaking of the same phenomenon—medical or sociological—in each successive era. Moreover, it is not impossible that the dissociative disorders will take on new configurations in the coming decade and that the special case of multiple personality will follow in train. Dissociation does not, at present, lend itself well to medication; it has not been successfully shown to have a distinct biological basis or to be amenable to specific drug treatment. Hence, it will not be a favored type of pathology for public health care but may be expected to become an increasingly central type of diagnosis in the private sector of psychotherapy. This will, in itself, have substantial socioeconomic consequences for patients with DID. Such considerations can be expected to play a larger part in the future of multiple personality than is commonly discussed in more strictly medical approaches.

References

American Psychiatric Association: Diagnostic and Statistical Manual of Mental Disorders, 3rd Edition. Washington, DC, American Psychiatric Association, 1980

American Psychiatric Association: Diagnostic and Statistical Manual of Mental Disorders, 3rd Edition, Revised. Washington, DC, American Psychiatric Association, 1987

American Psychiatric Association: Diagnostic and Statistical Manual of Mental Disorders, 4th Edition. Washington, DC, American Psychiatric Association, 1994

Angell EB: A case of double consciousness—amnesic type, with fabrication of memory. J Abnorm Psychol 1:155–169, 1910

Azam EE: Amnésie périodique, ou dédoublement de la vie [Periodic amnesia or doubling of life]. Revue Scientifique 10:481–487, 1876

Bean N: My life as a dissociated personality. J Abnorm Psychol 3:240–260, 1908

Beaune J-C: Le Vagabond et la Machine. Essaie sur le Médecine, Technique et Societé en France 1880–1910 [The Vagrant and the Machine. Essay on Medicine, Technology, and Society in France]. Seyssel, France, Champ Vallon, 1987

Berman E: Multiple personality: theoretical approaches. Journal of the Bronx State Hospital 2:99–107, 1974

Bernstein EM, Putnam FW: Development, reliability, and validity of a dissociation scale. J Nerv Ment Dis 174:727–735, 1986

Bliss EL: Multiple personalities: a report of 14 cases with implications for schizophrenia and hysteria. Arch Gen Psychiatry 37:1388–1397, 1980

Bliss EL: A symptom profile of patients with multiple personalities, including MMPI results. J Nerv Ment Dis 172:197–202, 1984

Boor M: The multiple personality epidemic: additional cases and inferences regarding diagnosis, dynamics and cure. J Nerv Ment Dis 170:302–304, 1982

Branscomb LP: Dissociation in combat-related post-traumatic stress disorder. Dissociation 4:13–20, 1992

Braude SL: First Person Plural: Multiple Personality and the Philosophy of Mind. London, Routledge, 1991

Breuer J, Freud S: Studies on hysteria (1893–1895), in The Standard Edition of the Complete Psychological Works of Sigmund Freud, Vol 2. Translated and edited by Strachey J. London, Hogarth Press, 1955

Briquet P: Traité Clinique et Thérapeutique de l'Hystérie [Clinical and Therapeutic Treatise of Hysteria]. Paris, J B Bailliére, 1859

Brodie F: When "the Other Woman" Is His Mother. Tacoma, WA, Winged Eagle Press, 1992

Camuset L: Un cas de dédoublement de la personnalité, periode amnésique d'une année chez un jeune homme hystérique [A case of doubling of personality, periodic amnesia lasting one year in a young man with hysteria]. Revue Philosophique 13:676–678, 1882

Charcot J-M: Maladie comitiale—automatisme ambulatoire, in Leçons du Mardi à la Salpêtrière I [Epilepsy—ambulatory automatism in Tuesday lessons at the Salpêtrière I]. Paris, Progrès Medicale, 1888, pp 155–169

Charcot J-M: Cas d' automatisme comitiale ambulatoire, in Leçons du Mardi à la Salpêtrière II [A case of epileptic ambulatory automatism]. Paris, Progrès Medicale, 1889, pp 303–327

Coons PM: Commentary: ICD-10 and beyond. Dissociation 3:216–217, 1990

Crabtree A: Multiple Man. Explorations in Possession and Multiple Personality. Toronto, Collins, 1985

Dell PF, Eisenhower JW: Adolescent multiple personality disorder: a preliminary study of 11 cases. J Am Acad Child Adolesc Psychiatry 29:357–365, 1990

Dennett D: Consciousness Explained. Boston, MA, Little, Brown, 1991

Despine A: De L'emploi du Magnétisme Animal et des Eaux Minérales Dans le Traitement des Maladies Nerveuses, Suivi D'une Observation Très Curieuse de Guérison de Névropathie [On the Use of Animal Magnetism and Mineral Waters in the Treatment of Nervous Diseases, Followed by a Remarkable Cure of Neuropathy]. Paris, Germer Ballière, 1844

Dewar H: Report on a communication from Dr. Dyce of Aberdeen, to the Royal Society of Edinburgh, "On uterine irritation, and its effects on the female constitution." Transactions of the Royal Society of Edinburgh 9:365–369, 1823

Dewey R: A case of disordered personality. J Abnorm Psychol 2:142–154, 1907

Ellenberger HF: The Discovery of the Unconscious. New York, Basic Books, 1970

Franz SI: Persons One and Three. A Study in Multiple Personalities. New York, McGraw-Hill, 1933

Garcia FO: The concept of dissociation and conversion in the new edition of The International Classification of Diseases (ICD-10). Dissociation 3:204–208, 1990

Gmelin E: Materialen für die Anthropologie [Materials for Anthropology]. Tübingen, Cotte, 1791

Goddard HH: A case of dual personality. The Journal of Abnormal and Social Psychology 21:170–191, 1926

Goldstein J: The wandering Jew and the problem of psychiatric antisemitism in fin de siécle France. Journal of Contemporary History 20:521–551, 1985

Hacking I: Double consciousness in Britain, 1815–1875. Dissociation 4:134–147, 1991a

Hacking I: The making and molding of child abuse. Critical Inquiry 17:253–288, 1991b

Hacking I: Multiple personality disorder and its hosts. History of the Human Sciences 5:23–31, 1992

Herman JL: Father-Daughter Incest. Cambridge, MA, Harvard University Press, 1981

Herman JL: Trauma and Recovery. New York, Basic Books, 1992

Hodgson R: A case of double consciousness. Proceedings of the Society for Psychical Research 7:221–257, 1891

Horevitz RP, Braun BG: Are multiple personalities borderline? An analysis of 33 cases. Psychiatr Clin North Am 7:69–88, 1984

Janet P: L'Automatisme Psychologique [Psychological Automatism]. Paris, Alcan, 1889

Janet P: The Major Symptoms of Hysteria. New York, Macmillan, 1906

Kempe CH, Silverman FN, Steele FN, et al: The battered-child syndrome. JAMA 181:17–24, 1962

Kluft RP: Treatment of multiple personality disorder: a study of 33 cases. Psychiatr Clin North Am 7:69–88, 1984

Kluft RP: An update on multiple personality disorder. Hosp Community Psychiatry 38:363–373, 1987

Kluft RP: The phenomenology and treatment of extremely complex multiple personality disorder. Dissociation 1:47–58, 1988

Kluft RP: Iatrogenic creation of new alter personalities. Dissociation 2:83–90, 1989

Lewis AJ: Hysterical dissociation in dementia paralytica. Monatsschrift für Psychiatrie und Neurologie 125:589–604, 1953

Leys R: The real Miss Beauchamp: gender and the subject of imitation, in Feminists Theorize the Political. Edited by Butler J, Scott J. London, Routledge, 1992, pp 167–214

Loewenstein RJ: The clinical psychology of males with multiple personality disorder: a report of 21 cases. Dissociation 3:135–143, 1990

MacKinnon C: Feminism Unmodified. Discourses on Life and Law. Cambridge, MA, Harvard University Press, 1987

McDougall W: The case of Sally Beauchamp. Proceeding of the Society for Psychical Research 19:410–431, 1907

McHugh PR: Psychiatric misadventures. American Scholar, Autumn 1992, pp 497–510

Merskey H: The manufacture of personalities: the production of multiple personality disorder. Br J Psychiatry 160:327–340, 1992

Mitchill SL: A double consciousness, or a duality of person in the same individual. The Medical Repository of Original Essays and Intelligence Relative to Physic, Surgery, Chemistry and Natural History n.s. 3:185–186, 1817

Pitres A: Leçons Cliniques sur l'Hystérie et l'Hypnotisme Faites a l'Hôpital Saint André de Bordeaux [Clinical Lessons on Hysteria and Hypnotism at the St. André Hospital in Bordeaux]. Paris, Doin, 1891

Prince M: The Dissociation of a Personality. New York, Longman Green, 1905

Putnam FW: Diagnosis and Treatment of Multiple Personality Disorder. New York, Guilford, 1989

Putnam FW: Altered states: peeling away the layers of multiple personality. The Sciences, November/December 1992, pp 30–38

Putnam FW, Guroff JJ, Silberman EK, et al: The clinical phenomenology of multiple personality disorder. a review of 100 recent cases. J Clin Psychiatry 47:285–293, 1986

Richer P: Etudes Cliniques sur l'Hystéro-épilepsie ou Grande Hystérie [Clinical Studies of Hysteroepilepsy or Major Hysteria]. Paris, Delehaye and Lecrosnier, 1881

Rivera M: Am I a boy or a girl? multiple personality as a window on gender differences. Resources for Feminist Research/Documentation sur la Recherche Féministe 17:41–43, 1987

Rivera M: Multiple personality disorder and the social systems: 185 cases. Dissociation 4:79–82, 1991

Rose J: Sexuality in the Field of Vision. London, Verso, 1986

Rosenbaum M: The role of the term schizophrenia in the decline of multiple personality. Arch Gen Psychiatry 37:1383–1385, 1980

Rosenzweig S: Sally Beauchamp's career: a psychoarchaeological key to Morton Prince's classic case of multiple personality. Genet Soc Gen Psychol Monogr 113:5–60, 1987

Ross C: Inpatient treatment of MPD. Can J Psychiatry 33:524–529, 1987

Ross CA, Norton GR, Wozney K: Multiple personality disorder: an analysis of 236 cases. Can J Psychiatry 34:413–418, 1989

Ross CA, Heber S, Anderson G: The Dissociative Disorders Interview Schedule. Am J Psychiatry 147:1698–1699, 1990

Ross CA, Ryan L, Vaught L, et al: High and low dissociators in a college student population. Dissociation 4:147–151, 1992

Rowan J: Subpersonalities. The People Inside You. London, Routledge, 1990

Rush F: The Best Kept Secret. Sexual Abuse of Children. New York, McGraw-Hill, 1980

Schreiber FR: Sybil. New York, Regnery, 1973

Spiegel D: Multiple personality as a post-traumatic stress disorder. Psychiatr Clin North Am 7:101–110, 1984

Spiegel D: Dissociating dissociation: a commentary on Dr. Garcia's article. Dissociation 3:214–216, 1990

Stern CR: The etiology of multiple personalities. Psychiatr Clin North Am 7:149–160, 1984

Tardieu A-A: Etude médico-légale sur les sévices et mauvais traitements exercés sur des enfants [Medical-legal study on torture and maltreatment of children]. Annales d'hygiène publique et de médecine légale [Annals of Public Health and Forensic Medicine] 2 sér 13:361–398, 1860

Taylor WS, Martin MF: Multiple personality. J Abnorm Soc Psychol 39:281–300, 1944

Thigpen CH, Cleckly HM: The Three Faces of Eve. New York, McGraw-Hill, 1957

Thigpen CH, Cleckly HM: On the incidence of multiple personality disorder: a brief communication. Int J Clin Exp Hypn 32:63–66, 1984

Tissié P: Les Alienés Voyageurs. Paris, Doin, 1887

Torem MS: Covert multiple personality underlying eating disorders. Am J Psychother 44:357–368, 1990

Tyson GM: Childhood multiple personality disorder/dissociative identity disorder: applying and extending current diagnostic checklists. Dissociation 5:20–27, 1992

Van der Hart O, Faure H, van Gerven M, et al: Unawareness and denial of pregnancy in patients with multiple personality disorder. Dissociation 4:65–73, 1991

Wessley S: Old wine in new bottles: from neurasthenia to chronic fatigue syndrome. Psychol Med 20:35–53, 1990

Wholey CC: A case of multiple personality. Am J Psychiatry 12:653–688, 1933

Wilbur CB: The effect of child abuse on the psyche, in Childhood Antecedents of Multiple Personality. Edited by Kluft RP. Washington, DC, American Psychiatric Press, 1985, pp 21–35

World Health Organization: The ICD-10 Classification of Mental and Behavioural Disorders. Geneva, World Health Organization, 1992

Young WC: Comments on Dr. Garcia's article. Dissociation 3:209–210, 1990

CHAPTER 3

Psychopathology and Non-Mendelian Inheritance

William C. Friend, M.Sc., M.D., C.M., F.R.C.P.C.

In 1865, Gregor Mendel presented his paper "Experiments in Plant Hybridization" to the Natural Science Association in Brunn, Czechoslovakia (Mendel 1959). In that paper, he enumerated three laws, each of which has remained a cornerstone of the science of genetics in this century: 1) the *law of unit inheritance,* which states that the characteristics of the parent do not, as had been supposed, blend in the offspring, but may skip generations, only to reappear in a form unchanged from the parent generation; 2) the *law of segregation,* which notes that two copies of a single gene segregate randomly and never appear in the same child; and 3) the *law of independent assortment,* which indicates that each single gene pair segregates in the offspring independently from other gene pairs. These three laws have had an extraordinary impact on our ability to understand the transmission of genetic disease in humans. By 1902, Garrod was able to report the first example of a mendelizing pattern of inheritance in humans—alkaptonuria (Garrod 1902)—and this century has seen a host of genetic disorders identified and categorized by the application of Mendelian principles.

For centuries, it has been observed that psychiatric disorders are familial. In recent decades, twin and adoption studies have pointed to a genetic basis for this familial transmission. Unfortunately, despite the insight offered by Mendel's laws, no clear inheritance pattern has been delineated for any of the functional psychiatric disorders. For instance, no single major gene locus explains the mode of transmission of schizophrenia (Baron 1982; Elston et al. 1978), and analyses of affective disorder pedigrees (Bucher and Elston 1981; Goldin et al. 1983) have suggested that a single major locus model cannot account for transmission of this illness either.

Although a number of reports over the last two decades have suggested X-linkage of bipolar affective disorder (Baron 1977; Del Zompo et al. 1984; Gershon et al. 1980; Mendlewicz and Fleiss 1974; Mendlewicz et al. 1979, 1980; Winokur et al. 1969), X-linkage is by no means present in all bipolar pedigrees. For X-linked traits, father-to-son transmission does not normally occur, and if it does, X-linkage can be excluded. But male-to-male transmission has been observed in some bipolar pedigrees (Gershon 1990). Also, close linkage between bipolar illness and red-green color blindness can be ruled out, indicating that bipolar illness is not generally transmitted by a single major gene in the proximity of the protan/deutan region of the X chromosome (Gershon et al. 1979). Therefore, at most, only a subgroup of bipolar patients appear to carry an X-linked gene, and substantial genetic heterogeneity seems to exist in bipolar disorder (Risch et al. 1986).

The difficulty experienced in establishing a Mendelian pattern of inheritance for psychiatric disorders has directed the attention of investigators to the hypothesis that these disorders are multifactorially inherited. Psychiatric disorders have several features suggestive of multifactorial inheritance. Typically, in multifactorial inheritance, the risk of illness for first-degree relatives of the proband is much higher than for second-degree relatives, for whom the risk is, in turn, substantially greater than for the general population. The risk for first-degree relatives is higher still when more than one family member is affected. Schizophrenia follows this pattern. The morbid risk for first-degree relatives of individuals with schizophrenia is about 10 times higher than the risk for the general population, and the risk is greater yet when two members of a kindred are affected. For second-degree relatives, morbid risk lies between that of the general population and that of first-degree relatives (Gottesman and Shields 1982).

Non-Mendelian Patterns of Inheritance

Recent advances in genetics have provided still other explanations for patterns of inheritance that do not have Mendelian characteristics. These nonclassical forms of inheritance include mosaicism, uniparental disomy, genomic imprinting, unstable deoxyribonucleic acid (DNA) sequences, and mitochondrial inheritance. They have only been observed recently, and their mechanisms are just now being elucidated, but they currently are receiving much attention. Already these forms of inheritance have greatly increased our knowledge of the molecular basis of some neurological disorders. They may prove increasingly instructive of the molecular genetics of behavior and may help to explain the gender differences that are observed in some psychiatric disorders.

Mosaicism

With only a few exceptions, every cell of an organism carries the same genetic information. What differentiates an epithelial cell from a neuron is not the content of the DNA but each cell's specific gene expression. Although generally true, this concept has in recent years begun to appear simplistic. An individual's cells, even those of the same type, may actually contain different genetic information and yet be derived from the same parental chromosomes. This phenomenon is referred to as *mosaicism.*

Several different types of mosaicism have been detected. One type of mosaicism, hypothesized by Mary Lyon (1961), is inactivation of one of the X chromosomes in females. Geneticists had hitherto been puzzled about the expression of X-linked genes. They wondered why females, who, of course, have two copies of X-linked genes, do not produce twice as much X-linked gene product as do males. Some mechanism of dosage compensation must be present. Lyon's explanation was that in the somatic cells of female mammals, one X chromosome in each cell is randomly inactivated in early embryonic life. The final result is that approximately half of the cells of the organism have one active X chromosome, while the other half have the other active X chromosome. Today we know that X inactivation occurs in the mouse at the stage of transition from morula to blastocyst. Once a cell has inactivated a particular X chromosome, all of its daughter cells inactivate the same X chromosome. Hence, although initially random, X inactivation, once established in the early embryo, is fixed in all somatic cells and follows characteristic patterns.

There are exceptions to the rule of randomness, however. For instance, in females bearing one normal X chromosome and one X chromosome with a partial deletion, in general, the abnormal chromosome is inactivated in all cells. Such an effect contributes to the fitness of the organism. Alternatively, in the case of one normal X chromosome and one X chromosome translocated to an autosome, the *normal* X chromosome is generally inactivated. Inactivation of the X portion of the translocation would spread onto the autosome, producing a hemizygous state and the possibility of nonviability (Gartler and Riggs 1983).

The behavioral disorder Lesch-Nyhan syndrome may involve nonrandom X-chromosome inactivation. This serious disorder, characterized by compulsive, self-destructive biting, hyperuricemia, mental retardation, choreoathetosis, and cerebral palsy, is transmitted as an X-linked recessive trait (Lesch and Nyhan 1964). Patients have complete inactivity of the enzyme hypoxanthine-guanine phosphoribosyltransferase (HGPRT) in erythrocytes (Seegmiller et al. 1967). Based on the strict Lyon hypothesis, mothers of boys with the disorder would be expected to have an inactivated X chromosome containing the normal HGPRT gene half the time. If that were so, their erythrocytic HGPRT enzyme activity would be expected to be 50% of normal. However, this is not the case. Carrier mothers have normal erythrocytic HGPRT enzyme activity. One explanation is that nonrandom inactivation of the X chromosome bearing the HGPRT-deficient gene is occurring in erythrocytes. An alternative proposal involves initial random inactivation, followed by selection against those cells with HGPRT deficiency. In either case, females with this mutation are phenotypically and biochemically normal, yet half of their sons have Lesch-Nyhan syndrome (Nyhan et al. 1970). However, the situation is even more complex. Individual clones of skin fibroblasts from carrier mothers often have deficient HGPRT activity, indicating that the X chromosome carrying the Lesch-Nyhan locus is not inactivated in *all* cell types of the mother (Migeon 1970).

Mosaicism can occur in autosomes. In Down's syndrome, mosaicism of chromosome 21 occurs occasionally. This could arise in several ways. A mosaic individual could develop from a normal zygote through mitotic nondisjunction of chromosome 21 in an early stage of division, producing a 21 trisome and a monosome. This is followed by loss of the monosomic cell line. However, most mosaic patients with Down's syndrome probably develop from a trisomy 21 zygote, which subsequently loses one chromosome 21 in one or more somatic cell lines. Nondisjunction events occurring late in development might produce mosaics with only a small proportion of trisomy 21 cells, and for such individuals, the syndrome might be relatively less severe. Nevertheless, individuals whose germ cells are trisomic for chromosome 21 may have a disproportionally high rate of children with Down's syndrome (Nielsen et al. 1988).

Somatic mosaicism—that is, mosaicism arising in somatic cells—can occur not only at the chromosomal level but also from a mutation in a single gene. Such events may be common. During growth, humans develop from a single cell to, perhaps, 10^{14} cells. Because this figure far exceeds the spontaneous mutation rate of most genes, there is ample opportunity for individual cells to acquire mutations during clonal expansion (Hall 1988). Neurofibromatosis type 1 (NF1) may be an example of somatic mosaicism involving a single gene. Occasionally, NF1 affects only one part of the body. This segmental form probably arises as a spontaneous somatic cell mutation and does not involve all somatic cells. However, when a segmental NF1 parent produces an affected child, the child's phenotype is non-segmental. In this situation, the parental mutation likely arose early enough in development to involve the germ cells but only a portion of the somatic cells. Thus, the disorder is transmitted to the offspring in a nonsegmental pattern (Riccardi and Lewis 1988).

Occasionally, phenotypically normal parents will have a child with genetic disease. If the mutation is not carried in the parent's somatic cells or is carried in too low a proportion of somatic cells to be detected, one might conclude that the child is carrying a new mutation, in which case the likelihood of recurrence in a second child would be low. Although such an explanation may be valid, it is also possible that a parent is a germ-line mosaic (i.e., a carrier of both normal and mutant germ cells). Unfortunately, if a parent is a germline mosaic, the risk of a second affected child developing from a mutant germ cell is much higher than the risk of a second spontaneous mutation.

Uniparental Disomy

Uniparental disomy refers to the generation of a diploid organism from the union of a gamete from one parent containing a pair of chromosomes with a gamete from the other parent missing the homologous chromosome. These two chromosomes might arise through duplication of one chromosome (a situation referred to as isodisomy) or from the presence of both homologues of one parent (heterodisomy). Although unknown until recently, several instances of this event have been documented because the parental source of chromosomes can now be determined. Two groups (Spence et al. 1988; Voss et al. 1989) have reported children with cystic fibrosis and short stature who had inherited two identical copies of one maternal chromosome 7 (isodisomy). Heterodisomy can also occur. Nicholls and colleagues (1989) reported two patients with Prader-Willi syndrome who had inherited from their mothers both homologues of chromosome 15 but no paternal chromosome 15 (maternal heterodisomy). Uniparental disomy involving the sex chromosomes has also been detected. Vidaud and co-workers (1989) reported the case of a boy who had inherited hemophilia A from his hemophiliac father. The mother, however, was well. X chromosome DNA markers showed that the proband had inherited not only the Y chromosome from his father but also the X chromosome carrying the gene for hemophilia. The autosomes, however, had segregated normally.

The actual frequency of uniparental disomy at present is not clear. Nevertheless, the potential impact of this phenomenon is substantial. For instance, inheritance of an XY pair of chromosomes from the father would allow father-to-son transmission of X-linked traits. In females, X-chromosome isodisomy could provide one explanation for manifestation of an X-linked recessive disorder in women. Isodisomy of autosomes could also result in the production of recessive phenotypes despite only one parent carrying the recessive allele. Finally, disomy, in and of itself, without a deletion or mutation, can produce disease through the mechanism of genomic imprinting.

Genomic Imprinting

Imprinting is a term familiar to psychiatrists and psychologists. It was first used by Konrad Lorenz to refer to the modification of behavior by environmental exposures or events. Lorenz was referring specifically to his observations that greylag goslings accept as their mother the first living being they encounter after hatching (Lorenz 1952). In recent years, it has become clear that the expression of some genes in an individual may also be modified by environment. Gene expression may vary depending on whether the genetic material has been inherited from the mother or the father. This phenomenon, referred to as *genomic imprinting,* is thought to involve modification of the DNA during gamete differentiation in the parents.

Genomic imprinting might occur in a variety of ways. The addition of methyl (CH_3) groups to the nitrogenous bases of DNA is probably one mechanism. The presence of methyl groups on DNA can result in inactivation of a gene, and, under some circumstances, the pattern of DNA methylation is stably maintained and inherited (Holliday 1987). Some forms of DNA are more methylated than others. Sperm DNA, for instance, is more methylated than egg DNA (Monk et al. 1987). Methylation may provide a way for gene activity to be modulated during growth by providing a switch mechanism to turn particular genes on or off in certain cells at critical times during development.

To demonstrate how a pedigree manifesting an imprintable gene might appear, consider the case of an autosomal, dominant allele (Figure 3–1). The allele is transmitted in a normal Mendelian fashion, with inheritance by half the children in the pedigree. However, in the case of maternal imprinting, the gene is inactivated in the mother's children, and, although inherited, it is not expressed in her offspring. Although those daughters inheriting the gene pass it on, their children do not express it either. However, in the sons, who have inherited but do not express the gene (nonmanifesting carriers), the imprint in their

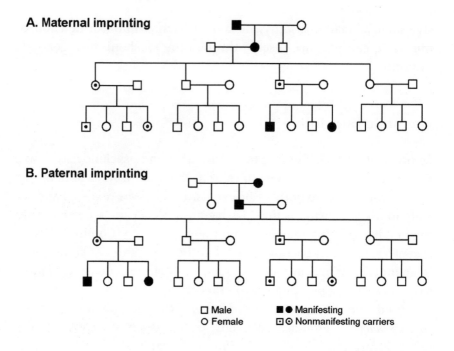

Figure 3–1. Hypothetical pedigrees demonstrating *(A)* maternal and *(B)* paternal imprinting. Maternal imprinting refers to the situation in which an allele is not phenotypically expressed when maternally inherited. However, after passing through a son, it is reactivated in his offspring. Paternal imprinting refers to the situation in which an allele is not phenotypically expressed when paternally inherited. However, after passing through a daughter, it is reactivated in her offspring.

germ line is erased (Surani et al. 1986) and the gene reactivated, and half of their children are affected. Such a pedigree would be characterized by skipped or nonmanifesting generations in the female lines, but in the male lines, there would be a greater likelihood of manifestation in each generation. The converse would occur in the case of paternal imprinting.

Genomic imprinting was noted in 1959 by Janice B. Spofford, who observed a gene in *Drosophila* that had differing effects, depending on whether the gene was inherited from the male or female parent. Until then, it had been thought that the source of the genetic material, whether from the mother or father, did not alter gene expression. In recent years, however, a substantial body of information has accrued, suggesting that the imprinting phenomenon does occur in mammals and can influence the presentation of some genetic disorders (Hall 1990). For instance, genomic imprinting appears to be involved in the development of Wilms' tumor and rhabdomyosarcoma (Sapienza 1989). In addition, several genetic disorders involving marked behavioral changes appear to be subject to gene imprinting effects. During the last several years, evidence has suggested that Angelman syndrome, Prader-Willi syndrome, Huntington's disease, and Alzheimer's disease may be subject to modification through imprinting mechanisms.

Perhaps the most unusual case of genomic imprinting involves the Prader-Willi and Angelman syndromes. Prader-Willi syndrome is characterized by mental retardation, hypotonia, hypogonadism, and obesity. Other behavioral features of this syndrome include rage behavior, depression, hyperactivity, and unusual behavior associated with food such as an insatiable appetite, stealing, gorging, and pica (Holm and Pipes 1976). Angelman syndrome is also associated with mental retardation but differs from Prader-Willi syndrome in that patients have seizure disorders, paroxysms of laughter, and peculiar repetitive ataxic symmetrical movements (Williams and Frias 1982).

Although these syndromes have different phenotypes, both are associated with deletions of the proximal long arm of chromosome 15 (15q11q13). Genetically, however, there is a difference. In Prader-Willi syndrome, the deletion occurs on the *paternally* inherited chromosome 15, whereas in Angelman syndrome, the deletion occurs on the *maternally* inherited chromosome 15 (Knoll et al. 1989). Thus, patients with Prader-Willi syndrome derive all genetic information encoded in the 15q11q13 region from their mothers, whereas patients with Angelman syndrome inherit such information from their fathers. Because the two syndromes are phenotypically so different, gene expression must be different between the maternally and paternally inherited regions.

Of course, it is possible that Prader-Willi and Angelman syndromes do not involve precisely the same chromosomal deletions, although the two regions share a large overlap. However, even if the deletions are not identical, other evidence suggests that the parental source of genetic information can affect the phenotype in these two conditions. Nicholls and associates (1989) studied two patients with Prader-Willi syndrome who lacked deletions of chromosome 15. Both patients had maternal heterodisomy of chromosome 15, with no chromosome 15 contribution from the father. Cytogenetically, neither patient appeared to have a deletion. The presence of only maternal alleles in Prader-Willi syndrome has been observed to occur in another way. Somatic recombination of the 15q region was seen in three patients with Prader-Willi syndrome, producing only a maternal contribution of genes to the 15q11q13 region, with no paternal contribution (Gregory et al. 1991). It appears then that Prader-Willi syndrome, whether resulting from a partial deletion, uniparental disomy, or somatic recombination, is associated with exclusive inheritance of genes from the 15q region of maternal chromosomes. Similarly, Angelman syndrome is associated with inheritance of genes from the 15q region of the paternal chromosome (Malcolm et al. 1991). For normal development to occur, regardless of the mechanism, it appears that 15q11q13 genes deriving from both the mother and the father must be present. Without that balance, both physical and behavioral development goes awry.

The genes responsible for Prader-Willi and Angelman syndromes are unknown. Nevertheless, the human γ-aminobutyric acid ($GABA_A$) receptor β_3 subunit has been mapped to chromosome 15q11q13 (Wagstaff et al. 1991). It is currently unknown whether a mutation or a complete lack of this receptor subunit contributes to the behavioral disorders of Prader-Willi and Angelman syndromes.

Several other behavioral disorders may also be subject to an imprinting effect. Huntington's disease is normally considered to be a dominantly inherited illness with a variable age at onset. The average age at onset is 38 years but can range from childhood to the senium (Ridley et al. 1988). About 10% of cases are juvenile in onset, beginning before age 20 years. Although juvenile onset can occur in cases of maternal inheritance, most juvenile-onset patients inherit the gene from their fathers, whereas the late-onset form is more frequently maternally inherited (Farrer and Conneally 1985). In addition, paternal age at time of conception is inversely correlated with age at onset of Huntington's disease (Farrer et al. 1992).

Several explanations have been proposed for these observations.

An X-linked recessive modifier may account for differences in age at onset when the gene is inherited from the mother rather than the father (Laird 1990). On the other hand, an imprinting mechanism based on DNA methylation may explain the paternal age effect. Farrer and co-workers (1992) suggested that Huntington's disease occurs as a result of inappropriate activation of one or more modifier genes. In young fathers, with more methylated sperm DNA, these genes may be inactivated, whereas in older fathers, whose sperm DNA is less methylated, these genes might be passed on to their offspring in a more active state, resulting in earlier onset of the disease.

Recently, genomic imprinting has been proposed as a mechanism in the inheritance of Alzheimer's disease. In one study of 127 patients, the late-onset form of the disease (age > 67.2 years) was associated with a decreased paternal age at conception (Farrer et al. 1991). These investigators hypothesized that the child of a young father would have more methylated genes and hence more inactive genes than the child of an older father. The inability to activate one or more genes at a critical developmental stage, they reasoned, might lead to Alzheimer's disease. Very little is currently known about gene activity in Alzheimer's disease; therefore, this hypothesis is speculative.

Heritable, Unstable DNA and Fragile X Syndrome

Fragile X syndrome is a common cause of chromosomally determined mental retardation occurring in 1 in 2,000 males and 0.4 in 2,000 females. Phenotypically, the illness is characterized by mental retardation, large ears, an elongated face with a prominent jaw, and large testes. Individuals affected may have schizoaffective syndromes and autistic disorders (Brown et al. 1982; Reiss et al. 1986). The fragile site appears as a break or gap in the q27.3 band of the X chromosome when lymphocytes are cultured under conditions of deoxycytidine or thymidine deprivation. The fragile site is not always apparent, however. It is seen in less than half of mentally retarded males, even less frequently in mentally retarded and carrier females, and almost never in carrier males (Nussbaum and Ledbetter 1986).

Because the chromosomal defect is located on the X chromosome, one might expect inheritance to follow a relatively straightforward X-linked pattern. Oddly, it does not. Fragile X syndrome is unusual in several ways. For example, some men are cytogenetically and intellectually normal yet transmit the gene to all their daughters. In such cases, the daughters are almost always phenotypically normal but may have sons and daughters who are affected. All mutations must pass through a female before having a phenotypic effect, and affected females always receive the fragile X from their mothers, never from their fathers. Sherman (1991) noted that fragile X carrier mothers of normal transmitting males are less likely to bear affected children than the daughters of normal transmitting males. This is paradoxical, because for X-linked disease, rates of transmission for carrier mothers and carrier daughters should be identical.

Recently, an explanation has been proposed for this paradox (Richards and Sutherland 1992). The fragile X mutation belongs to a class of sequences known as microsatellite repeats. The repeat, consisting of three repeating bases, $p(CCG)_n$, may be amplified over successive generations to produce hundreds of tandem copies. Apparently, when large numbers (hundreds) of the repeat sequence are present, they disrupt expression of a gene for the ubiquitous brain protein FMR-1. Most affected fragile X males do not express this protein, and the number of repeat sequences carried by an individual correlates with degree of morbidity. Amplification of the repeat is much more likely to occur when transmitted by females than males. Hence, the normal transmitting male has a relatively low proportion of repeats, and so do his offspring, who are usually unaffected. However, once the repeat sequence is inherited by a female, amplification occurs, and her offspring are more likely to be affected. The Sherman paradox is thus explicable. Mothers and daughters of normal transmitting males have different rates of affected children because different stages of amplification of the repeat sequences are expressed.

This amplification of a simple three-base repeat sequence within the genome has a pronounced effect on psychopathology. Reiss and colleagues (1989) compared adult fragile X female carriers (who inherited the fragile X chromosome from their mothers and demonstrated positive fragility) with fragile X women who inherited the chromosome from their fathers (had negative fragility). The group with maternal inheritance and positive fragility showed greater social and educational impairment and disturbances in communication, socialization, thought, and affect. Specifically, they had a higher frequency of schizophrenia spectrum disorders, social disability in adolescence, more time away from work for psychological problems, and a tendency toward depression.

Mitochondrial Inheritance

Normally, the mechanism of inheritance involves transmission of nuclear DNA from one generation to the next. However, nuclei are not the only cellular organelles with DNA. Mitochondria also contain DNA molecules. Mitochondrial DNA comprises a separate genome coding for ribosomal ribonucleic acids (RNAs), transfer RNAs, and 13 subunits of the oxidative phosphorylation (OXPHOS) enzymes involved in adenosine triphosphate (ATP) production: subunits of NADH dehydrogenase, ubiquinol-cytochrome C oxidoreductase, cytochrome C oxidase, and ATP synthase. The extent to which cell function is determined by mitochondrial DNA depends on the extent to which the cell type utilizes mitochondrial energy; brain, heart, kidney, liver, and skeletal muscle are particularly sensitive to energy deficits. Each cell has thousands of mitochondrial DNA molecules, and possibly as much as 0.3% of total cellular DNA is mitochondrial.

The genetics of mitochondrial DNA differ in several ways from that of nuclear DNA. First, because ova contain cytoplasmic elements but sperm do not, mitochondrial DNA can only be maternally inherited. Second, mitochondrial DNA appears to be considerably more prone to deleterious mutations than nuclear DNA. Third, in those cells containing a mixture of normal and mutant DNA, the mutant and normal DNA will partition during replication, randomly resulting in daughter cells of varying mitochondrial DNA constitution. Over time, some lineages may maintain a mixture of DNA types (heteroplasmic), whereas others may drift toward a pure type (homoplasmic). Finally, in those cells containing mutant DNA, the phenotype will depend on the proportion of mutant and wild (normal) DNA in the mitochondria (Wallace 1989).

The key to recognizing mitochondrial DNA–transmitted disease is transmission exclusively through the mother. The presence of a single case of paternal transmission excludes mitochondrial inheritance. None of the typical psychiatric disorders has been shown to be associated with mitochondrial DNA. However, several neurological diseases are inherited in this manner and, as might be expected, are associated with higher central nervous system dysfunction. Leber's hereditary optic neuropathy (LHON) is characterized by blindness associated with optic nerve death, cardiac dysrhythmias, dystonias, myopathy of skeletal muscle, and mental retardation. LHON results from a missense mutation (arginine to histidine) at nucleotide 11778 in the gene for NADH dehydrogenase subunit 4. This particular arginine residue is evolutionarily conserved in mitochondrial DNA and is critical for efficient electron transport. Even this subtle mutation may lower the efficiency of electron transport, reducing neuronal ATP production and producing a gradual decline in cellular function over time (Wallace et al. 1988a).

Several other genetic diseases are inherited through mitochondrial DNA. LHON is sometimes associated with infantile bilateral striatal necrosis (IBSN). The IBSN mutation may be caused by a heteroplasmic deleterious point mutation in mitochondrial DNA. Myoclonic epilepsy and ragged red muscle fiber (MERRF) disease, which also includes cerebellar ataxia, dementia, cardiomyopathy, and hypoventilation, is also maternally inherited as a result of a deleterious heteroplasmic point mutation that leads to OXPHOS dysfunction. Strikingly, in this disorder, variation in individual mitochondrial respiratory deficiency correlates closely with severity of clinical manifestations (Wallace et al. 1988b). Another disorder characterized by mitochondrial myopathy, encephalomyopathy, lactic acidosis, and strokelike episodes (MELAS) is likely transmitted by mitochondrial DNA. Kearns-Sayre syndrome provides an interesting example of a sporadic yet genetic disease. This illness is characterized by dementia, ophthalmoplegia, retinopathy, seizures, strokelike symptoms, and deafness. The illness usually occurs sporadically but is associated with deletions of 2–7 kilobases of mitochondrial DNA. The sporadic nature of the disorder indicates that the deletions are likely new mutations that result in heteroplasmic DNA (Lestienne and Ponsot 1988).

Hormonal Effects on Gene Expression

Until recently, genes were considered to be heritable units giving rise to phenotypic variation, but little was known about their physical structure or how they exerted their effects. However, the development of molecular biology has made it possible to understand, in unprecedented detail, the physical characteristics of genes and the factors controlling gene transcription. Several classes of hormones can directly act on the genome to alter the transcription rates of some genes. For example, because steroid and thyroid hormones are highly fat soluble, they easily diffuse through the plasma membrane of target cells and bind to specific receptor proteins in the cytoplasm or cell nucleus. Once bound, this hormone-receptor complex binds with high affinity to specific DNA regulatory sequences upstream of the protein coding region of certain genes. The hormone-receptor complex acts either to enhance or to repress gene expression. Occasionally, a cascade effect develops in which the product of an enhanced gene may, in turn, activate other genes, further extending the effect of the hormone on gene expression. The intracellular receptors for steroid and thyroid hormones form a superfamily of proteins, each member recognizing a specific hormone and binding to specific DNA sequences (Evans 1988).

It would be misleading to suggest that the locus of steroid action is exclusively on the genome. As lipophilic molecules, steroids are capable of exerting some effects at the cell surface. For instance, pregnenolone can rapidly induce secretion of luteinizing hormone releasing hormone (LHRH), and some steroids facilitate GABA-receptor activation (McEwen 1991).

Nevertheless, the effects of steroids on gene expression are remarkable. One illustration involves the effects of steroids on neural plasticity. Of these, the effects of estradiol have been most studied. Estradiol can induce dendritic spine formation, increasing spine density in brain, because dendritic spines are the site of synapse formation; synaptogenesis is thus regulated via estradiol. This effect has been observed in the ventromedial nucleus (VMN) of the hypothalamus, an important site for induction of rodent female sexual behavior. Furthermore, these effects are seen with physiological levels of estradiol because, when spine density in the VMN is measured throughout the estrous cycle, spine density is significantly greater at proestrus than at diestrus (Frankfurt et al. 1990). Because these effects take hours or days to occur and are observed only in brain regions containing intracellular estrogen receptors, they are likely mediated through modulation of gene expression.

Estradiol can also induce several neurochemical changes in the brain, likely by altering gene expression. This hormone can induce the enzyme choline acetyltransferase, the major synthetic enzyme for acetylcholine, in the female rat basal forebrain. In the VMN, estradiol induces synthesis of oxytocin receptors, increasing both the number and the immunostaining of oxytocin fibers. In rats, estradiol induces progesterone-receptor synthesis in the hypothalamus and pituitary gland. This induction by estradiol is required for activation of female mating behaviors such as lordosis. That estradiol is acting through modulation of progesterone-receptor gene expression is suggested by the finding that inhibitors of RNA and protein synthesis block induction of mating behavior (Terkel et al. 1973). Estrogens also induce increases in serotonin receptors, $GABA_A$ receptors, and enkephalin messenger RNA. The time course of this induction and its location exclusively in regions containing intracellular estrogen receptors suggest a genomic mechanism of action (McEwen et al. 1991).

Undoubtedly, there are many more examples of estrogens, progesterones, and androgens acting on the genome to induce or inhibit gene transcription in the central nervous system. The effects of estradiol on progesterone-receptor induction and synaptogenesis provide just one example of how a change in hormonal concentration can modulate gene expression leading to formation of a new set of behaviors. An ultimate understanding of the genetics of behavior will not merely consist of matching genes with their respective behavioral repertoires but will involve an analysis of the physiological and environmental factors controlling regulation of gene transcription.

Conclusion

As noted at the beginning of this chapter, none of the functional psychiatric disorders fit any recognized Mendelian pattern of inheritance. Yet several psychiatric disorders have an undisputable genetic basis. These disorders might be explained by multifactorial and/or polygenic inheritance. Nevertheless, in the past decade, advances in genetics have identified several new modes of genetic transmission of disease. Each type has already been shown to affect central nervous system function. For example, genomic imprinting, as demonstrated in the Prader-Willi and Angelman syndromes, quite clearly can produce behavioral changes. The unstable microsatellite repeats of the fragile X syndrome evidently produce psychopathology. Both mosaicism and uniparental disomy are involved in the Lesch-Nyhan and Prader-Willi syndromes. The central nervous system is particularly sensitive to mutations in mitochondrial DNA, and mitochondrial disease frequently produces pathology in the central nervous system. Steroid and thyroid hormones can produce some of their behavioral effects by action on the genome.

Could functional psychiatric disorders also be subject to one or more of these genetic mechanisms? As yet, no association has been found. Nevertheless, it seems reasonable to consider the possibility. It would be worthwhile to review the segregation of psychiatric disorders in pedigrees to determine whether these disorders are consistent with one of these mechanisms. Further knowledge of factors regulating gene transcription will be helpful. Perhaps in some psychiatric disorders, the regulatory elements of one or more genes have mutated, producing abnormal gene transcriptional responses to hormonal or environmental stimuli. With the exponential increase in our knowledge of genetics currently under way, other unrecognized mechanisms of inheritance may be detected. If so, perhaps one of them will shed light on the familial segregation and molecular biology of these puzzling disorders and may explain the sometimes striking gender differences seen in psychiatric illness.

References

Baron M: Linkage between an X-chromosome marker (deutan color blindness) and bipolar affective illness: occurrence in the family of a lithium carbonate-responsive schizo-affective proband. Arch Gen Psychiatry 34:721–725, 1977

Baron M: Genetic models of schizophrenia. Acta Psychiatr Scand 65:263–275, 1982

Brown WT, Friedman E, Jenkins EC, et al: Association of fragile X syndrome with autism (letter). Lancet 1:100, 1982

Bucher KD, Elston RC: The transmission of manic depressive illness, I: theory, description of the model and summary of results. J Psychiatr Res 16:53–63, 1981

Del Zompo M, Bocchetta A, Goldin LR, et al: Linkage between X-chromosome markers and manic-depressive illness, two Sardinian pedigrees. Acta Psychiatr Scand 70:282–287, 1984

Elston RC, Namboodiri KK, Spence MA, et al: A genetic study of schizophrenia pedigrees, II: one locus hypotheses. Neuropsychobiology 4:193–206, 1978

Evans RM: The steroid and thyroid hormone receptor superfamily. Science 240:889–895, 1988

Farrer LA, Conneally PM: A genetic model for age at onset in Huntington disease. Am J Hum Genet 37:350–357, 1985

Farrer LA, Cupples LA, Connor L, et al: Association of decreased paternal age and late-onset Alzheimer's disease, an example of genetic imprinting? Arch Neurol 48:599–604, 1991

Farrer LA, Cupples LA, Kiely DK, et al: Inverse relationship between age at onset of Huntington disease and paternal age suggests involvement of genetic imprinting. Am J Hum Genet 50:528–535, 1992

Frankfurt M, Gould E, Woolley C, et al: Gonadal steroids modify dendritic spine density in ventromedial hypothalamic neurons: a Golgi study in the adult rat. Neuroendocrinology 51:530–535, 1990

Garrod AE: The incidence of alkaptonuria: a study in chemical individuality. Lancet 2:1616–1620, 1902

Gartler SM, Riggs AD: Mammalian X-chromosome inactivation. Annu Rev Genet 17:155–190, 1983

Gershon ES: Genetics, in Manic-Depressive Illness. Edited by Goodwin FK, Jamison KR. New York, Oxford University Press, 1990, pp 373–401

Gershon ES, Targum SD, Matthyse S, et al: Color blindness not closely linked to bipolar illness: report of a new pedigree series. Arch Gen Psychiatry 36:1423–1430, 1979

Gershon ES, Mendlewicz J, Gastpar M, et al: A collaborative study of genetic linkage of bipolar manic-depressive illness and red/green colorblindness. Acta Psychiatr Scand 61:319–338, 1980

Goldin LR, Gershon ES, Targum SD, et al: Segregation and linkage analyses in families of patients with bipolar, unipolar and schizoaffective mood disorders. Am J Hum Genet 35:274–287, 1983

Gottesman II, Shields J: Schizophrenia, The Epigenetic Puzzle. Cambridge, MA, Cambridge University Press, 1982

Gregory CA, Schwartz J, Kirkilionis AJ, et al: Somatic recombination rather than uniparental disomy suggested as another mechanism by which genetic imprinting may play a role in the etiology of Prader-Willi syndrome. Hum Genet 88:42–48, 1991

Hall JG: Review and hypothesis: somatic mosaicism: observations related to clinical genetics. Am J Hum Genet 43:355–363, 1988

Hall JG: Genomic imprinting: review and relevance to human diseases. Am J Hum Genet 46:857–873, 1990

Holliday R: The inheritance of epigenetic defects. Science 238:163–170, 1987

Holm VA, Pipes PL: Food and children with Prader-Willi syndrome. Am J Dis Child 130:1063–1067, 1976

Knoll JHM, Nicholls RD, Magenis RE, et al: Angelman and Prader-Willi syndromes share a common chromosome 15 deletion but differ in parental origin of the deletion. Am J Med Genet 32:285–290, 1989

Laird CD: Proposed genetic basis of Huntington's disease. Trends Genet 6:242–247, 1990

Lesch M, Nyhan WL: A familial disorder of uric acid metabolism and central nervous system function. Am J Med 36:561–570, 1964

Lestienne P, Ponsot G: Kearns-Sayre syndrome with muscle mitochondrial DNA deletion (letter). Lancet 1:885, 1988

Lorenz KZ: King Solomon's Ring, New Light on Animal Ways. New York, Time Inc Book Division, 1952

Lyon MF: Gene action in the X-chromosome of the mouse (Mus musculus L.) (letter). Nature 190:372–373, 1961

Malcolm S, Clayton-Smith J, Nichols M, et al: Uniparental disomy in the Angelman syndrome. Lancet 337:694–697, 1991

McEwen BS: Non-genomic and genomic effects of steroids on neural activity. Trends Pharmacol Sci 12:141–147, 1991

McEwen BS, Coirini H, Westlind-Danielsson A, et al: Steroid hormones as mediators of neural plasticity. J Steroid Biochem Mol Biol 39:223–232, 1991

Mendel G: Experiments in plant hybridization, in Classic Papers in Genetics. Edited by Peters JA. New York, Prentice-Hall, 1959, pp 1–20

Mendlewicz J, Fleiss JL: Linkage studies with X-chromosome markers in bipolar (manic-depressive) and unipolar (depressive) illnesses. Biol Psychiatry 9:261–294, 1974

Mendlewicz J, Linkowski P, Guroff JJ, et al: Color blindness linkage to bipolar manic-depressive illness: new evidence. Arch Gen Psychiatry 36:1442–1447, 1979

Mendlewicz J, Linkowski P, Wilmotte J: Linkage between glucose-6-phosphate dehydrogenase deficiency and manic-depressive psychosis. Br J Psychiatry 137:337–342, 1980

Migeon BR: X-linked hypoxanthine-guanine phosphoribosyl transferase deficiency: detection of heterozygotes by selective medium. Biochem Genet 4:377–383, 1970

Monk M, Boubelik M, Lehnert S: Temporal and regional changes in DNA methylation in the embryonic, extraembryonic and germ cell lineages during mouse development. Development 99:371–382, 1987

Nicholls RD, Knoll JH, Butler MG, et al: Genetic imprinting suggested by maternal heterodisomy in non-deletion Prader-Willi syndrome. Nature 342:281–285, 1989

Nielsen KG, Poulsen H, Mikkelsen M, et al: Multiple recurrence of trisomy 21 Down syndrome. Hum Genet 78:103–105, 1988

Nussbaum RL, Ledbetter DH: Fragile X syndrome: a unique mutation in man. Annu Rev Genet 20:109–145, 1986

Nyhan WL, Bakay B, Connor JD, et al: Hemizygous expression of glucose-6-phosphate dehydrogenase in erythrocytes of heterozygotes for the Lesch-Nyhan syndrome. Proc Natl Acad Sci U S A 65:214–218, 1970

Reiss AL, Feinstein C, Toomey KE, et al: Psychiatric disability associated with the fragile X chromosome. Am J Med Genet 23:393–401, 1986

Reiss AL, Freund L, Vinogradov S, et al: Parental inheritance and psychological disability in fragile X females. Am J Hum Genet 45:697–705, 1989

Riccardi VM, Lewis RA: Penetrance of von Recklinghausen neurofibromatosis: a distinction between predecessors and descendants. Am J Hum Genet 42:284–289, 1988

Richards RI, Sutherland GR: Fragile X syndrome: the molecular picture comes into focus. Trends Genet 8:249–255, 1992

Ridley RM, Frith CD, Crow TJ, et al: Anticipation in Huntington's disease is inherited through the male line but may originate in the female. J Med Genet 25:589–595, 1988

Risch N, Baron M, Mendlewicz J: Assessing the role of X linked inheritance in bipolar-related major affective disorder. J Psychiatr Res 20:275–288, 1986

Sapienza C: Genome imprinting and dominance modification. Ann N Y Acad Sci 564:24–38, 1989

Seegmiller JE, Rosenbloom FM, Kelley WN: Enzyme defect associated with a sex-linked human neurological disorder and excessive purine synthesis. Science 155:1682–1684, 1967

Sherman SL: Genetic epidemiology of the fragile X syndrome with special reference to genetic counselling, in Fragile X Cancer Cytogenetics. Edited by Willey AM, Murphy PD. Prog Clin Biol Res 368:79–99, 1991

Spence JE, Perciaccante RG, Greig GM, et al: Uniparental disomy as a mechanism to human genetic disease. Am J Hum Genet 42:217–226, 1988

Spofford JB: Parental control of position effect variegation, I: parental heterochromatin and expression of the white locus in compound X Drosophila melanogaster. Proc Natl Acad Sci U S A 45:1003–1007, 1959

Surani MAH, Reik W, Norris ML, et al: Influence of germline modifications of homologous chromosomes in mouse development. Journal of Embryology and Experimental Morphology 97 (suppl):123–136, 1986

Terkel AS, Shryne J, Gorski RA: Inhibition of estrogen facilitation of sexual behaviour by the intracerebral infusion of actinomycin-D. Horm Behav 4:377–386, 1973

Vidaud D, Vidaud M, Plassa F, et al: Father-to-son transmission of hemophilia A due to uniparental disomy (abstract). Am J Hum Genet 45:A226, 1989

Voss R, Ben-Simon E, Avital A, et al: Isodisomy of chromosome 7 in a patient with cystic fibrosis: could uniparental disomy be common in humans? Am J Hum Genet 45:373–380, 1989

Wagstaff J, Chaillet JR, Lalande M: The GABA$_A$ receptor β3 subunit gene: characterization of a human cDNA from chromosome 15q11q13 and mapping to a region of conserved synteny on mouse chromosome 7. Genomics 11:1071–1078, 1991

Wallace DC: Mitochondrial DNA mutations and neuromuscular disease. Trends Genet 5:9–13, 1989

Wallace DC, Singh G, Lott MT, et al: Mitochondrial DNA mutation associated with Leber's hereditary optic neuropathy. Science 242:1427–1430, 1988a

Wallace DC, Zheng X, Lott MT, et al: Familial mitochondrial encephalomyopathy (MERRF): genetic, pathophysiological, and biochemical characterization of a mitochondrial DNA disease. Cell 55:601–610, 1988b

Williams CA, Frias JL: The Angelman ("happy puppet") syndrome. Am J Med Genet 11:453–460, 1982

Winokur G, Clayton PJ, Reich T: Manic depressive disease and linkage with a genetic marker, in Manic Depressive Illness. St. Louis, MO, CV Mosby, 1969, pp 122–125

CHAPTER 4

Epidemiology and Theories of Gender Differences in Unipolar Depression

Susan Nolen-Hoeksema, Ph.D.

M ajor depression is one of the most common forms of psychopathology, and it is much more common in women than in men (Paykel 1991). In this chapter, I briefly review the epidemiology of gender differences in depression and then review the most prominent theories for why women are more vulnerable to depression.

Definitions and Rates of Depression

Depressive Disorders

The common symptoms of depression include loss of motivation, sadness, low self-esteem, physical aches and pains, difficulty in concentration, anhedonia, appetite and sleep disturbances, fatigue, psychomotor retardation or agitation, and suicidal ideation. According to DSM-IV (American Psychiatric Association 1994), to receive a diagnosis of a major depressive episode, an individual must experience anhedonia or sadness plus four of the other symptoms of depression for at least a 2-week period. DSM-IV also recognizes a more chronic and less severe form of depression, dysthymic disorder, in which individuals experience depressed mood plus at least two depressive symptoms consistently for at least 2 years. (The criteria for diagnoses of major depression and dysthymic disorder in the two previous editions of the DSM were almost identical to the criteria in DSM-IV.)

As can be seen in Table 4-1, the rates of people treated for major depression and dysthymic disorder are higher in women than in men across all age groups of adults. The treatment statistics presented in Table 4-1 are for people treated for any type of affective disorder (as defined by DSM-III [American Psychiatric Association 1980]) in inpatient mental health facilities in 1980 (National Institute of Mental Health, Survey and Reports Branch, Division of Biometry and Applied Sciences, unpublished data, September 1987). Across all age groups, 206 of 100,000 women and 138 of 100,000 men in the general population were treated for a unipolar depression. The data in Table 4-2 are from a study conducted by the National Institute of Mental Health of 9,543 adults in three United States cities (Myers et al. 1984). In this study, the Diagnostic Interview Schedule (Robins et al. 1981) was administered to a representative sample of each city, and the information was used to make DSM-III diagnoses as warranted. The rates in Table 4-2 represent the percentages of people estimated to

Table 4-1. Rate of people treated for depressive disorders, per 100,000 population (1980)

Age group (years)	Females	Males
18–24	151	123
25–44	266	178
45–64	251	141
65+	154	110

Source. National Institute of Mental Health: "Psychiatric Hospitalizations in 1980," unpublished data. Survey and Reports Branch, Division of Biometry and Applied Sciences, 1987.

meet the criteria for a diagnosis of major depression during the 6 months before the interview. Across all age groups, 4.0% of the women and 1.7% of the men were diagnosed with a major depressive disorder.

The sex difference in rates of depressive disorders does not emerge until early to midadolescence. In studies of preadolescent children, equal rates of depression in boys and girls have been reported; boys may even have higher rates of depression than girls (see Nolen-Hoeksema 1990 and Nolen-Hoeksema and Girgus 1994 for reviews). For example, Anderson and colleagues (1987) administered the Diagnostic Interview Schedule for Children (Herjanic and Reich 1982) to 792 children aged 11 years. They found that 2.5% of the boys, but only 0.5% of the girls, met the criteria for a major depressive disorder or dysthymic disorder. In contrast, when Kashani and colleagues (1987) administered the Diagnostic Interview Schedule for Children and Adolescents (Herjanic and Reich 1982) to 150 adolescents, ages 14–16 years, they found that 13.3% of the girls but only 2.7% of the boys met the criteria for a major depressive disorder or dysthymic disorder. This developmental trend in the emergence of sex differences in depressive disorders is not well understood, but it provides an important backdrop against which to view any theory of why females are more prone to depression than males.

Depressive Symptoms

One of the biggest debates in research on depression is whether periods of depressive symptoms that do not quite meet the criteria for

Table 4–2. Rates of depressive disorders in the general population diagnosed using structured clinical interviews (DSM-III criteria)

Age group (years)	Female (%)	Male (%)
18–24	6.9	3.8
25–44	10.8	4.8
45–64	7.8	3.3
65+	3.2	1.2

Source. Adapted from Myers et al. 1984.

a depressive disorder differ in *kind* or only in *severity* from "true" depressive disorders. There is no definitive answer to this question. However, even moderate levels of depression interfere with functioning in occupational, school, and social settings (e.g., Hirschfeld and Cross 1982; Kandel and Davies 1986). Thus, sex differences in these milder forms of depression should also be of interest. One of the largest studies of depressive symptoms in the United States was conducted by Comstock and Helsing (1976). In this study, 3,845 adults completed the Center for Epidemiological Studies Depression Scale (CESD; Radloff 1977), a widely used self-report measure of depressive symptoms. More women than men scored in the "depressed" range of the CESD at all age levels.

As stated earlier, the sex difference in rates of more severe depressive symptoms does not emerge until early to midadolescence. In a study of depressive symptoms in elementary-school children, we found that boys consistently showed higher levels of symptoms than girls on a self-report measure through age 12 years (Nolen-Hoeksema et al. 1991; see also Petersen et al. 1991). However, in a study of 762 adolescents, ages 15–16 years, Kandel and Davies (1986) found that 23% of the girls and only 10% of the boys reported depressive symptoms that were at moderate-to-severe levels.

Cross-Cultural Studies of Gender Differences in Depression

The higher rate of depression in women than in men is found across a variety of cultures, despite variations in the definition and measurement of depression (Nolen-Hoeksema 1990). The female-to-male ratio varies considerably, but, across countries, about twice as many women have depression (Paykel 1991).

Biological Explanations for the Gender Difference in Depression

Several investigators have suggested that depression in women is brought about by changes or imbalances in levels of estrogen, progesterone, or other female hormones (Harris et al. 1989; O'Hara 1987; Parry 1994). This hypothesis is fueled by evidence that women are particularly prone to depression during times in their lives when their bodies experience significant hormonal changes—specifically, the premenstrual period, the postpartum period, and menopause—and by the fact that the gender differences in depression appear to start during or after puberty, when pronounced sex differences in tonic levels of gonadal hormones (e.g., estrogens, progestins, and androgens) emerge. These hormones enter the brain and may influence mood by modulating the release of certain neurotransmitters associated with mood, especially norepinephrine and serotonin.

Nevertheless, the very notion that women often experience depression during periods of hormonal flux has been severely challenged by empirical research. The most clear-cut case is menopausal depression. Several studies indicate that women are no more likely to show depression around the time of menopause than at any other time in their lives (Matthews et al. 1990; Weissman 1979).

Postpartum Depression

The prevalence of mild postpartum "blues" has been estimated to be very high. When standardized depression questionnaires, such as the Beck Depression Inventory (Beck 1978), are used to assess depressive symptoms, about 30% of women score above the cutoff for mild depression at about 2 weeks after delivery (Cutrona 1982; O'Hara et al. 1984). O'Hara et al. (1984) found, however, that postpartum women score higher than matched control groups only on somatic symptoms associated with depression (e.g., appetite loss, fatigue) and actually score lower than control groups on the cognitive/affective symptoms of depression (e.g., sadness, guilt, pessimism).

Estimates of the prevalence of major depressive episodes in women during the postpartum period range from 3% to 33%, depending on the stringency of the criteria used to diagnose depression (Cutrona 1982). Cutrona interviewed 85 first-time mothers in their third trimester of pregnancy, 2 weeks after delivery, and 8 weeks after delivery and found that 8.2% of the women met the criteria for a diagnosis of major depressive disorder (as defined by DSM-III) in at least one of the interviews. This figure is higher than the rate of depression in women who are neither pregnant nor in the postpartum period (Weissman and Myers 1978), suggesting that the risk for this disorder is increased during pregnancy and the postpartum period. (For similar results, see O'Hara et al. 1984 and Webster et al. 1994.)

However, researchers who have attempted to link postpartum depression to specific imbalances in hormones have found few consistent differences between postpartum women with and without depression. One of the biggest problems for a hormonal explanation of postpartum depression is that many, perhaps most, women who are depressed postpartum were depressed during pregnancy, and hormonal levels during these two periods differ greatly (O'Hara et al. 1982). Other researchers have searched inconclusively for evidence that disturbances in specific neurotransmitters can be correlated with postpartum depression (Harris et al. 1989).

On the other hand, there is evidence that psychosocial factors affect a woman's vulnerability to postpartum depression. Women who are undergoing chronic stress (e.g., financial strain or marital difficulties) or isolated stress (e.g., bereavement) at the time of childbirth may be more likely to develop postpartum depression than women not undergoing such stress. Women who have conflictual relationships with their parents, no close confidants, or no close relatives living nearby may be more prone to postpartum depression. Finally, women who interpret the difficult situations in their lives in pessimistic self-defeating ways appear more likely to develop postpartum depressive symptoms (O'Hara 1987).

Thus, some evidence suggests that the quality of social support and the existence of additional stressors at the time of childbirth predict postpartum depression. The argument that environmental factors may be more relevant than biological factors is buttressed by evidence that adoptive mothers and natural fathers are also at increased risk for depression after the arrival of a new baby (Rees and Lutkins 1971).

Premenstrual Depression

The belief that women often experience significant depression during their premenstrual period is very strongly held by laypeople, clinicians, and researchers. One of the most popular assessment tools in studies of premenstrual symptoms has been the Moos Menstrual Distress Questionnaire (Moos 1968). This questionnaire lists 47 symptoms, divided into eight categories: pain, trouble concentrating, lowered daily activity, autonomic reactions (dizziness, vomiting), water retention, negative affect (depression, anxiety), arousal (affectionate feelings or well-being), and control (heart pounding, feeling of suffocation). Women are asked to rate, on a six-point scale, the extent to which they experienced each symptom during each of the premenstrual, menstrual, and intermenstrual phases of their last cycle. Reviews of the older literature on premenstrual symptoms tend to conclude that "the general consensus based on questionnaire data is that 70% to 90% of the female population will admit to recurrent premenstrual symptoms and that 20% to 40% report some degree of temporary mental or physical incapacitation" (Reid and Yen 1981, p. 86).

However, several studies show that the information women provide on retrospective questionnaires bears no resemblance to their actual experience of mood during the menstrual cycle (Gallant et al. 1992; Parlee 1982, 1994; Schnurr et al. 1994). As a result, investigators and clinicians have required that a diagnosis of premenstrual depression be made on the basis of prospective charting of a woman's mood throughout the menstrual cycle, for at least two menstrual cycles. Indeed, the criteria for late luteal phase dysphoric disorder set forth in the DSM-III-R (American Psychiatric Association 1987) require prospective evidence of elevations in depressive symptoms occurring during the late luteal phase, followed by decreases in depressive symptoms after the onset of the follicular phase.

Prospective studies have found that it is possible to identify women who have elevated depressive symptoms during the late luteal phase and women who meet the criteria for late luteal phase dysphoric disorder as defined in the DSM-III-R (see review by Endicott 1994). Almost all of these studies used samples of women who had sought treatment for premenstrual complaints or who had responded to advertisements for women who have premenstrual mood changes. To date, however, we do not know the prevalence of serious depressive episodes during the late luteal phase in the general population of women. In addition, as Endicott (1994) notes, studies of women seeking treatment for premenstrual complaints have found that many of these women "will not be found to have a clear-cut and distinct condition that meets the proposed criteria for late luteal phase dysphoric disorder because the symptoms are not present, are not severe enough, or cannot be differentiated from some other chronic medical condition" (p. 12). It has been especially difficult to differentiate the diagnosis of premenstrual depression from depression not related to the menstrual cycle or other psychiatric disorders. Most studies have found that the majority of women who meet the criteria for late luteal phase dysphoric disorder have a history of either major depressive episodes with no connection to the menstrual cycle or other psychiatric disorders (usually anxiety disorder) (Harrison et al. 1989; Pearlstein et al. 1990; Severino et al. 1989).

Parry (1994) reviewed recent studies of biological correlates of premenstrual complaints. With regard to the role of estrogen and progesterone in premenstrual mood changes, Parry concluded that "no consistent or identifiable pattern has been established that can differentiate women with PMS from control subjects" (p. 50). With regard to neurovegetative signs and symptoms (sleep and appetite) during the menstrual cycle, some studies provide evidence suggesting differences between women with premenstrual syndrome (PMS) and control subjects, but these have been small-scale pilot studies. With regard to neuroendocrine differences between women with PMS and control subjects, there are no consistent findings on thyroid, cortisol, prolactin, or glucose abnormalities. One study found differences in melatonin secretion between women with PMS and control subjects (Parry et al. 1990), but this study has yet to be replicated. A few small studies have found differences between women with PMS and control subjects in premenstrual levels of serotonin. Finally, studies have shown that plasma β-endorphin levels are lower in women with PMS than in control subjects during the luteal phase. Parry (1994) concluded that the existing research suggests that women with PMS have a biological vulnerability manifested in the serotonergic and melatonin systems that is unmasked premenstrually. Clearly, however, a great deal more research using large samples and careful diagnostic criteria is necessary before firm conclusions about the biological correlates of premenstrual mood changes can be made.

Puberty

Whether the hormonal changes girls experience at puberty account for the increase in their vulnerability to depression at this time has been examined in a limited number of studies. The few existing studies of the relationship between the hormonal changes at puberty and depression in early adolescent girls suggest that the emergence of the sex difference in depression is not directly related to hormonal changes (Brooks-Gunn and Warren 1989; Paikoff et al. 1991; Sussman et al. 1987, 1991). For example, in a study of 103 girls, ages 10–14 years, Brooks-Gunn and Warren (1989) found no relationship between degree of depression and levels of any of five different hormones. In an analysis of follow-up data on 72 of these girls, Paikoff and colleagues (1991) found a positive linear relationship between levels of estradiol and one self-report measure of depression, but estradiol levels were not significantly correlated with maternal reports of the girls' depression levels or with a second self-report measure of depression. Sussman and colleagues (1987, 1991) found no significant relationships between estradiol levels (or levels of several other hormones) and depression in either early adolescent girls or boys.

Brooks-Gunn (1988) has suggested that another biological change of adolescence—the development of secondary sex characteristics— may have a greater influence on the emotional development of girls and boys than hormonal development because these characteristics affect male and female self-esteem differently. Girls appear to value the physical changes that accompany puberty much less than boys do. Girls dislike the weight gained in fat and their loss of the long, lithe prepubescent look that is idealized in modern fashions; in contrast, boys like the increase in muscle mass and other pubertal changes their bodies undergo (Dornbusch et al. 1984; Simmons and Blyth 1987; Tobin-Richards et al. 1983). In turn, body satisfaction appears to be more closely related to self-esteem and well-being in girls than in boys (Allgood-Merten et al. 1990). Thus, girls' attitudes toward their physical changes at puberty are more negative than boys' attitudes, and, at the same time, girls' self-esteem is more closely associated with body image than is boys' self-esteem. Several studies have shown that the more negative body image in girls is associated with increased levels of depression in girls compared with boys (Allgood-

Merten et al. 1990; Teri 1982). In addition, girls who enter puberty significantly earlier than their peers are at particularly high risk for body dissatisfaction and for developing major depressive episodes (Hayward et al. 1993).

Conclusions

The hormonal explanations of sex differences in depression have not, thus far, been well supported. First, the increase in risk for depression during periods of hormonal change does not seem to be as great as is commonly believed. Even among women who do clearly experience serious depression during periods of hormonal fluctuation, there has been no consistent evidence of a particular hormonal or biochemical abnormality that distinguishes them from women who do not experience such depression.

Personality Theories

Two personality characteristics are thought to be more common in women than in men and may, theoretically, contribute to women's greater vulnerability to depression. First, women are said to be more likely than men to base their self-esteem on their relationships with others (Kaplan 1986). Second, women are thought to be less assertive and to lack self-confidence compared with men and to have low expectations for their ability to control important events (Radloff 1975).

Relationship With Others ("Dependency")

One of the major problems in investigating sex differences in "dependency" has been in operationalizing the construct (Maccoby and Jacklin 1974). In studies of children, dependency has been defined as the tendency to seek help, consolation, reassurance, or protection; the tendency to remain near others; and the tendency to touch or cling to others. When Maccoby and Jacklin (1974) tallied the results of 32 studies of infants and preschoolers, they found no consistent sex differences in these various operationalizations of dependency.

Steinberg and Silverberg (1986) assessed dependency in adolescents through a self-report questionnaire given to 865 adolescents, ages 10–16 years. The questionnaire asked subjects about their emotional dependence or autonomy in their relationships with their parents and with their peers and their sense of self-reliance. At all age levels, girls rated themselves as *more* autonomous and *less* dependent than boys rated themselves. Similarly, Levit (1991) found that adolescent girls (ages 14–19) described themselves as more "communal" (e.g., helpful and friendly) than did adolescent boys, but there were no sex differences in scores on a "passivity-dependency" scale (see also Allgood-Merten et al. 1990).

In the adult literature, there is some evidence that men's emotional well-being is actually more at risk than women's well-being when they lose a close relationship. After divorce and after the death of a spouse, men are as likely or more likely than women to experience depression and physical illness (Stroebe and Stroebe 1987). Moreover, whereas married men clearly are at lower risk for depression than unmarried men, marriage does not afford the same protection against depression for women (Gove 1972). Indeed, some studies show that married women are more likely to be depressed than unmarried women.

Thus, there is little evidence that women are more dependent than men on relationships for their emotional well-being and that this contributes to women's higher rate of depression. Women may describe themselves as more communal and people oriented than men, but this does not appear to put them at risk for depression. Indeed, having a strong social network may act as a buffer against depression (Belsher and Costello 1991; Brugha et al. 1987, 1990; Kessler et al. 1985).

Assertiveness

Perhaps the most popular personality-based explanation for why women are more prone to depression is that they tend to be unassertive, have a low opinion of their competence, and blame themselves for adverse events. As in studies of dependency, it has been difficult for researchers to find a satisfactory operationalization of assertiveness. Much of the evidence pertinent to the assertiveness hypothesis comes from studies of the causal attributions children and adults make for achievement-related successes and failures and their subsequent tendencies toward helplessness or mastery orientation.

Meta-analyses of the literature on sex differences in attributions for events have shown that the evidence for such differences is mixed at best (Frieze et al. 1982; Sohn 1982). Some studies find that females make more self-defeating attributions than males (e.g., Basow and Medcalf 1988; Frey and Ruble 1987; Licht et al. 1989; Ryckman and Peckman 1987). Other studies find no sex differences (Winfield 1988).

When researchers have directly observed males' and females' tendencies to show learned helplessness deficits, defined as lowered motivation and persistence, passivity, and lowered self-esteem in response to uncontrollable events, there also have been mixed results. Some studies of preadolescents have found that girls show more learned helplessness deficits compared with boys after unsuccessfully completing unsolvable tasks. Other studies of preadolescents and adolescents or college students (Baucom and Danker-Brown 1984; Roberts and Nolen-Hoeksema 1989) have found no sex differences in learned helplessness after unsuccessful completion of tasks. Furthermore, several of the studies that have shown females to make more self-defeating attributions and to be more prone to helplessness than males have been conducted with children; yet, among preadolescent children, boys are more likely than girls to show actual achievement problems and to become depressed. Thus, the hypothesis that sex differences in attributional tendencies and perceived control lead to more helplessness and depression in females than males has not been consistently supported.

Some self-report studies have used the Masculinity Scale of the Bem Sex Role Inventory (BSRI; Bem 1974) as a measure of assertiveness. This scale includes several items that index instrumentality and assertive behaviors, such as "willingness to take risks" and "has leadership abilities." Correlational studies have shown that the more masculine-type traits males or females endorse, the less likely they are to be depressed (Allgood-Merten et al. 1990; Craighead and Green 1989; Petersen et al. 1991). In addition, two studies have found that endorsement of masculine-type traits is a better predictor of depression levels in adolescents than several other variables and seems to account substantially for observed sex differences in depression (Allgood-Merten et al. 1990; Petersen et al. 1991).

Thus, the evidence suggests that the lower level of masculine attributes, such as independence and instrumentality, in girls compared with boys might help to explain their greater likelihood of depression. In contrast, there is little evidence that the presence of feminine attributes, such as sociability, leads to higher levels of depression in girls. One problem with the studies cited above, however, is that they all relied on self-report measures of attributes and depression. Common method variance, or more specifically the overlap in the content of the items measuring instrumentality, self-esteem, and depression, may account for the relationships observed.

Reviews of studies of aggression show a consistent trend for males to be more likely to engage in aggression than females (Nolen-Hoeksema 1990). The distributions of data on aggression, however, show that males are overrepresented in that small group of people who are very aggressive, but generally the distributions in males and females overlap (Maccoby and Jacklin 1980).

Perhaps a more acceptable operationalization of assertiveness is found in studies of dominance and submissiveness in group interactions. In a number of studies of male and female styles of interacting in same-sex and mixed-sex groups, the members of the group are working toward a goal or deciding how to share a scarce resource (see reviews by Maccoby 1990 and Maltz and Borker 1983). In samples ranging in age from preschoolers to adults, sex differences in styles of interacting exist. In same-sex groups, males tend to be concerned with issues of dominance: they interrupt one another, use commands or boasts of authority, harass and heckle one another, and refuse to comply with others' demands. Females in same-sex groups are more concerned with reciprocity and maintaining positive relations between members: they express agreement with one another, pause to allow each member her chance to speak, and work to ensure that each person receives a share of the scarce resource. It is *not* the case that females are generally more passive or unassertive in their interactions with other females than men are in their interactions with other men; there are no sex differences in simple level of activity in same-sex groups. There simply seem to be different goals and styles of interacting in female groups than in male groups.

In mixed-sex groups, however, males' more competitive and aggressive interacting style sometimes seems to overwhelm females' more cooperative, polite style (Fagot 1985; Lockheed 1985; Pugh and

Wahrman 1983). In studies of preschoolers, Jacklin and Maccoby (1978) found that, in mixed-sex groups, girls would stand on the sidelines watching the boys play, even though these same girls had earlier been very active in all-girl groups. Boys in mixed-sex groups are not responsive to girls' attempts to influence them verbally and tend to take more than their share of scarce resources, leaving the girls with less than their share (Powlishta and Maccoby 1990). Among adults, men's and women's behavior in mixed-sex groups is more complex (Maccoby 1990). Men talk more than women in mixed-sex groups (e.g., interrupting, offering their opinions, and directing the group) (Eagly 1987). In some studies, women appear to become more assertive in interactions with men than they are in interactions with women (e.g., raising their voices and interrupting) (Carli 1989). In other studies, women appear to focus their behaviors on maintaining and supporting the group process; for example, by reflecting others' comments and giving praise rather than providing their own opinions and suggestions as men do (Eagly 1987).

Are females unhappy about their roles and outcomes in mixed-sex interactions? A few laboratory studies of adults have found that women are less satisfied and more uncomfortable after working on a problem with a man than men are after working with a woman (Hogg and Turner 1987). In general, however, studies have focused on documenting differences in male and female interaction styles and not on each group member's emotional reaction to the interactions. Although one might argue that "losing" in interactions with males is demoralizing for females and could contribute to low self-esteem and perhaps even to depression, none of the studies described above were designed to test this hypothesis.

Nolen-Hoeksema (1990) has argued that a specific type of passivity is especially significant to the development and maintenance of depression. Some people, when they feel depressed or distressed, tend to focus on their distress and passively ruminate about it rather than take action to distract themselves or change their situations. Laboratory and naturalistic studies have shown that people with such a passive, ruminative style of coping with depression and distress have longer and more severe periods of depression (see Nolen-Hoeksema 1991). Moreover, studies of adults have shown that this style is more prevalent in women than in men (Nolen-Hoeksema et al. 1993).

Our ongoing self-report studies of rumination and depression in older children and adolescents suggest that girls demonstrate a more ruminative style than boys (Girgus et al. 1991). The girls in these studies were more depressed than the boys at every grade level (the youngest grade level was the sixth grade). Regression analyses showed that the gender differences in depression become nonsignificant when ruminative response styles are entered into the equation, suggesting that the gender differences in depression may be accounted for, in part, by gender differences in ruminative response styles.

In summary, there is some evidence that women describe themselves as less instrumental, less aggressive, and less domineering in mixed-sex interactions. They have a greater tendency toward a ruminative style of handling their moods than men. However, these sex differences are present in preadolescent children, perhaps even to a greater extent than they are in adolescents and adults. In contrast, the gender differences in depression do not emerge until adolescence. It is therefore questionable whether gender differences in assertiveness, aggressiveness, or instrumentality can fully explain the gender difference in rates of depression.

Nolen-Hoeksema and Girgus (1994) suggest that if a tendency toward less instrumentality, less assertiveness, or less aggressiveness contributes to females' tendency toward depression, it must do so in interaction with other forces emerging in early adolescence. We argue that girls face certain challenges in early adolescence that boys do not face. These challenges, combined with their less aggressive interaction styles and perhaps with their more ruminative style of coping with their emotions, increase girls' risk for depression, relative to boys, in early adolescence and then into adulthood (see also Nolen-Hoeksema 1990 and Petersen et al. 1991). These challenges may include hormonal dysregulation, which first arises as girls enter puberty, and a variety of social challenges, described in the next section.

Social Conditions

Several psychologists and sociologists have argued that the restrictive social role prescribed for females and the secondary status of women in society result in a greater likelihood of depression in females than in males (Gove and Herb 1974; McGrath et al. 1990; Radloff 1975). In early adolescence—the time when gender differences in depression emerge—girls may confront the restrictions of their sex roles.

Parents allow their sons to have more independence than their daughters (Block 1991). For example, in their study of sixth- through tenth-grade students, Simmons and Blyth (1987) found that boys were more likely than girls to report that their parents' permission was not needed for going places after dark, that they were left at home alone, and that their parents expected them to act older. Interestingly, the girls actually said they valued independence more than the boys. This may be because they were not given the independence they wanted. Also, even though the girls were more likely than the boys to want to go to college and to have a high-status job, the boys were more likely than the girls to report that their parents expected them to have a career. This suggests that parents' expectations were lower and their encouragement was less than the girls' aspirations, at least from the girls' point of view.

One result of parents' messages to girls about girls' abilities may be their choices of subjects to study and careers to pursue. In high school, the percentage of girls in math courses declines precipitously, whereas girls make up nearly the entire class in feminine-stereotyped courses, such as home economics. In addition, girls' actual performance in math decreases relative to boys' in high school (Grant and Eiden 1982). In college, the percentage of women who are majoring in math and science is quite small. For example, in 1986–1987, women received only 15% of the bachelor's degrees awarded in engineering (National Center for Educational Statistics 1989). In contrast, women received 76% of the bachelor of arts degrees in education and 84% of the bachelor's degrees in nursing and home economics. Although girls may enter female-dominated fields voluntarily (Eccles et al. 1984), they may also set themselves up for jobs that are low paying, resulting in low status and, perhaps, frustration.

A woman who attempts to assert her expertise or authority in a situation is often seen as being "out of place." In a recent review of studies of perceptions of male and female leaders, Eagly and colleagues (1992) found that female leaders were generally perceived less favorably than male leaders, but this was particularly true if the woman had a "masculine" style of leading.

Do the social consequences of showing one's competence and otherwise violating the feminine stereotype lead to depression in females? We do not know. Block and co-workers (1991) found a significant positive correlation between intelligence and depression in adolescent girls. Thus, the more intelligent girls were more depressed than the less intelligent girls. In contrast, in boys there was a small negative correlation between intelligence and depression, indicating that being intelligent was associated with somewhat less depression in the boys. These data support the suggestions of Gove and Herb (1974) that females who are intelligent and who reject demands to conceal their competence and assertiveness are at increased risk for depression.

Increases in Sexual Abuse in Adolescent Females

There is one additional explanation for the increase in rates of depression in girls in adolescence that cannot be ignored. Rates of sexual abuse in girls increase substantially in early adolescence, and many girls continue to be abused throughout their adolescent years (Russell 1984). In a random sample of 930 adult women, Russell found that 12% of the women had experienced some type of serious intrafamilial sexual abuse (e.g., an incestuous relationship with a father or stepfather; unwanted fondling by an uncle) before age 17 years; 26% of the women had experienced serious abuse from someone outside the family before age 17. The greatest increase in rates of abuse occurred between ages 10 and 14 years. Girls are two to three times more likely than boys to be the victims of sexual abuse (Finkelhor et al. 1990).

Females who have been raped and sexually abused show high levels of depression just after an assault (Wirtz and Harrell 1987) and perhaps for many months thereafter (Kilpatrick et al. 1981). One study found that more than half of the women who sought therapy for depression as adults in one clinic were sexually abused as children (Carmen et al. 1984). Cutler and Nolen-Hoeksema (1991) attempted to calculate the extent to which childhood sexual abuse accounts for sex differences in depression among adults from studies that assessed depression in randomly selected abused patients and control groups using well-accepted standardized clinical interviews (e.g., Stein et al. 1988). They estimated that up to 35% of the difference in rates of depression in adult men and women might be attributable to the higher rate of childhood sexual abuse (and subsequent depression) in women compared with men. Thus, it seems very plausible that at least some of the increases in depression rates in girls as they progress through adolescence can be attributed to increases in the fear of abuse and in actual rates of abuse (see also Beitchman et al. 1992).

Conclusion

Several of the explanations for women's greater vulnerability to depression have not been supported. Despite strong popular belief that women's moods are linked to their hormones, there has been little consistent evidence that the gender differences in depression are hormonally mediated. Similarly, the notion that women are more dependent on others for their well-being and that this contributes to their greater vulnerability to depression is not supported by the existing research. Women do appear to be less aggressive and domineering than men and may have a more passive, ruminative coping style than men. The extent to which these characteristics contribute to the gender differences in depression is not well known yet. Finally, women face a number of obstacles and threats, such as discrimination and violence, that may contribute to their tendencies toward depression. Clearly, much more research is required to understand the sources of gender differences in depression. Based on the very large number of women (and men) with depression, this is an important area for future study.

References

Allgood-Merten B, Lewinsohn PM, Hops H: Sex differences and adolescent depression. J Abnorm Psychol 99:55–63, 1990

American Psychiatric Association: Diagnostic and Statistical Manual of Mental Disorders, 3rd Edition. Washington, DC, American Psychiatric Association, 1980

American Psychiatric Association: Diagnostic and Statistical Manual of Mental Disorders, 3rd Edition, Revised. Washington, DC, American Psychiatric Association, 1987

American Psychiatric Association: Diagnostic and Statistical Manual of Mental Disorders, 4th Edition. Washington, DC, American Psychiatric Association, 1994

Anderson JC, Williams S, McGee R, et al: DSM-III disorders in preadolescent children. Arch Gen Psychiatry 44:69–76, 1987

Basow SA, Medcalf KL: Academic achievement and attributions among college students: effects of gender and sex-typing. Sex Roles 19:555–567, 1988

Baucom DH, Danker-Brown P: Sex role identity and sex-stereotyped tasks in the development of learned helplessness in women. J Pers Soc Psychol 46:422–430, 1984

Beck AT: Depression Inventory. Philadelphia, PA, Philadelphia Center for Cognitive Therapy, 1978

Beitchman JH, Zucker K, Hood E, et al: A review of the long-term effects of child sexual abuse. Child Abuse Negl 16:101–118, 1992

Belsher G, Costello CG: Do confidants of depressed women provide less social supports than confidants of non-depressed woman? J Abnorm Psychol 100:516–525, 1991

Bem SL: The measurement of psychological androgyny. J Consult Clin Psychol 42:155–162, 1974

Block JH, Gjerde PF, Block JH: Personality antecedents of depressive tendencies in 18-year-olds: a prospective study. J Pers Soc Psychol 60:726–738, 1991

Brooks-Gunn J: Antecedents and consequences of variations in girls' maturational timing. J Adolesc Health Care 9:365–373, 1988

Brooks-Gunn J, Warren MP: Biological contributions to affective expression in young adolescent girls. Child Dev 60:372–385, 1989

Brugha TS, Bebbington PE, MacCarthy B, et al: Social networks, social support and the type of depressive illness. Acta Psychiatr Scand 76:664–673, 1987

Brugha TS, Bebbington PE, MacCarthy B, et al: Gender, social support and recovery from depressive disorders: a prospective clinical study. Psychol Med 20:147–156, 1990

Carli LL: Gender differences in interaction style and influence. J Pers Soc Psychol 56:565–576, 1989

Carmen E, Rieker PP, Mills T: Victims of violence and psychiatric illness. Am J Psychiatry 141:378–383, 1984

Comstock GW, Helsing KJ: Symptoms of depression in two communities. Psychol Med 6:551–563, 1976

Craighead LW, Green BJ: The relationship between depression and sex-typed personality characteristics in adolescents. Journal of Youth and Adolescence 18:467–474, 1989

Cutler SE, Nolen-Hoeksema S: Accounting for sex differences in depression through female victimization: childhood sexual abuse. Sex Roles 24:425–438, 1991

Cutrona CE: Non-psychotic postpartum depression: a review of recent research. Clinical Psychology Review 2:487–503, 1982

Dornbusch SM, Carlsmith JM, Duncan PD, et al: Sexual maturation, social class, and the desire to be thin among adolescent females. J Dev Behav Pediatr 5:308–314, 1984

Eagly AH: Sex Differences in Social Behavior: A Social Role Interpretation. Hillsdale, NJ, Erlbaum, 1987

Eagly AH, Makhijani MG, Klonsky BG: Gender and the evaluation of leaders: a meta-analysis. Psychol Bull 111:3–22, 1992

Eccles J, Adler T, Meece JL: Sex differences in achievement: a test of alternate theories. J Pers Soc Psychol 46:26–43, 1984

Endicott J: Differential diagnoses and comorbidity, in Premenstrual Dysphorias: Myths and Realities. Edited by Gold JH, Severino SK. Washington, DC, American Psychiatric Press, 1994, pp 3–17

Fagot BI: Beyond the reinforcement principle: another step toward understanding sex roles. Developmental Psychology 21:1097–1104, 1985

Finkelhor D, Hotaling G, Lewis IA, et al: Sexual abuse in a national survey of adult men and women: prevalence, characteristics, and risk factors. Child Abuse Negl 14:19–28, 1990

Frey KS, Ruble DN: What children say about classroom performance: sex and grade differences in perceived competence. Child Dev 58:1066–1078, 1987

Frieze IH, Whitley B, Hanusa B, et al: Assessing the theoretical models for sex differences in causal attributions for success and failure. Sex Roles 3:333–343, 1982

Gallant SJ, Popiel DA, Hoffman DM, et al: Using daily ratings to confirm premenstrual syndrome/late luteal phase dysphoric disorder, II: what makes a "real" difference? Psychosom Med 54:167–181, 1992

Girgus JS, Nolen-Hoeksema S, Seligman MEP: Why do girls become more depressed than boys in early adolescence? Paper presented to the American Psychological Association, San Francisco, CA, August 1991

Gove W: The relationship between sex roles, marital status, and mental illness. Social Forces 51:34–44, 1972

Gove W, Herb T: Stress and mental illness among the young: a comparison of the sexes. Social Forces 53:256–265, 1974

Grant WF, Eiden LJ: Digest of Educational Statistics. Washington, DC, National Center for Educational Statistics, U.S. Department of Education, 1982

Harris B, Johns S, Fung H, et al: The hormonal environment of post-natal depression. Br J Psychiatry 154:660–667, 1989

Harrison WM, Endicott J, Nee J, et al: Characteristics of women seeking treatment for premenstrual syndrome. Psychosomatics 30:405–411, 1989

Hayward C, Killen JD, Gandy S, et al: Timing of puberty and onset of psychiatric symptoms. Presented to the American Academy of Child and Adolescent Psychiatry, San Antonio, TX, October 1993

Herjanic B, Reich W: Development of a structured psychiatric interview for children: agreement between child and parent on individual symptoms. J Abnorm Child Psychol 10:307–324, 1982

Hirschfeld RMA, Cross CK: Epidemiology of affective disorders: psychosocial risk factors. Arch Gen Psychiatry 39:35–46, 1982

Hogg MA, Turner JC: Intergroup behavior, self-stereotyping and the salience of social categories. Br J Soc Psychol 26:325–340, 1987

Jacklin CN, Maccoby EE: Social behavior at 33 months in same-sex and mixed-sex dyads. Child Dev 49:557–569, 1978

Kandel DB, Davies M: Adult sequelae of adolescent depressive symptoms. Arch Gen Psychiatry 43:255–262, 1986

Kaplan A: The "self-in-relation": implications for depression in women. Psychotherapy 23:234–242, 1986

Kashani JH, Beck NC, Hoeper EW, et al: Psychiatric disorders in a community sample of adolescents. Am J Psychiatry 144:584–589, 1987

Kessler RC, Price RH, Wortman CB: Social factors in psychopathology: stress, social support, and coping processes. Annu Rev Psychol 36:531–572, 1985

Kilpatrick D, Resick P, Veronen L: Effects of a rape experience: a longitudinal study. Social Issues 37:105–122, 1981

Levit DB: Gender differences in ego defenses in adolescence: sex roles as one way to understand the differences. J Pers Soc Psychol 61:992–999, 1991

Licht BG, Stader SR, Swenson CC: Children's achievement-related beliefs: effects of academic area, sex, and achievement level. Journal of Educational Research 82:253–260, 1989

Lockheed ME: Sex and social influence: a meta-analysis guided by theory, in Status, Attributions, and Rewards. Edited by Berger J, Zelditch M. San Francisco, CA, Jossey-Bass, 1985, pp 406–429

Maccoby EE: Gender and relationships: a developmental account. Am Psychol 45:513–520, 1990

Maccoby EE, Jacklin CN: The Psychology of Sex Differences. Stanford, CA, Stanford University Press, 1974

Maccoby EE, Jacklin CN: Sex differences in aggression: a rejoinder and reprise. Child Dev 51:964–980, 1980

Maltz DN, Borker RA: A cultural approach to male-female miscommunication, in Language and Social Identity. Edited by Gumperz JA. New York, Cambridge University Press, 1983, pp 195–216

Matthews KA, Wing RR, Kuller LH, et al: Influences of natural menopause on psychological characteristics and symptoms of middle-aged women. J Consult Clin Psychol 58:345–351, 1990

McGrath E, Keita GP, Strickland BR, et al: Women and Depression: Risk Factors and Treatment Issues: Final Report of the American Psychological Association's National Task Force on Women and Depression. Washington, DC, American Psychological Association, 1990

Moos RH: The development of a menstrual distress questionnaire. Psychosom Med 30:853–867, 1968

Myers JK, Weissman MM, Tischler GL, et al: Six-month prevalence of psychiatric disorders in three communities: 1980 to 1982. Arch Gen Psychiatry 41:959–967, 1984

National Center for Educational Statistics: Digest of Education Statistics. Washington, DC, U.S. Department of Education, Office of Education Research and Improvement, 1989

Nolen-Hoeksema S: Sex Differences in Depression. Stanford, CA, Stanford University Press, 1990

Nolen-Hoeksema S: Responses to depression and their effects on the duration of depressive episodes. J Abnorm Psychol 100:569–582, 1991

Nolen-Hoeksema S, Girgus JS: The emergence of sex differences in depression in adolescence. Psychol Bull 115:424–443, 1994

Nolen-Hoeksema S, Girgus JS, Seligman MEP: Sex differences in explanatory style and depression in children. Journal of Youth and Adolescence 20:233–245, 1991

Nolen-Hoeksema S, Morrow J, Fredrickson BL: Response styles and the duration of episodes of depressed mood study. J Abnorm Psychol 102:20–28, 1993

O'Hara M: Post-partum "blues," depression, and psychosis: a review. Journal of Psychosomatic Obstetrics and Gynecology 7:205–227, 1987

O'Hara M, Rehm LP, Campbell SB: Predicting depressive symptomatology: cognitive-behavioral models and postpartum depression. J Abnorm Psychol 91:457–461, 1982

O'Hara MW, Neunaber DJ, Zekoski EM: Prospective study of postpartum depression: prevalence, course, and predictive factors. J Abnorm Psychol 93:158–171, 1984

Paikoff RL, Brooks-Gunn J, Warren MP: Effects of girls' hormonal status on depressive and aggressive symptoms over the course of one year. Journal of Youth and Adolescence 20:191–215, 1991

Parlee MB: Changes in moods and activation levels during the menstrual cycle in experimentally naive subjects. Psychology of Women Quarterly 7:119–131, 1982

Parlee MB: Commentary on the literature review, in Premenstrual Dysphorias: Myths and Realities. Edited by Gold JH, Severino SK. Washington, DC, American Psychiatric Press, 1994, pp 149–167

Parry BL: Biological correlates of premenstrual complaints, in Premenstrual Dysphorias: Myths and Realities. Edited by Gold JH, Severino SK. Washington, DC, American Psychiatric Press, 1994, pp 47–66

Parry BL, Berga SL, Kripke DF, et al: Altered waveform of plasma nocturnal melatonin secretion in premenstrual depression. Arch Gen Psychiatry 47:1139–1146, 1990

Paykel ES: Depression in women. Br J Psychiatry 158:22–29, 1991

Pearlstein TH, Frank E, Rivera-Tovar A, et al: Prevalence of Axis I and Axis II disorders in women with late luteal phase dysphoric disorder. J Affect Disord 20:129–134, 1990

Petersen AC, Sarigiani P, Kennedy RE: Adolescent depression: why more girls? Journal of Youth and Adolescence 20:247–271, 1991

Powlishta KK, Maccoby EE: Resource utilization in mixed-sex dyads: the influence of adult presence and task type. Sex Roles 23:223–240, 1990

Pugh MD, Wahrman R: Neutralizing sexism in mixed-sex groups: do women have to be better than men? American Journal of Sociology 88:746–761, 1983

Radloff LS: Sex differences in depression: the effects of occupation and marital status. Sex Roles 1:249–267, 1975

Radloff LS: The CES-D Scale: a self-report depression scale for research in the general population. Applied Psychological Measurement 1:385–401, 1977

Rees WD, Lutkins SG: Parental depression before and after childbirth: an assessment with the Beck Depression Inventory. J R Coll Gen Pract 21:26–31, 1971

Reid RL, Yen SSC: Premenstrual syndrome. Am J Obstet Gynecol 1:85–104, 1981

Roberts T-A, Nolen-Hoeksema S: Sex differences in reactions to evaluative feedback. Sex Roles 21:725–747, 1989

Robins LN, Helzer JE, Croughan J, et al: National Institute of Mental Health Diagnostic Interview Schedule: its history, characteristics, and validity. Arch Gen Psychiatry 38:381–389, 1981

Russell DEH: Sexual Exploitation. Beverly Hills, CA, Sage Library of Social Research, 1984

Ryckman DB, Peckman P: Gender differences in attributions for success and failure situations across subject areas. Journal of Educational Research 81:120–125, 1987

Schnurr PP, Hurt SW, Stout AL: Consequences of methodological decisions in the diagnosis of late luteal phase dysphoric disorder, in Premenstrual Dysphorias: Myths and Realities. Edited by Gold JH, Severino SK. Washington, DC, American Psychiatric Press, 1994, pp 19–46

Severino SK, Hurt SW, Shindledecker RD: Late luteal phase dysphoric disorder: spectral analysis of cyclic symptoms. Am J Psychiatry 146:1155–1160, 1989

Simmons RG, Blyth DA: Moving Into Adolescence: The Impact of Pubertal Change and School Context. New York, Aldine DeGruyter, 1987

Sohn D: Sex differences in achievement self-attributions: an effect-size analysis. Sex Roles 8:345–357, 1982

Stein JA, Golding JM, Siegel JM, et al: Long-term psychological sequelae of child sexual abuse: the Los Angeles epidemiologic catchment area study, in Lasting Effects of Child Sexual Abuse. Edited by Wyatt GE, Powell GJ. Newbury Park, CA, Sage, 1988, pp 135–154

Steinberg L, Silverberg SB: The vicissitudes of autonomy in early adolescence. Child Dev 57:841–851, 1986

Stroebe W, Stroebe MS: Bereavement and Health. Cambridge, England, University Press, 1987

Sussman EJ, Nottelmann ED, Inoff-Germain GE, et al: Hormonal influences on aspects of psychological development during adolescence. J Adolesc Health Care 8:492–504, 1987

Sussman EJ, Dom LD, Chrousos GP: Negative affect and hormone levels in young adolescents: concurrent and predictive perspectives. Journal of Youth and Adolescence 20:167–190, 1991

Teri L: Depression in adolescence: its relationship to assertion and various aspects of self-image. Journal of Clinical Child Psychology 11:101–106, 1982

Tobin-Richards M, Boxer A, Petersen AC: The psychological significance of pubertal change: sex differences in perceptions of self during early adolescence, in Girls at Puberty: Biological and Psychosocial Perspectives. Edited by Brooks-Gunn J, Petersen AC. New York, Plenum, 1983, pp 127–154

Webster ML, Thompson JMD, Mitchell EA, et al: Postnatal depression in a community cohort. Aust N Z J Psychiatry 28:42–49, 1994

Weissman MM: The myth of involutional melancholia. JAMA 242:742–744, 1979

Weissman MM, Myers JK: Affective disorders in a United States community: the use of research diagnostic criteria in an epidemiological survey. Arch Gen Psychiatry 35:1304–1311, 1978

Winfield A: Children's attributions for success and failure: effects of age and attentional focus. Journal of Educational Psychology 80:76–81, 1988

Wirtz PW, Harrell AV: Effects of post-assault exposure to attack—similar stimuli on long-term recovery of victims. J Consult Clin Psychol 55:10–16, 1987

CHAPTER 5

Gender Differences in Mood Disorders

A Clinical Focus

Jennifer Shaw, M.D.
Sidney H. Kennedy, M.D., F.R.C.P.C.
Russell T. Joffe, M.D.

The study of gender issues in psychiatric illness has recently assumed increasing importance and may be especially applicable to the mood disorders. Although mood disorders have traditionally, but not necessarily universally, been regarded as disorders of women, only a limited number of empirical studies have specifically evaluated gender differences in these disorders. Such studies may have important clinical implications. First, they may clarify whether the preponderance of women seen in the clinic reflects a generally higher rate of depression in the population or whether this can be explained by other gender-related issues. Second, empirical studies may be able to identify clinical subtypes or symptom clusters specific to each sex, which may have diagnostic and treatment implications. Last, such studies may shed light on general pathophysiological mechanisms involved in affective illness. Gender differences in peptide biology, neurotransmitter function, and hormonal regulation have been identified in animal and human studies. Because all of these neurochemicals have been implicated in the biology of depression, the study of gender differences and their clinical correlates is of obvious importance. In this chapter, we focus on the clinical and epidemiological studies of gender issues in mood disorders. We examine studies pertaining to both bipolar and unipolar illness and their various subtypes and gender differences in prevalence estimates, clinical symptomatology, course of illness, and treatment outcome.

Unipolar Disorder

Epidemiology

It is a consistent finding in epidemiological studies of unipolar depression that women are more commonly affected than men (Boyd and Weissman 1981; Merikangas et al. 1985b; Nolen-Hoeksema 1987; Regier et al. 1988; Weissman and Klerman 1977, 1985; Weissman et al. 1984). Several investigators have described the methodological difficulties associated with epidemiological investigations of depression, particularly the inconsistency of a case definition across studies (Nolen-Hoeksema 1987; Weissman and Klerman 1977). Weissman and Klerman (1977) reviewed more than 40 studies from 30 countries involving both clinical populations of depressed patients and community surveys. With few exceptions, women predominated over men for depressive disorder by a ratio of 2–3:1. The exceptions were 1) studies of less industrialized countries, 2) studies of bereavement, and 3) a study of the Amish population.

In the first exception, data from developing countries (India, Iraq, New Guinea) were confined to treated cases of depression. The data may be profoundly affected by differences in the utilization of health care by women and men in these cultures (Nolen-Hoeksema 1987). Studies of bereavement were included in the review by Weissman and Klerman as sources of epidemiological data on depression. Clayton and colleagues (1971) were the first to demonstrate that there were no sex differences in the rate of depression during the first year after the death of a spouse, but the relationship of bereavement to depressive disorder is unclear, and, therefore, the epidemiology of bereavement may not be helpful in understanding depression. In the last exception, Egeland and Hostetter (1983) found no sex difference in the prevalence of unipolar depression in their study of the Amish population. This study has been criticized methodologically on several counts. First, case finding of subjects in the community was done by community informants who may have been biased by the norms of a community where sex roles are sharply differentiated. The visibility of symptoms and the amount of community disruption that they caused (greater in men) may have influenced the identification of subjects (Klerman 1983). In light of these concerns, it is uncertain whether the finding in the Amish population of an equal sex ratio is a result of methodological bias or whether it is less contaminated than other studies of affective disorder in which alcohol, substance abuse, and antisocial behavior mask true male prevalence (Clayton 1983).

An unresolved issue in epidemiological studies of depression is whether the predominance of depressive disorder in women represents a "true" difference or whether it may be explained by other factors. These factors include sociocultural issues considered under the "artifact hypothesis" (Nolen-Hoeksema 1987; Weissman and Klerman 1977), biases created by different diagnostic systems (Angst and Dobler-Mikola 1984a, 1984b), and concepts of depressive spectrum disease (Van Valkenburg and Winokur 1979; Winokur 1979).

The artifact hypothesis proposes that the rate of depression is equal among men and women but that women express and report more symptoms, seek help more frequently, and are subject to sex biases in diagnosis, thereby providing a false elevation in the measurement of the rate of depression in women. It has been suggested that, compared with women, men report fewer symptoms, suppress their depressive responses, are more reluctant to disclose symptoms, and are less willing to seek help (Funabiki et al. 1980). However, these findings have been disconfirmed by others. It has also been suggested that mental health clinicians differentially diagnose depression in women (Broverman et al. 1970; Potts et al. 1991). Amensohn and Lewinsohn (1981) attempted to address many of these aspects of the artifact hypothesis in a prospective, longitudinal study focusing on the occurrence of depressive symptoms and episodes of illness in a community sample. They showed that men, as compared with women, were as likely to report symptoms, to seek help for depression at the same level of symptom severity, and to receive a diagnosis of depression from clinicians at the same level of self-reported symptoms.

It should be mentioned that many of the studies collectively contributing to the artifact hypothesis used nonclinical samples, and case detection was by self-report instruments rather than by structured interviews. It is therefore difficult to compare these studies with studies of clinical populations of depressed patients (Clark et al. 1981; Myers and Weissman 1980). Evidence of the higher prevalence of depressed women in community surveys challenges the argument that sex differences in utilization of health care lead to overdetection of depression in women (Blazer et al. 1994; Eaton et al. 1989).

Angst and Dobler-Mikola (1984a, 1984b) suggested that the increased prevalence of depression in women is a function of the diagnostic criteria used. Women report more *symptoms* of depression than men; thus, they are more frequently diagnosed with the depressive syndrome by diagnostic criteria that require an arbitrary minimal number of symptoms. Further, these investigators suggested that if diagnosis was based primarily on social and occupational dysfunction, the female preponderance would be reduced. This hypothesis was not supported by Young and co-workers (1990a), who examined the sex ratio of depression based on various diagnostic criteria, using a cutoff from one to more than eight symptoms. Although women did report more symptoms of depression, more women were still diagnosed with depression when only the criteria of depressed mood and impairment of functioning were used. The findings of Young and co-workers supported a true sex difference in the rates of depression.

Winokur (Van Valkenburg and Winokur 1979; Winokur 1979) hypothesized that women and men may manifest different phenotypic expressions of the same genetic diathesis to depression. This concept of *depressive spectrum disease* suggests that, based on the same vulnerability, men are more likely to have alcoholism, and women are more likely to have unipolar depression. Although this concept evolved in an attempt to subclassify unipolar depression rather than to explain epidemiological differences, the inference was that this view contributed to the higher rates of depression seen in women (Winokur 1979). Although an association between mood disorders and alcoholism is frequently reported, several genetic studies have demonstrated that depression and alcoholism are not alternate manifestations of the same disorder (Cloninger et al. 1978; Merikangas et al. 1985a).

Notwithstanding these alternative explanations, methodologically sound studies consistently report a female predominance of depressive disorder. Boyd and Weissman (1981), in a review of community surveys of unipolar depression, reported a point prevalence of nonbipolar depression to be 3.2 per 100 men and 4.0–9.3 per 100 women, with a lifetime risk of 8%–12% for men and 20%–26% for women. Results from the five sites of the National Institute of Mental Health Epidemiologic Catchment Area (ECA) Program (Regier et al. 1984) indicate that the 1-month prevalence of major depressive disorder (MDD) in adults older than age 18 years was 2.6%–3.9% for women and 1.2%–2.2% for men. The increased female prevalence was maintained across all age groups (Regier et al. 1988).

The findings of a preponderance of women with major depression are also supported by a 5-year prospective study by Coryell and associates (1992a) of 965 never-ill first-degree relatives and spouses of probands with mood disorders. The prospective nature of the investigation minimized the effects of forgetting or denial of symptoms, which might contribute to underdetection of depression in males (Angst and Dobler-Mikola 1984b). The relatively long duration of the study (the cohort was followed for 5 years) provided a unique opportunity to identify the onset of major depression. Seventy-nine (8.2%) individuals, of whom 10.4% were women and 5.5% were men, developed a major depressive episode with significant role disruption. There was no sex difference in treatment-seeking behavior.

Clinical Issues

Age at onset. The age at onset of unipolar depression does not appear to be different in men and women (Regier et al. 1988; Weissman et al. 1984). Coryell and colleagues (1992a) identified age under 40 years to be a risk factor for the onset of major depression for both sexes, with a tendency for women under age 20 years to be at even greater risk. Women may have more episodes of depression than men (Amensohn and Lewinsohn 1981; Coryell et al. 1992a).

Response to antidepressants.   An early report to the British
Medical Research Council by its Clinical Psychiatry Committee
(1965) suggested that women responded less effectively to imipramine and phenelzine than men. This finding has not been replicated
in subsequent studies, and the initial observation that phenelzine was
inferior to placebo has not been confirmed in more recent investigations. The treatment-resistant nature of the sample, the absence of a
diagnosis using currently accepted criteria, and the use of relatively
low doses of antidepressants may have affected both the subject selection and the results of the British Medical Research Council trial.

Nonresponse to tricyclic antidepressants (TCAs) has been correlated with advanced age, marital disharmony, lower socioeconomic
status, and a series of clinical variables. These variables include
chronicity, double depression (a depressive episode superimposed on
dysthymia), delusions, and antecedent nonaffective psychiatric disorders such as antisocial personality disorder, drug dependence, alcoholism, and panic disorder (Coryell et al. 1990, 1992a; Thase and
Kupfer 1987). When these variables are controlled, there is no evidence that gender predicts treatment response (Coryell et al. 1990;
Thase and Kupfer 1987). A subgroup of females with atypical
neurovegetative depressive symptoms, nonautonomous or reactive
mood, and characterological features of rejection sensitivity or histri-
onic interpersonal style may show a poorer response to TCAs but
show a response to monoamine oxidase inhibitors (MAOIs) (Thase
and Kupfer 1987). This will be elaborated on further in the discussion
of atypical depression.

Frank and associates (1988) observed that men were more likely
to show a rapid response within 8 weeks to treatment with antidepressants and/or psychotherapy. However, because response was measured by self-report measures of depression (which are subjective),
this finding awaits confirmation by other studies.

Phenomenology.   In general, studies have shown few differences in
the clinical symptoms of depression between women and men. Several investigators have reported no gender difference in the severity
of symptoms using clinician-rated measures (Frank et al. 1988; Perugi
et al. 1990; Young et al. 1990a). However, women have been shown
to have higher severity of self-reported symptoms on the Beck De-

pression Inventory (Beck 1978; Frank et al. 1988; Young et al. 1990b). It has been hypothesized that this could relate to certain features of the depressed state in women, such as a higher level of anxiety, which may influence the self-reporting of other symptoms (Young et al. 1990b). Akiskal and co-workers (1983) and other researchers have suggested that sociocultural factors or personality factors may interact with depression and influence the expression of symptoms in women (Gjerde et al. 1988; Paykel 1991; Perugi et al. 1990). When symptom differences have been reported, it can be assumed that those found by clinician-rated measures would be subject to less interpatient differences and less gender-influenced reporting styles and would therefore be more reliable.

Frank and colleagues (1988) and Young and associates (1990b) found that, of all clinical features examined, women were significantly more likely to report increased appetite and weight gain (Angst and Dobler-Mikola 1984a). Earlier studies have suggested that women report more anxiety, although Frank and colleagues (1988) found, using both clinician-rated and self-report measures, that there was only a trend for women to demonstrate more somatic anxiety, hypochondriasis, and expressed anger. In the study by Young and associates, women showed a trend toward a relative increase in phobias and insomnia.

Subtypes

Atypical depression.   Atypical depression is thought of as a disorder primarily of women, with the gender ratio more pronounced than that of depression as a whole. However, this is not specifically addressed in most of the literature on atypical depression. To determine whether this clinical lore has any validity, a post-hoc reexamination of earlier studies of atypical depression with this specific issue in mind is required.

Such a review is limited by the fact that the focus of earlier studies was to determine the validity of this subtype of depression, with no specific attention to gender differences. Furthermore, this is complicated by the variety of uses of the term *atypical,* which is now used to describe a group of MAOI-responsive patients rather than a symptom cluster (Davidson et al. 1982).

Given these limitations, the purpose of this section is to review from a historical perspective the three most common descriptions of atypical depression while focusing on gender: 1) depression with a prominent anxiety component, 2) depression with a reversal of vegetative symptoms, and 3) hysteroid dysphoria. We then review more recent studies showing different pharmacotherapeutic responses of women.

The term *atypical depression* was first used by West and Dally (1959) to describe a group of patients who responded to the MAOI iproniazid phosphate and who had not shown a response to previous antidepressants or to electroconvulsive therapy (ECT). Clinically, these patients were described as having hysterical features, somatic complaints, phobic anxiety, and fatigue and were observed to have a more chronic condition. They displayed initial rather than terminal insomnia and an absence of the classical "endogenous" features of depression. Because they differed from those with typical endogenous depression, this MAOI-responsive group was called atypical.

Several investigators subsequently used the term atypical to refer to affectively ill patients, either with anxiety and phobias or physiological symptoms referred to as the *reversed functional shift* (Pollitt 1960). These were vegetative symptoms of increased appetite, increased weight, increased libido, diurnal mood changes with a decline in the evening, and initial insomnia. In addition, patients with phobic anxiety states who were responsive to MAOIs were included in this group (Tyrer 1976). Pollitt and Young (1971) attempted to subdivide clinical features of MAOI-responsive patients into anxiety states and depression. Their sample had a female-to-male ratio of 2.2:1 and 1.5:1 for anxious and depressed groups, respectively. They described the presence of atypical physiological symptoms as a function of age, with both male and female subjects having increased frequency of atypical symptoms in younger age and increased frequency of typical symptoms with advancing age. Paykel and co-workers (1983) addressed the reliability of the term atypical by studying the interrelationship of three concepts of atypical depression: 1) presence of anxiety or phobias, 2) nonendogenous, and 3) reversed functional shift. However, patient gender was not identified.

Robinson and colleagues (1973) treated subjects matched for age, sex, and degree of atypicality with either medication or placebo. Although they reported a female-to-male ratio of 1.8:1 in both groups, gender differences specific to atypical depression are obscured by the study design.

Davidson and co-workers (1982), in a review of atypical depression, reported that the female-to-male ratio in previous studies ranged from 2.3:1 to 2.5:1. Liebowitz and colleagues (1988) reported on a large sample of patients with atypical depression, of whom 62% were female and 38% were male.

In summary, a post-hoc review of atypical depression indicates that the ratio of women to men is comparable to other studies of unipolar depression, with no clear indication that atypical depression is more of a disorder of women than unipolar depression as a whole.

Hysteroid dysphoria.   Quitkin and associates (1979) suggested that previous investigators were combining at least two disorders under one label—panic/phobic disorders and hysteroid dysphoria. Hysteroid dysphoria, as described by Klein and his group (1980), is the one subtype of atypical depression that has been identified as occurring almost exclusively in women. This is a syndrome of unipolar depression characterized by repeated episodes in response to real or perceived rejection. Patients are described as attention seeking and showing the hallmark of rejection sensitivity. In the face of such rejection, they experience depressive symptoms including overeating, carbohydrate craving, oversleeping, and fatigue (a contrast to typical endogenous symptoms). In addition, their mood remains responsive to their environment (Liebowitz and Klein 1979). Klein and his investigators (1980) distinguished between these female patients with rejection sensitivity (hysteroid dysphoria) and the group of both males and females who had atypical vegetative symptoms but no rejection sensitivity. The identification of hysteroid dysphoria as a disorder of women seems to emanate from Klein's clinical experience and original description of the syndrome, although there are no published studies to date. Of interest, however, is a study by Liebowitz and others (1984, 1988) examining antidepressant efficacy in subtypes of atypical depression, including a group with panic symptoms and a group with hysteroid dysphoria. They report no sex differences between the groups, but the sample size was small. Based on Klein and colleagues, one would have anticipated subjects in the hysteroid dysphoria group to be all women.

MAOI responsiveness. Investigators have attempted to identify a group of patients with selective response to MAOIs compared with TCAs (Liebowitz et al. 1984; Quitkin et al. 1988, 1989, 1990, 1991; Ravaris et al. 1980; Stewart et al. 1989). Although the focus of these studies has been to further delineate the features of an MAOI-responsive subtype, some gender-related findings have emerged. In a panic subgroup of patients with atypical depression treated with either phenelzine or imipramine, a gender effect was seen. Women showed a preferential response to phenelzine, and men showed a preferential response to imipramine (Liebowitz et al. 1988).

Davidson and Pelton (1986) also found that women with depression and panic attacks showed a significantly better response to MAOIs than to TCAs, with the opposite effect in men. Small sample size is a limiting factor in both of these studies. A short duration of treatment of only 3 weeks and comparatively low maximum treatment doses of imipramine (150 mg imipramine versus up to 90 mg phenelzine) limit the conclusions from this study. However, it can be argued that the clinical picture of atypical depression and panic symptoms in females is predictive of an MAOI response. Preliminary data also suggest superior efficacy of fluoxetine over imipramine in this type of depression (Reimherr et al. 1984).

Dysthymia. Information on gender issues in this subtype of depression is limited. Akiskal (1983) suggests that dysthymia or chronic low-grade depression is composed of a heterogeneous group of disorders, including a subgroup that represents a subsyndromal affective disorder rather than character pathology. He studied a group of patients with chronic depressive symptoms that appeared to be a habitual trait (characterological depression) as distinct from patients who had previously been well but who now had a residuum of clearly defined major depression (Akiskal et al. 1980). The purpose of the study was to identify a subgroup of patients who *appeared* to have characterological depression but who, in fact, showed features of a primary affective disorder. After treatment with a TCA, groups of responders and nonresponders emerged. The former showed similarities in clinical characteristics and rapid eye movement (REM) latency to patients with primary affective disorder and were identified as having subaffective dysthymia, a subsyndromal version of primary affective disorder. Akiskal and coinvestigators referred to the nonresponder group as having *character spectrum disorder*. The sex ratio of the nonresponders was no different from the unipolar depressed control subjects, with the usually reported 2:1 female-to-male ratio. The reported sex ratio of the group of responders was almost 1:1. It would be erroneous to interpret this as evidence for a gender difference in the response of dysthymic patients to TCAs. The group of responders included a high percentage of individuals who became hypomanic with treatment and reported a high frequency of hypersomnic retarded episodes (Akiskal et al. 1980). This suggests, as the authors acknowledge, that the group of responders could have included bipolar II patients, which would account for the approximately equal sex ratio. Incidentally, the 1-month prevalence of dysthymia has been reported in the ECA study as 3.3%, with a female-to-male ratio of 2:1 (Regier et al. 1988).

Recurrent brief depression. Recurrent brief depression (RBD) has been proposed primarily by Angst and co-workers (1990) as a new subtype of affective disorder. The diagnostic criteria suggested are similar to DSM-IV (American Psychiatric Association 1994) criteria for major depression but with a duration of less than 2 weeks and 1–2 episodes per month over a year. In studying the validity of this subtype, Angst and co-workers (1990) identified a female-to-male ratio similar to that of MDD. They reported a significantly high female-to-male ratio of combined RBD and MDD (e.g., 6.0:1.7). Of note, in this group of combined RBD and MDD, they reported a higher incidence of comorbid psychiatric disorders, including panic disorder, mania, hypomania, and substance abuse. Their inclusion of subjects with the latter three states in the group of combined RBD and MDD raises diagnostic confusion that interferes with the interpretation of their finding.

Seasonal affective disorder. Seasonal affective disorder is a subtype of unipolar or bipolar disorder characterized by recurrent episodes of illness with a regular temporal relationship to season of the year. The symptoms of this depressive subtype are the same as those of a major depressive episode with the frequent characteristics of the more atypical neurovegetative features such as hypersomnia, hyperphagia, weight gain, and anergia. The winter pattern prevalence rate of seasonal affective disorder in North America is 4.3%, of whom 68% are females. For the summer pattern, the prevalence is 0.7%–1.4%, of whom 66% are females (Kasper et al. 1989; Rosen et al. 1990). The female-to-male ratio for this disorder is 3.5:1. In women, it most commonly affects individuals between ages 21 and 30 years, and incidence declines with age. There appears to be a similar incidence across age groups in men (Kasper et al. 1989; Rosen et al. 1990). No published data have demonstrated any sex difference in treatment response to either light therapy or pharmacotherapy in patients with seasonal affective disorder.

Bipolar Disorder

Epidemiology

The lifetime risk of bipolar disorder is less than 1%, with reports ranging from 0.6% to 0.9% in industrialized nations (Goodwin and Jameson 1990). It is important to clarify that this is the reported risk for bipolar I disorder as defined by the presence of mania. Bipolar II disorder is defined by the presence of major depression with periods of hypomania rather than mania. Boyd and Weissman (1981) report a lifetime risk of 0.6% for both bipolar I and bipolar II disorder, providing a combined prevalence of 1.2%. The findings from the ECA program revealed 1-month, 6-month, and 1-year prevalence rates per 100 subjects of 0.8%, 0.9%, and 1.0%, respectively (Goodwin and Jameson 1990; Regier et al. 1988). A consistent observation is that there have been no sex differences in the incidence of bipolar I disorder (Boyd and Weissman 1981; Regier et al. 1988; Weissman and Klerman 1977; Weissman et al. 1984). The highest prevalence is in the 18- to 44-year-old group in both sexes (Goodwin and Jameson 1990; Regier et al. 1988).

Clinical Issues

Course of illness.   Combined data from 22 studies indicate that the age at onset of bipolar disorder peaks in the 15- to 24-year-old group, followed closely by the 25- to 29-year-old group (Goodwin and Jameson 1990). No sex difference in the age at onset was apparent from these data. It has been frequently observed that women with bipolar disorder are more prone to depression than are men (Goodwin and Jameson 1990). The predominance of depressive episodes in women has also been found by Coryell and colleagues (1989) and Roy-Byrne and associates (1985) but not by Kukopulos and co-workers (1980).

Outcome. In studies examining treatment response to lithium and other mood stabilizers in bipolar illness, no gender differences have emerged. An important difference between the sexes in the course of illness and subsequent outcome is the female preponderance of rapid cycling disorder.

Rapid cycling. Rapid cycling, defined as four or more episodes of mania and/or depression in a 12-month period, is said to occur in approximately 15% of bipolar patients who present for treatment (Coryell et al. 1992b). This bipolar subtype has been reported to have an inadequate response to lithium treatment (Dunner and Fieve 1974) and a poor long-term prognosis (Wehr et al. 1988). Recent data suggest that, at least in some cases, rapid cycling may be a transient phenomenon occurring during the normal life course of bipolar illness (Coryell et al. 1992b). Although the clinical characteristics of rapid cycling remain to be clarified, the most consistent correlate is female gender, reported in most studies to date (Coryell et al. 1992b; Nurenberger et al. 1988; Wehr et al. 1988). The reason for this female preponderance is unclear. There may be a relationship between various degrees of hypothyroidism, female gender, and rapid cycling, although a recent study found no association (Maj et al. 1994). This may, however, be related to duration of lithium treatment rather than to frequency of cycling. The relationship of rapid cycling to the menstrual cycle has also been examined; only preliminary case studies have suggested a relationship between perimenstrual difficulties and rapid cycling (MacKenzie et al. 1986; Price and DiMarzio 1986). Rapid cycling is, however, also seen in postmenopausal women and in men.

Treatment Issues

Antidepressants

Despite the many effects of menstrual cycle fluctuations on antidepressant blood levels (Yonkers et al. 1992), there are no data on preferential responses of men or women to specific antidepressants. There are no consistent sex-specific dose requirements.

Lithium

There are some case reports of possible fluctuations in lithium levels related to the menstrual cycle (Kukopulos et al. 1985). Chamberlain and co-workers (1990), however, demonstrated no difference in lithium levels across the menstrual cycle after a 300-mg loading dose in 14 healthy female volunteers both on and off oral contraceptives.

Gonadal Hormones

There are inconclusive data on the efficacy of estrogen therapy in the treatment of depression. The possible role of estrogen in the treatment of depression arises from observations of gender-specific mood syndromes, including premenstrual syndrome, postpartum depression, and perimenopausal depression. These syndromes occur during fluctuations of sex steroids, particularly during periods of decreasing levels of estradiol. Estrogen enhances central norepinephrine availability and in animal models has been shown to induce changes in β-adrenergic–, serotonergic-, and dopaminergic-receptor mechanisms (Oppenheim 1983; Oppenheim et al. 1987; Sherwin 1991). Although this suggests a biological rationale for estrogen treatment of depression, there are few controlled investigations to date.

The literature reviewed in this section is confined to studies using estrogen in the treatment of mood disorders. It includes studies using estrogen alone and in combination with progestational agents in oral contraceptives.

Klaiber and colleagues (1979) assessed estrogen therapy alone versus placebo in a group of severely depressed inpatient females who had been ill for at least 2 years and who had been refractory to an average of three treatments for depression. Previous treatments had included standard antidepressants, psychotherapy, and/or ECT. Twenty-three women received 15–25 mg of conjugated estrogen (Premarin) daily for a 3-month period. In the 15 premenopausal subjects, 2.5 mg daily of a progestin was given on day 21 of estrogen treatment for 5 days. Although the estrogen-treated patients showed a significantly greater reduction in their mean depression scores on the Hamilton Rating Scale for Depression (M. Hamilton 1960), they remained in a moderately depressed state, with an average score of 22.0. There was a considerable range of response to estrogen therapy, with 2 patients worsening and 6 subjects showing improvement to a mild level of depression. Those patients with more chronic illness showed the least improvement. In comparison, none of the placebo group showed appreciable improvement, and 8 became worse. There was some improvement in a few subjects, but it is difficult to generalize treatment principles from this study. The high dose of estrogen and the lack of robust changes in the level of the depression over a long treatment period of 3 months limit definitive conclusions. Prange and associates (1976) investigated estrogen as an augmenting agent to 150 mg of imipramine in a group of depressed female inmates at a correctional institution. Significant improvement was seen in all of the imipramine-treated subjects, but there was no additional benefit or significant acceleration of response with the addition of 25 or 50 μg of estradiol. In fact, women receiving 50 μg (but not 25 μg) of estradiol showed symptoms of toxicity by the seventh day of treatment. These symptoms resolved after discontinuation of estradiol. The toxic symptoms included hypotension, drowsiness, tremor, dry mouth, and urinary retention and were attributed to a pharmacokinetic interaction with imipramine.

Shapira and associates (1985) failed to show overall improvement with estrogen versus placebo augmentation of imipramine in 11 treatment-resistant depressed women. Although there was no overall effect, there were some individual responses. One patient showed remission of depressive symptoms after 1 week of estrogen augmentation and remained in remission for 3 months. Another patient with bipolar depression developed symptoms of mania.

The remainder of the literature is limited to case reports. Oppenheim (1984) reported induction of rapid cycling, depression, and hypomania in a 72-year-old woman with a history of severe recurrent depression after treatment with Premarin. This cycling disorder remitted with discontinuation of the estrogen.

Although there is no general support for estrogen treatment in depression, there are reports of individual beneficial responses. The clinician should be aware of the effect that the menstrual cycle, oral contraceptive use, pregnancy, the postpartum period, and menopause has on a female patient's mood (J. A. Hamilton et al. 1988). Attention should be paid to any contribution of reproductive events to an affective syndrome.

Thyroid Hormones

The thyroid hormone triiodothyronine (T_3) has been used to modify the effects of antidepressants in two ways: 1) by *acceleration* of antidepressant response and 2) by *augmentation* of the therapeutic effect in antidepressant nonresponders.

Prange and collaborators (1969; Wilson et al. 1970) were the first to observe that the addition of small amounts of T_3 would accelerate and enhance the response to imipramine in depressed women (but not men), regardless of whether they had a retarded or agitated depression. These findings were replicated in some (Koppen et al. 1972; Wheatley 1972) but not other (Feighner et al. 1972; Steiner et al. 1978) studies.

The mechanism of action of T_3 is unknown. It has been suggested from these data that the gender difference in response to T_3 acceleration may imply a gender difference in the hormonal basis of depression that is unrelated to gonadal hormones (Wilson et al. 1970). Note that studies reporting this T_3 acceleration effect have observed no difference in baseline thyroid indices between depressed men and women (Koppen et al. 1972; Prange et al. 1969; Wheatley 1972; Wilson et al. 1970).

Both open and controlled studies suggest that between 50% and 60% of antidepressant nonresponders will be converted to responders by the addition of small amounts of T_3 (Joffe et al. 1993). The antidepressant augmentation effect of T_3 is comparable to that of lithium in unipolar depressed patients. Unlike the T_3 acceleration effect, no gender difference in the T_3 augmentation effect has been observed (Joffe et al. 1993).

The studies that suggest a gender difference in T_3 acceleration of the antidepressant response were carried out more than 20 years ago. If confirmed in studies using current research methodology, the use of T_3 to accelerate antidepressant response may be a useful means of further studying the potential gender differences in the biological basis of depression. In bipolar affective disorder, case studies (Stancer and Persad 1982) provide preliminary evidence that high doses of thyroxine (T_4) may ameliorate the frequency and severity of mood cycles. This may be particularly applicable to the rapid-cycling form of the illness, which is probably more common in women.

Conclusion

Our selective review reveals that the epidemiological data consistently find a higher prevalence of depressive, but not manic-depressive, illness in women. However, with few exceptions, the clinical studies show limited gender differences in clinical features, course of illness, and response to treatment. Some subtypes of these disorders, particularly the hysteroid dysphoria subtype of unipolar depression and the rapid-cycling form of bipolar illness, appear to be especially common in women. Further studies of the clinical and biological features of these subtypes of illness may be important in understanding the pathophysiology of these disorders in general and may explain the biological basis of the gender difference in reported prevalence.

Our review of the literature is limited by the fact that most studies evaluated were not intended to examine gender differences but to report them in the overall description of the sample studied. To eliminate biases inherent in the results of such studies, future investigations should focus primarily on gender issues if they are to be replicable and if they are to lead to researchable questions.

References

Akiskal HS: Dysthymic disorder: psychopathology of proposed chronic depressive subtypes. Am J Psychiatry 40:11–20, 1983

Akiskal HS, Rosenthal TL, Haykal RF, et al: Characterological depressions: clinical and sleep EEG findings separating "sub-affective dysthymias" from "character spectrum disorders." Arch Gen Psychiatry 37:777–783, 1980

Akiskal HS, Hirschfeld RMA, Yerevanian BI: The relationship of personality to affective disorders: a critical review. Arch Gen Psychiatry 40:801–810, 1983

Amensohn CS, Lewinsohn PM: An investigation into the observed sex difference in prevalence of unipolar depression. J Abnorm Psychol 90:1–13, 1981

American Psychiatric Association: Diagnostic and Statistical Manual of Mental Disorders, 4th Edition. Washington, DC, American Psychiatric Association, 1994

Angst J, Dobler-Mikola A: Do the diagnostic criteria determine the sex ratio in depression? J Affect Disord 7:189–198, 1984a

Angst J, Dobler-Mikola A: The definition of depression. J Psychiatr Res 18:401–406, 1984b

Angst J, Merikangas K, Scheidegger P, et al: Recurrent brief depression: a new subtype of affective disorder. J Affect Disord 19:87–98, 1990

Beck AT: Depression Inventory. Philadelphia, PA, Philadelphia Center for Cognitive Therapy, 1978

Blazer DG, Kessler RC, McGonagle KA, et al: The prevalence and distribution of major depression in a national community sample: the national comorbidity survey. Am J Psychiatry 151:979–986, 1994

Boyd JH, Weissman MM: Epidemiology of affective disorders, a re-examination and future directions. Arch Gen Psychiatry 38:1039–1046, 1981

Broverman IK, Broverman DM, Clarkson FE, et al: Sex-role stereotypes and clinical judgements of mental health. J Consult Clin Psychol 34:1–7, 1970

Chamberlain S, Hahn PM, Cassan P, et al: Effect of menstrual cycle phase and oral contraceptive use on serum lithium after a loading dose of lithium in normal women. Am J Psychiatry 147:907–909, 1990

Clark VA, Aneshensel CS, Frerichs RR, et al: Analysis of effects of sex and age in response to items on the Capital CES-D Scale. Psychiatry Res 5:171–181, 1981

Clayton PJ: Gender and depression, in The Origins of Depression: Current Concepts and Approaches. Edited by Angst J. Berlin, Springer-Verlag, 1983, pp 77–89

Clayton PJ, Halikes JA, Maurice ML: The bereavement of the widowed. Diseases of the Nervous System 32:597–604, 1971

Cloninger CR, Christiansen KO, Reich T, et al: Implications of sex differences in the prevalences of antisocial personality, alcoholism, and criminality for familial transmission. Arch Gen Psychiatry 35:941–951, 1978

Coryell W, Keller M, Endicott J, et al: Bipolar II illness: course and outcome over a 5-year period. Psychol Med 19:129–141, 1989

Coryell W, Endicott J, Keller M: Outcome of patients with chronic affective disorder: a 5-year follow-up. Am J Psychiatry 147:1627–1633, 1990

Coryell W, Endicott J, Keller M: Major depression in a non-clinical sample. Arch Gen Psychiatry 49:117–125, 1992a

Coryell W, Endicott J, Keller M: Rapid cycling affective disorder. Arch Gen Psychiatry 49:126–131, 1992b

Davidson J, Pelton S: Forms of atypical depression and their response to antidepressant drugs. Psychiatry Res 17:87–95, 1986

Davidson JRT, Miller RD, Turnbull CP, et al: Atypical depression. Arch Gen Psychiatry 39:527–534, 1982

Dunner DL, Fieve RR: Clinical factors in lithium carbonate prophylaxis failure. Arch Gen Psychiatry 30:229–233, 1974

Eaton WW, Kramer M, Anthony JC, et al: The incidence of specific DIS/DSM-III mental disorders: data from the NIMH epidemiological catchment area program. Acta Psychiatr Scand 79:163–178, 1989

Egeland JA, Hostetter AM: Amish study, I: affective disorders among the Amish, 1976-1980. Am J Psychiatry 140:56–61, 1983

Feighner AP, King LJ, Schuckit MA, et al: Hormonal potentiation of imipramine and ECT in primary depression. Am J Psychiatry 128:1230–1234, 1972

Frank E, Carpenter LL, Kupfer DJ: Sex differences in recurrent depression: are there any that are significant? Am J Psychiatry 145:41–45, 1988

Funabiki D, Bologna NC, Pepping M, et al: Revisiting sex differences in the expression of depression. J Abnorm Psychol 89:194–202, 1980

Gjerde PF, Block J, Block JH: Depressive symptoms and personality during late adolescence: gender differences in the externalization-internalization of symptom expression. J Abnorm Psychol 97:475–486, 1988

Goodwin FK, Jameson KR: Manic-Depressive Illness. New York, Oxford University Press, 1990

Hamilton JA, Parry BL, Blumenthal S: The menstrual cycle in context, I: affective syndromes associated with reproductive hormonal changes. J Clin Psychiatry 49:474–480, 1988

Hamilton M: A rating scale for depression. J Neurol Neurosurg Psychiatry 23:56–62, 1960

Joffe RT, Singer W, Levitt AJ, et al: A placebo-controlled comparison of lithium and triiodothyronine (T3) augmentation in unipolar refractory depression. Arch Gen Psychiatry 50:387–393, 1993

Kasper S, Wehr TA, Bartko JJ, et al: Epidemiological findings of seasonal changes in mood and behaviour: a telephone survey of Montgomery County, Maryland. Arch Gen Psychiatry 46:823–833, 1989

Klaiber E, Broverman DM, Vogel W, et al: Estrogen therapy for severe persistent depressions in women. Arch Gen Psychiatry 36:550–554, 1979

Klein DF, Gittelman R, Quitkin FM, et al: Diagnosis and Drug Treatment of Psychiatric Disorders: Adults and Children, 2nd Edition. Baltimore, MD, Williams & Wilkins, 1980

Klerman GL: On the Amish study (letter). Am J Psychiatry 140:1262, 1983

Koppen A, Whybrow PC, Noguera R, et al: The comparative antidepressant value of L-tryptophan and imipramine with and without attempted potentiation by iodothyronine. Arch Gen Psychiatry 26:234–241, 1972

Kukopulos A, Reginaldi D, Laddomada P, et al: Course of the manic-depressive cycle and changes caused by treatments. Pharmakopsychiatrica Neuropsychopharmakologia 13:156–167, 1980

Kukopulos A, Minnai G, Muller-Oerlinghauser B: The influence of mania and depression on the pharmacokinetics of lithium: a longitudinal single-case study. J Affect Disord 8:159–166, 1985

Liebowitz MR, Klein DF: Hysteroid dysphoria. Psychiatr Clin North Am 2:555–575, 1979

Liebowitz MR, Quitkin FM, Stewart JW, et al: Psychopharmacologic validation of atypical depression. J Clin Psychiatry 45:22–25, 1984

Liebowitz MR, Quitkin FM, Stewart JW, et al: Antidepressant specificity in atypical depression. Arch Gen Psychiatry 45:129–137, 1988

MacKenzie TB, Wilcox K, Baron H: Lifetime prevalence of psychiatric disorders in women with perimenstrual difficulties. J Affect Disord 10:15–19, 1986

Maj M, Magliano L, Pirozzi R, et al: Validity of rapid cycling as a course specifier for bipolar disorder. Am J Psychiatry 151:1015–1019, 1994

Merikangas KR, Leckman JF, Prusoff BA, et al: Familial transmission of depression and alcoholism. Arch Gen Psychiatry 42:367–372, 1985a

Merikangas KR, Weissman MM, Pauls DL: Genetic factors in the sex ratio of major depression. Psychol Med 15:63–69, 1985b

Myers JK, Weissman MM: Use of a self-report systems scale to detect depression in a community sample. Am J Psychiatry 137:1081–1084, 1980

Nolen-Hoeksema S: Sex differences in unipolar depression: evidence and theory. Psychol Bull 101:259–282, 1987

Nurenberger J, Guroff JJ, Hamovit J, et al: A family study of rapid cycling bipolar illness. J Affect Disord 15:87–91, 1988

Oppenheim G: Estrogen in the treatment of depression: neuropharmacological mechanisms. Biol Psychiatry 18:721–725, 1983

Oppenheim G: A case of rapid mood cycling with estrogen: implications for therapy. J Clin Psychiatry 45:34–35, 1984

Oppenheim G, Zohar J, Shapiro B, et al: The role of estrogen in treating resistant depression, in Treating Resistant Depression. Edited by Zohar J, Belmaker R. New York, PMA Publishers, 1987, pp 357–365

Paykel ES: Depression in women. Br J Psychiatry 158:22–29, 1991

Paykel ES, Parker RR, Rowan PR, et al: Nosology of atypical depression. Psychol Med 13:131–139, 1983

Perugi G, Musetti ES, Piagentini F, et al: Gender-mediated clinical features of depressive illness: the importance of temperamental differences. Br J Psychiatry 157:835–841, 1990

Pollitt J: Depression and the functional shift. Compr Psychiatry 1:381–390, 1960

Pollitt J, Young T: Anxiety states or masked depression? A study based on the action of monoamine oxidase inhibitors. Br J Psychiatry 119:143–149, 1971

Potts MK, Burnam MA, Wells KB: Gender differences in depression detection: a comparison of clinical diagnosis and standardized assessment. J Consult Clin Psychol 3:609–615, 1991

Prange AJ Jr, Wilson IC, Rabon AM, et al: Enhancement of imipramine antidepressant activity by thyroid hormone. Am J Psychiatry 126:457–469, 1969

Prange AJ Jr, Wilson IC, Breese GR, et al: Hormonal alteration of imipramine response: a review, in Hormones, Behaviour and Psychopathology. Edited by Sachar EJ. New York, Raven, 1976, pp 41–67

Price WA, DiMarzio L: Premenstrual tension syndrome in rapid cycling bipolar affective disorder. J Clin Psychiatry 47:415–417, 1986

Quitkin F, Rifkin A, Klein DF: Monoamine oxidase inhibitors: a review of antidepressant effectiveness. Arch Gen Psychiatry 36:749–760, 1979

Quitkin FM, Stewart JW, McGrath PJ, et al: Phenelzine vs. imipramine in the treatment of probably atypical depression: defining syndrome boundaries of selective MAOI responders. Am J Psychiatry 145:306–311, 1988

Quitkin FM, McGrath PJ, Stewart JW, et al: Phenelzine and imipramine in mood reactive depressives: further delineation of the syndrome of atypical depression. Arch Gen Psychiatry 46:787–793, 1989

Quitkin FM, McGrath PJ, Stewart JW, et al: Atypical depression, panic attacks, and response to imipramine and phenelzine: a replication. Arch Gen Psychiatry 47:935–941, 1990

Quitkin FM, Harrison W, Stewart JW, et al: Response to phenelzine and imipramine in placebo non-responders with atypical depression: a new replication of a crossover design. Arch Gen Psychiatry 48:319–323, 1991

Ravaris CL, Robinson DS, Ives JO, et al: Phenelzine and amytriptyline in the treatment of depression: a comparison of present and past studies. Arch Gen Psychiatry 37:1075–1080, 1980

Regier DA, Myers JK, Kramer M, et al: The NIMH epidemiological catchment area program: historical context, major objectives, and study population characteristics. Arch Gen Psychiatry 41:934–941, 1984

Regier DA, Boyd JH, Burke JD Jr, et al: One-month prevalence of mental disorders in the United States. Arch Gen Psychiatry 45:977–985, 1988

Reimherr FW, Wood DR, Byerley B, et al: Characteristics of responders to fluoxetine. Psychopharmacol Bull 20:70–72, 1984

Report to the British Medical Research Council by its Clinical Psychiatry Committee: Clinical trial of the treatment of depressive illness. BMJ 1:881–886, 1965

Robinson DS, Nies A, Ravaris CL, et al: The monoamine oxidase inhibitor, phenelzine, in the treatment of depressive–anxiety states: a controlled clinical trial. Arch Gen Psychiatry 29:407–413, 1973

Rosen LN, Targum SG, Terman M, et al: Prevalence of seasonal affective disorder at four latitudes. Psychiatry Res 31:131–144, 1990

Roy-Byrne P, Post RM, Uhde TW, et al: The longitudinal course of recurrent affective illness: lifechart data from research patients at the NIMH. Acta Psychiatr Scand 71 (suppl 317):1–34, 1985

Shapira B, Oppenheim G, Zohar J, et al: Lack of efficacy of estrogen supplementation to imipramine in resistant female depressives. Biol Psychiatry 20:570–583, 1985

Sherwin B: Estrogen and refractory depression, in Advances in Neuropsychiatry and Psychopharmacology, Vol 2: Refractory Depression. Edited by Amsterdam J. New York, Raven, 1991, pp 209–218

Stancer HC, Persad E: Treatment of intractable rapid-cycling manic-depressive disorder with levothyroxine. Arch Gen Psychiatry 39:311–312, 1982

Steiner M, Radgin M, Elizur A, et al: Failure of L-triiodothyronine (T3) to potentiate tricyclic antidepressant response. Current Therapeutic Research 23:655–659, 1978

Stewart JW, McGrath PJ, Quitkin FM, et al: Relevance of DSM-III depressive subtype and chronicity of antidepressant efficacy in atypical depression: differential response to phenelzine, imipramine and placebo. Arch Gen Psychiatry 46:1080–1087, 1989

Thase ME, Kupfer DJ: Characteristics of treatment-resistant depression, in Treating Resistant Depression. Edited by Zohar J, Belmaker RH. New York, PMA Publishing, 1987, pp 23–45

Tyrer P: Towards rational therapy with monoamine oxidase inhibitors. Br J Psychiatry 128:25–31, 1976

Van Valkenburg C, Winokur G: Depressive spectrum disease. Psychiatr Clin North Am 2:469–482, 1979

Wehr T, Sack D, Rosenthal M, et al: Rapid cycling affective disorder: contributing factors and treatment responses in 51 patients. Am J Psychiatry 145:179–184, 1988

Weissman MM, Klerman GL: Sex differences and the epidemiology of depression. Arch Gen Psychiatry 34:98–111, 1977

Weissman MM, Klerman GL: Gender and depression. Trends Neurosci 8:416–420, 1985

Weissman MM, Leaf PJ, Holzer CE III, et al: The epidemiology of depression—an update on sex differences in rates. J Affect Disord 7:179–188, 1984

West ED, Dally PJ: Effect of iproniazid in depressive symptoms. BMJ 1:1491–1494, 1959

Wheatley D: Potentiation of amytriptyline by thyroid hormone. Arch Gen Psychiatry 26:229–233, 1972

Wilson IC, Prange AJ Jr, McClean TK, et al: Thyroid hormone enhancement of imipramine in non-retarded depression. N Engl J Med 282:1063–1067, 1970

Winokur G: Unipolar depression: is it divisible into autonomous subtypes? Arch Gen Psychiatry 36:47–52, 1979

Yonkers KA, Kando JC, Cole JO, et al: Gender differences in pharmacokinetics and pharmacodynamics of psychotropic medication. Am J Psychiatry 149:587–595, 1992

Young MA, Fogg LF, Scheftner WA, et al: Sex differences in the lifetime prevalence of depression: does varying the diagnostic criteria reduce the female/male ratio? J Affect Disord 18:187–192, 1990a

Young MA, Scheftner WA, Fawcett J, et al: Gender differences in the clinical features of unipolar major depressive disorder. J Nerv Ment Dis 178:200–203, 1990b

CHAPTER 6

Gender Differences in the Prevalence and Expression of Anxiety Disorders

Kimberly A. Yonkers, M.D.
George Gurguis, M.D.

Several psychiatric disorders show distinctive gender-related patterns of morbidity. As others in this book note, illnesses such as alcoholism and antisocial personality disorder, as currently defined, are more often found in men, whereas women are at increased risk for eating disorders, mood disorders, and some anxiety disorders (Robins et al. 1984). The distress associated with anxiety disorders, in particular, prompts women to seek medical and psychiatric care and is a leading cause of women's disproportionate use of minor tranquilizers (see Chapter 15). The magnitude of this sex-related effect is not inconsequential. Compared with men, women are three to four times more likely to have simple phobia, two to three times more prone to experience panic with agoraphobia, and one and one-half times more likely to develop social phobia. They are at twice the risk for developing posttraumatic stress disorder (PTSD) (Bourdon et al. 1988; Breslau et al. 1990; Schneier et al. 1992). Analyzing the causes for this asymmetrical expression of anxiety disorders in men and women would be helpful in understanding the psychological and

113

biological substrates that underlie anxiety disorders. Yet, as noted by Cameron and Hill (1989), little is known about gender-related features or mechanisms associated with anxiety disorders. In this chapter, we review the available information about gender differences in anxiety disorders and discuss hypothetical explanatory mechanisms. Sections of this chapter are based on a recent review of the treatment of women with anxiety disorders (Yonkers and Ellison, in press).

Gender-Related Features of Phobias

The three major phobias are specific phobia, social phobia, and agoraphobia. The gender ratio of each is shown in Table 6–1.

Specific Phobia

Specific phobias are marked and persistent fears of circumscribed objects or situations (Marks 1987). DSM-IV (American Psychiatric Association 1994) requires that the fear of the phobic object cause social or occupational impairment or significant emotional distress. Even with this diagnostic restriction, specific (simple) phobias are commonly found in community samples, with a 6-month prevalence of 9% in women and 4% in men (Bourdon et al. 1988). The age at onset is early, and more than 80% who develop the disorder will do so before age 25 years (Bourdon et al. 1988). In women, animal phobias appear to have the earliest onset and are the most heritable phobias (Kendler et al. 1992b). Treated prevalence may be low because most individuals do not seek treatment for specific phobia, but the

Table 6–1. Community rates of phobias in men and women

	Men (%)	Women (%)
Panic with agoraphobia	2.9	7.7
Specific phobia	4.0	9.0
Social phobia	2.0	3.1

Source. Robins et al. 1984; Schneier et al. 1992.

syndrome may be detected when patients present to a physician for treatment of another disorder such as depression. Specific phobias may, however, seriously affect an individual's work or lifestyle. For example, flying phobias inhibit or inconvenience a patient who would like to travel for work or for pleasure. A common tool used in psychiatry and psychology to assess the severity of phobias is the Fear Survey Schedule developed by Wolpe and Lang (1964). As reported by Thyer and colleagues (1985), women tend to score higher on this instrument than men, but this difference is not likely to be clinically significant. Several groups have compared the items men and women endorse as most fearful. Although the actual ranking of fears differs somewhat, men and women identify similar conditions (Bourdon et al. 1988; Thyer et al. 1985). Furthermore, men and women appear to have an analogous physiological response to these sources of fear (Katkin and Hoffman 1975).

Social Phobia

Social phobia, the persistent fear of situations in which an individual may be open to scrutiny by others (American Psychiatric Association 1994), causes greater morbidity than specific phobia. Patients will go to great lengths to evade the feared social situation, and their avoidance may impair daily functioning. Social phobia differs from agoraphobia in that patients are comfortable in large crowds if they are not being observed or examined. The Epidemiologic Catchment Area (ECA) survey found that social phobia begins by age 15 years in 56% of those afflicted and by age 25 years in more than 85% of cases identified (Schneier et al. 1992). The disorder may be broken down into two types: generalized social phobia and limited social phobia. In the generalized form of the disorder, patients have global fears of social situations such as attending parties or classes where they may receive attention. Limited social phobia includes difficulties with performance such as public speaking or playing a musical instrument. Women are less likely to experience social phobia than agoraphobia or specific phobia. However, social phobia occurs more frequently in women than in men. According to community data (Schneier et al. 1992), the lifetime prevalence rate for social phobia is about 2.4%, of whom 70% are women. A logistic regression analysis of patients with social phobia found that, in addition to female gender, other characteristics of patients with social phobia include being single, of younger age, of lower socioeconomic status, and of lesser education (Schneier et al. 1992). Only 5% of those with the disorder seek psychiatric treatment (Schneier et al. 1992). In clinical settings, men with social phobia predominate, perhaps because women experience relatively less social dysfunction associated with the illness (Marks 1987). Patients with social phobia frequently have comorbid conditions, in particular, concomitant specific phobia, agoraphobia, major depression, and alcohol abuse (Schneier et al. 1992). In clinical cohorts, depression and suicidal ideation are found in more than 90% of patients, and alcohol abuse is seen in as many as 40% (Liebowitz et al. 1985; Uhde et al. 1991).

Agoraphobia

Agoraphobia, which is derived from the Greek word *agora,* is a fear of public places, particularly crowded places (Marks 1987). In DSM-III (American Psychiatric Association 1980), agoraphobia applied to patients who had phobic avoidance with or without panic. DSM-III-R (American Psychiatric Association 1987) redefined this one category into two: panic with agoraphobia and agoraphobia without panic, and DSM-IV has maintained the distinction. This change reflects the view that agoraphobia develops as a consequence of panic attacks (Klein and Gorman 1987), although some maintain that the phobia occurs first and that panic is simply a common manifestation of exposure to a feared object (Marks 1987). The difference in prevalence rates for agoraphobia, with or without panic attacks (DSM-III definition), is striking in that nearly 8% of women in the ECA had agoraphobia, whereas only 3% of men appeared to have the syndrome. However, men were more likely to inform their physician about their illness than were women (Bourdon et al. 1988). In more than 70% of patients with agoraphobia, the illness begins before age 25 years, and in 50% of patients it may have begun before age 15 years. There does not appear to be a gender difference in the average age at illness onset (Bourdon et al. 1988). Ongoing work in our clinic indicates that after the illness begins, more than 80% of patients remain symptomatic over the next year. There is a trend toward women having a longer illness duration than men.

A role for developmental and sociological factors in the dispro-portionate expression of phobias among women has been proposed. The early onset of phobias and the longevity of these illnesses seem to implicate early developmental experiences. Fodor (1974) reviewed the contributions of sex-role socialization whereby women learn "helplessness, avoidance of mastery experiences, competition, and lack of assertiveness" (p. 140) and suggested that women are not taught mastery and assertiveness, tools that are helpful in overcoming fears and phobias. She went on to suggest that for women in unequal mar-riages, economic concerns and the traditional fears that accompany the female marital role may lead to agoraphobia. Although having such an illness further entraps the wife, it can be experienced as re-taliatory against the husband because he is burdened with caring for an agoraphobic partner. As noted by Bourdon and co-workers (1988), the early age at illness onset makes it unlikely that unhappy marriages are the predominant cause of agoraphobia. However, the notion that role socialization may be a factor in susceptibility to this illness was noted by another group, who found that the severity of agoraphobia in women is inversely correlated with their scores on masculinity scales (Chambless and Mason 1986).

Panic Disorder

As noted above, panic with agoraphobia is more frequently seen in women, and although uncomplicated panic is seen less often, the ra-tio is still two to three times higher in women. The community rate for uncomplicated panic in women ranges from 16 to 21 per 1,000, whereas in men it is 6 to 9 per 1,000 (Robins et al. 1984). Panic dis-order is commonly seen in medical and psychiatric treatment set-tings, and the first presentation may be of a woman who fears she is having a heart attack or other life-threatening illness. The panic at-tack itself is a sudden paroxysm of four or more of the following somatic symptoms: shortness of breath, sweating, trembling, chok-ing, nausea, dizziness, chills or flushes, feelings of unreality, numb-ness or tingling, heart palpitations, and chest discomfort. Patients also feel out of control or sense that something catastrophic is about to occur. Symptoms begin precipitously and dissipate gradually. DSM-IV criteria for panic disorder stipulate that the attacks be recurrent, unprovoked, and followed by 1 month or more of persistent concern or significant behavior change. In addition to frequently accompanying agoraphobia, panic disorder in women is also commonly seen with specific phobia, generalized anxiety disorder (GAD), and depression (Table 6–2) (Scheibe and Albus 1992).

Genetic studies show an increased risk for anxiety disorders in first-degree relatives of patients with panic disorder. Relatives of probands with panic disorder have five times the risk of developing panic with agoraphobia than relatives of subjects without panic disorder (Crowe et al. 1983). In addition, the rate of panic with agoraphobia is three times higher in female relatives than in male relatives, who are more likely to have alcoholism. Uncomplicated panic is also more prevalent in female relatives (Crowe et al. 1983).

The profile of panic symptoms does not differ between men and women (Chambless and Mason 1986; Scheibe and Albus 1992). However, many women complain of premenstrual worsening of panic. This has been assessed in three small cohorts. Cameron and colleagues (1988) found only small increases in panic among women who retrospectively complained of premenstrual worsening. Similarly, Cook and associates (1990) did not find an increase in panic but

Table 6–2. Co-occurrence of panic disorder and other anxiety disorders in a large clinical cohort

| | Lifetime risk | | |
| | Men (%) (n = 160) | Women (%) (n = 367) | P |
Comorbid diagnosis			
Agoraphobia	72	82	.013
Generalized anxiety disorder	19	27	.043
Obsessive-compulsive disorder	17	12	NS
Posttraumatic stress disorder	6	10	NS
Specific phobia	12	21	.015
Social phobia	20	20	NS

Note. NS = not significant.
Source. Data adapted from the Harvard Anxiety Research Program.

did find a rise in overall anxiety levels during the premenstrual phase. Luteal phase worsening of panic was not found by Stein and colleagues (1989) among patients with panic, but they did find greater anxiety premenstrually in a comparison group with documented late luteal phase dysphoric disorder. Of note, women with premenstrual disorders are prone to develop either lactate- or CO_2-induced panic, which approaches the susceptibility of those who have panic disorder (Facchinetti et al. 1992; Harrison et al. 1989). Premenstrual increases in anxiety among some women and the sensitivity of those with premenstrual dysphoria to panic suggest a role for ovarian hormones in modulating vulnerability to anxiety and panic. Analogous mechanisms may be responsible for postpartum anxiety and panic in women (Metz et al. 1988).

Differences in biological vulnerability may influence the gender difference in prevalence of panic disorder. As noted above, fluctuating levels of sex hormones may influence neurotransmitter systems or other physiological parameters and change the thresholds for symptom development. For example, progesterone causes a mild chronic hyperventilation (Damas-Mora et al. 1980). Carr and Sheehan (1984) suggested that this luteal phase increase in ventilation increases the likelihood of panic in susceptible people. On the other hand, Klein (1993), who maintains that panic develops from triggering of a "suffocation alarm," believes that the decrease in hyperventilation after progesterone withdrawal provokes panic.

Ovarian hormones and their metabolites have bioactive effects and can directly contribute to the occurrence of or susceptibility for panic. The A-ring reduced progesterone metabolites allopregnenolone and tetrahydrodeoxycorticosterone (THDOC) bind to the γ-aminobutyric acid ($GABA_A$) receptor in a partial agonist fashion (Majewska 1987). GABA and agents that bind to the GABA/benzodiazepine receptor affect anxiety, possibly via influences on adrenergic neurotransmission (Cameron et al. 1990). In a genetically prone individual, the repetitive binding and unbinding of these endogenous compounds may influence GABA's inhibitory action and hence the expression of panic and other forms of anxiety in women. It is likely that other factors are involved, however. Jones and colleagues (1983) found menstrual cycle variations in the amount of α_2-receptor binding. Furthermore, during the middle portion of the menstrual cycle, when estrogen levels peak and progesterone levels are low, noradrenergic sensitivity is increased, as shown by sensitivity to tyramine-induced blood pressure elevation (Ghose and Turner 1977; Hamilton 1991). Finally, if the neurotransmitter serotonin is involved in the expression of panic symptoms, progesterone may play a role in modulating serotonin neurotransmission. Recently, progesterone receptors have been found on serotonin neurons in the dorsal and ventral raphe nuclei of primates (Bethea 1993).

Additional biological contributions to the onset of panic may result from the co-occurrence of certain medical disorders (Table 6–3). Mitral valve prolapse and hyperthyroidism, which have been associated with panic disorder, occur more often in women (Lohr et al. 1986). Cognitive-behavioral theories suggest that some individuals with panic catastrophically misinterpret somatic sensations, which increases anxiety and eventually induces panic (Clark 1986).

These hypothetical explanations suggest fertile areas for investigation. Because extensive overlap is found among anxiety disorders, the same potential mechanisms may be relevant to many anxiety disorders.

Generalized Anxiety Disorder

As originally conceptualized, GAD was meant to describe the anticipatory anxiety seen in panic and phobic states, the anxious prodrome occurring before panic, and the residual anxiety that may

Table 6–3. Panic disorder and concurrent medical disorders in a large clinical cohort

Medical illness	Men (%) ($n = 160$)	Women (%) ($n = 367$)	P
Allergies	36	52	.001
Gastrointestinal ulcer	17	7	.001
Headache	30	45	.001
Low blood pressure	7	23	.000
Migraine	21	37	.000

Source. Data adapted from the Harvard Anxiety Research Program.

continue after discrete panic attacks cease. The DSM-IV criteria for GAD include physical manifestations of anxiety such as fatigue, restlessness, muscle tension, and sleep disturbance, as well as cognitions of worry and apprehension. The DSM-III definition for GAD included a number of hierarchical restrictions such that all other anxiety disorders and depression were considered above GAD in the hierarchy. DSM-III-R and DSM-IV retain the hierarchical exclusion of depression and stipulate that the worry experienced by individuals with generalized anxiety not be restricted to concerns about phobias, panic, obsessions, or compulsions.

The ECA survey prevalence data for GAD were based on 1 month of illness, as required by DSM-III. Results showed that GAD occurs twice as often in women as in men, with 1-year prevalence rates of 1.0%–2.4% for men and 2.4%–5.0% for women, depending on the exclusionary criteria used (Blazer et al. 1991). An epidemiological study specifically investigating this disorder in female twins found a lifetime prevalence, using the 1-month definition, of 23.5%; the prevalence rate was 5.9% according to a 6-month definition (Kendler et al. 1992a). ECA data do not show gender differences in the average age at onset or duration of symptoms. They do show that a diagnosis of GAD is associated with greater comorbidity for panic and depression and higher utilization of health care (usually primary care) services (Blazer et al. 1991). The co-occurrence of GAD and dysthymia in women is also seen frequently in clinical settings (Shores et al. 1992). Among patients with GAD, women predominate and thus experience a differential impact associated with this disorder.

The genetic basis of panic disorder has been adequately substantiated, but the same is not true of GAD. However, Kendler et al. (1992a) found that for women, genetic factors play a significant role in the etiology of GAD, regardless of whether the definition for length of illness is 1 or 6 months. These investigators also noted an essential role for individual life experiences in the genesis of GAD in women.

Obsessive-Compulsive Disorder

Patients with obsessive-compulsive disorder (OCD) experience obsessions, recurrent ego-dystonic ideas or thoughts, and/or compulsions, behaviors that are repeated in an attempt to ward off anxiety. OCD ranks fourth in lifetime prevalence among all psychiatric disorders (Robins et al. 1984). Until the ECA survey, OCD was thought to be more prevalent in men (Insel 1990; Rasmussen and Tsuang 1984). The ECA survey found similar prevalence rates for men and women (Robins et al. 1984), although the average age at onset differs by sex. As reviewed by Yonkers and Ellison (in press) and as shown in Table 6–4, several significant features differentiate OCD in men from that in women. One study found that males develop OCD early in life (ages 5–15 years), whereas females often develop the disorder between ages 26 and 35 years (Noshirvani et al. 1991). Perhaps confounded by the earlier age at onset, the length of illness is longer in males (Noshirvani et al. 1991). The later-onset type of OCD, which occurs more often in women, may begin with an episode of depression that improves, while the obsessions and compulsions remain (Welner et al. 1976). In contrast, a recent prospective study showed that the only subjects recovering from OCD were women with OCD and depression (K. White, D. Shera, G. Steketee, et al., unpubished manuscript, 1993). Others have noted that depression co-occurs with OCD more often in women (Noshirvani et al. 1991).

Early-onset OCD is associated with a poor prognosis, and males may be more treatment resistant. Because men seek treatment over longer periods and have greater treatment resistance (Rasmussen and Tsuang 1984), the pre-ECA finding of male predominance is partially explained. In addition to the length and severity of the disorder, other

Table 6–4.   Gender-divergent features of obsessive-compulsive disorder

Women
- ↦ Have older age at onset
- ↦ Frequently also experience depression and anorexia
- ↦ Engage in compulsive washing
- ↦ More often have the associated disorder of trichotillomania

Men
- ↦ Frequently engage in checking rituals
- ↦ Have longer and more severe illness

unique gender-related features include differences in symptoms expressed. Persons who compulsively wash tend to be women, and men are more likely to have checking rituals (Akhtar et al. 1975; Dawson 1977; Noshirvani et al. 1991). In addition, obsessions about food and weight, including diagnoses of anorexia, are more common in women (Kasvikis et al. 1986). A related disorder, trichotillomania, also appears to be more prevalent in women (Swedo 1993).

Posttraumatic Stress Disorder

PTSD is a distinctive symptom cluster that develops after an event so traumatic that it exceeds usual human experiences. PTSD is most often a sequela of combat exposure or natural disasters, although, in women, PTSD may occur as a result of rape, incest, or childhood sexual abuse. The symptoms of PTSD fall into three categories: 1) reexperiencing of the traumatic event, 2) avoidance or general numbing of responsiveness, and 3) increased sympathetic arousal. Symptoms should be present for at least 1 month to satisfy DSM-IV diagnostic criteria.

The age at onset for PTSD is not fixed; it depends on when the trauma is experienced. Two community studies provide prevalence estimates. A report based on the ECA survey found a surprisingly low lifetime rate of 1% for PTSD (Helzer et al. 1987). The two groups with the largest incidence were combat veterans (9%) and assault victims (3%). In contrast, a large health maintenance organization–based study showed an overall rate nine times higher than that of Helzer and colleagues' study, including 11% of women and 7% of men (Breslau et al. 1990). This group found that nearly 24% of those exposed to trauma developed symptoms of PTSD. Rates of trauma were also higher for men in this study, as in the Helzer report, but of those exposed to trauma, 31% of women and only 19% of men developed PTSD. A logistic regression model identified variables of female gender, neuroticism, and family history of anxiety or depression as risk factors for PTSD. A subsequent report compared groups with chronic PTSD and those with acute PTSD. The investigators found that although women constitute 65% of the acute PTSD group, they constitute 85% of the group with symptoms lasting at least 1 year (Breslau and Davis 1992). Other predictor variables for chronic PTSD are personal history of affective disorder and a family history of antisocial behavior (Breslau and Davis 1992).

Another group noted that after exposure to stressful events, women are more likely to develop "psychological distress" (Kessler and McLeod 1984). However, they demonstrated that women are exposed to a greater number of "network events" (i.e., events occurring to people who are intimate with the female subject). The combination of the subject's own traumatic experiences and network events leads to greater cumulative stress and higher psychological distress. Theoretical writings on the psychology of women complement the work of Kessler and McLeod by emphasizing the important role other individuals play in women's emotional health. Miller and Stiver (1993) posit the need women have to stay "in connection" with others. The loss of these integral relationships is the antecedent to anxiety and depressive reactions.

As noted above, PTSD in women has some distinctive features (Table 6–5). It may occur as a result of trauma, sexual abuse, or incest. Childhood trauma is associated with a variety of disturbances, including dissociative experiences, borderline personality disorder, and multiple personality disorder (Hamilton and Jensvold 1992; Herman et al. 1989; Putnam et al. 1986; Ross and Anderson 1988; Soloff and Millward 1983). Among women with borderline personality disorder, the reported rate of physical and sexual abuse ranges from 60% to 80% (Herman et al. 1989; Soloff and Millward 1983). The rate is at least as high in patients with multiple personality disorder (Ross and

Table 6–5.   Gender-related features of posttraumatic stress disorder

Community rate in women is 11%.

Community rate in men is 7%.

Chronic symptoms are more likely to develop in women.

Childhood sexual abuse is associated with borderline personality disorder in women.

Posttraumatic stress disorder symptoms may fluctuate across the menstrual cycle.

Anderson 1988). Studies conducted in children also have found elevated rates of physical and/or sexual abuse among those with a diagnosis of borderline personality disorder (Famularo et al. 1991; Goldman et al. 1992). Based on these findings, some question whether borderline personality disorder is a personality disorder or a variant of chronic PTSD (Hamilton and Jensvold 1992; Saunders and Arnold 1991). Childhood abuse is invasive and experienced as shameful. Because its secretive nature limits a child's access to help and protection, the opportunity for others to affirm that the abuse is not the child's fault is narrowed. Furthermore, childhood abuse may occur during a critical time in development when the impact of the trauma can cause pervasive and enduring impairment. Because of this longevity, PTSD may appear to be a personality disorder to clinicians.

In addition to developmental theories, biological theories may be helpful in understanding gender-related variability in the expression and course of PTSD. Neurobiological hypotheses on the mechanisms of PTSD invoke the role of various neurotransmitter systems in an attempt to understand the causes of PTSD. The most compelling theories focus on limbic system dysfunction and the interactions of catecholamines and endogenous opioid peptides (EOPs). Chronic arousal as manifested by a strong startle response and physical reactivity is a hallmark of PTSD and suggests overactivity of adrenergic and possibly dopaminergic systems (Charney et al. 1993). Noradrenergic supersensitivity occurs in the model of *inescapable shock* (van der Kolk et al. 1985). In this paradigm, an animal's repeated exposure to inescapable shock causes depletion of dopamine and serotonin, thus leading to noradrenergic and dopaminergic supersensitivity and autonomic hyperarousal. Repeated shock also leads to the release of endogenous opiates, as is seen in animal models of stress-induced analgesia (Charney et al. 1993). Again, after repeated administration of uncontrollable shock, the animals develop endogenous opiate-dependent analgesia to subsequent aversive stimuli. The stress response seen in these animals is believed to be similar to that experienced by humans exposed to trauma. In particular, reexperiencing the trauma or the pain of self-mutilation may lead to an increase in endogenous opiate activity; the soothing opiate response subsequently, perhaps, reinforces these behaviors (van der Kolk et al. 1985). Opioid (EOP) secretion may also lead to certain dissociative phenomena. Of note, levels of EOPs vary across the menstrual cycle such that levels increase during the follicular and early luteal phases and decrease just before menses (Chuong et al. 1985; Giannini et al. 1990).

Worsening of PTSD symptoms, particularly dissociative episodes during the luteal phase of the menstrual cycle, has been reported (Hamilton 1991). Whether fluctuations in levels of EOPs correlate with PTSD symptoms or with symptoms of dissociation is unknown. The fluctuations in symptoms noted by some clinicians suggest that it does seem judicious to monitor women for menstrual cycle entrainment of symptoms.

Summary

Anxiety disorders are especially prevalent in women. Current evidence suggests that for some anxiety disorders, such as agoraphobia and PTSD, the course of illness is longer in women, whereas men may have longer periods of illness and greater morbidity when they develop OCD. Symptom profiles are similar for men and women for panic disorder, phobias, and PTSD, but they may vary for OCD.

Ongoing research continues to uncover promising hypotheses for anxiety disorders. These theories should be able to explain gender differences in prevalence rates. It is hoped that research into these factors will provide increasing understanding of the biological, psychological, and developmental substrates for anxiety disorders.

References

Akhtar S, Wig NN, Varma VK: A phenomenological analysis of symptoms in obsessive-compulsive neurosis. Br J Psychiatry 127:342–348, 1975

American Psychiatric Association: Diagnostic and Statistical Manual of Mental Disorders, 3rd Edition. Washington, DC, American Psychiatric Association, 1980

American Psychiatric Association: Diagnostic and Statistical Manual of Mental Disorders, 3rd Edition, Revised. Washington, DC, American Psychiatric Association, 1987

American Psychiatric Association: Diagnostic and Statistical Manual of Mental Disorders, 4th Edition. Washington, DC, American Psychiatric Association, 1994

Bethea CL: Colocalizatin of progestin receptors with serotonin in raphe neurons of macaque. Neuroendocrinology 57:1–6, 1993

Blazer DG, Huges D, George LK, et al: Generalized anxiety disorder, in Psychiatric Disorders in America. Edited by Robins LN, Regier DA. New York, Free Press, 1991, pp 181–203

Bourdon KH, Boyd JH, Rae DS, et al: Gender differences in phobias: results of the ECA community survey. Journal of Anxiety Disorders 2:227–241, 1988

Breslau N, Davis G: Posttraumatic stress disorder in an urban population of young adults: risk factors for chronicity. Am J Psychiatry 149:671–675, 1992

Breslau N, Davis GC, Andreski P: Traumatic events and traumatic stress disorder in an urban population of young adults. Arch Gen Psychiatry 48:218–222, 1990

Cameron OG, Hill EM: Women and anxiety. Psychiatr Clin North Am 12:175–186, 1989

Cameron OG, Kuttesch D, McPhee K, et al: Menstrual fluctuation in the symptoms of panic anxiety. J Affect Disord 15:169–174, 1988

Cameron OG, Smith CB, Myung AL, et al: Adrenergic status in anxiety disorders: platelet alpha-2-adrenergic receptor binding, blood pressure, pulse, and plasma catecholamines in panic and generalized anxiety disorder patients and in normal subjects. Biol Psychiatry 28:3–20, 1990

Carr DB, Sheehan DV: Panic anxiety: a new biological model. J Clin Psychiatry 45:323–330, 1984

Chambless DL, Mason J: Sex, sex-role stereotyping and agoraphobia. Behav Res Ther 24:231–235, 1986

Charney DS, Deutch AY, Krystal JH, et al: Psychobiologic mechanisms of posttraumatic stress disorder. Arch Gen Psychiatry 50:294–305, 1993

Chuong CJ, Coulam CB, Kao PC, et al: Neuropeptide levels in premenstrual syndrome. Fertil Steril 44:760–763, 1985

Clark DMA: A cognitive approach to panic. Behav Res Ther 24:461–470, 1986

Cook BL, Noyes R, Garvey MJ, et al: Anxiety and the menstrual cycle in panic disorder. J Affect Disord 19:221–226, 1990

Crowe RR, Noyes R, Pauls DL, et al: A family study of panic disorder. Arch Gen Psychiatry 40:1065–1069, 1983

Damas-Mora J, Davies L, Taylor W, et al: Menstrual respiratory changes and symptoms. Br J Psychiatry 136:492–497, 1980

Dawson JH: The phenomenology of severe obsessive-compulsive neurosis. Br J Psychiatry 131:75–78, 1977

Facchinetti F, Romano G, Fava M, et al: Lactate infusion induces panic attacks in patients with premenstrual syndrome. Psychosom Med 54:288–296, 1992

Famularo R, Kinscherff R, Fenton T: Posttraumatic stress disorder among children clinically diagnosed as borderline personality disorder. J Nerv Ment Dis 179:428–431, 1991

Fodor IG: The phobic syndrome in women: implications for treatment, in Women in Therapy: New Psychotherapies for a Changing Society. Edited by Franks V, Burtle V. New York, Brunner/Mazel, 1974, pp 132–168

Ghose K, Turner P: The menstrual cycle and the Tyramine Pressor Response Test. Br J Clin Pharmacol 4:500–502, 1977

Giannini AJ, Martin DM, Turner CE: Beta-endorphin decline in late luteal phase dysphoric disorder. Int J Psychiatry Med 20:279–284, 1990

Goldman SJ, D'Angelo EJ, Demaso DR, et al: Physical and sexual abuse histories among children with borderline personality disorder. Am J Psychiatry 149:1723–1726, 1992

Hamilton JA: Clinical pharmacology panel report, in Forging a Women's Health Research Agenda (conference proceedings). Edited by Blumenthal SJ, Parry B, Sherwin B. Washington, DC, National Women's Health Resource Center, 1991, pp 1–27

Hamilton JA, Jensvold M: Personality, psychopathology and depression in women, in Personality and Psychopathology: Feminist Reappraisals. Edited by Brown LS, Ballou M. New York, Guilford, 1992, pp 116–143

Harrison W, Sandberg D, Gorman J, et al: Provocation of panic with carbon dioxide inhalation in patients with premenstrual dysphoria. Psychiatry Res 27:183–192, 1989

Helzer JE, Robins LN, McEvoy L: Post-traumatic stress disorder in the general population. N Engl J Med 317:1630–1634, 1987

Herman JL, Perry JC, van der Kolk BA: Childhood trauma in borderline personality disorder. Am J Psychiatry 146:490–495, 1989

Insel TR: Phenomenology of obsessive compulsive disorder. J Clin Psychiatry 51 (suppl):4–8, 1990

Jones SB, Bylund DB, Rieser CA, et al: Alpha adrenergic receptor binding in human platelets: alterations during the menstrual cycle. Clin Pharmacol Ther 34:90–96, 1983

Kasvikis JG, Tsakiris F, Marks IM: Women with obsessive-compulsive disorder frequently report a past history of anorexia nervosa. International Journal of Eating Disorders 5:1069–1075, 1986

Katkin ES, Hoffman LS: Sex differences in phobia and self-report of fear: a psychophysical assessment. J Abnorm Psychol 85:607–610, 1975

Kendler KS, Neale MC, Kessler RC, et al: Generalized anxiety disorder in women: a population-based twin study. Arch Gen Psychiatry 49:267–272, 1992a

Kendler KS, Neale MC, Kessler RC, et al: The genetic epidemiology of phobias in women. Arch Gen Psychiatry 49:273–281, 1992b

Kessler RC, McLeod JD: Sex differences in vulnerability to undesirable life events. American Sociological Review 49:620–631, 1984

Klein DF: False suffocation alarms and spontaneous panic: subsuming the CO_2 hypersensitivity theory. Arch Gen Psychiatry 50:306–317, 1993

Klein DF, Gorman JM: A model of panic and agoraphobic development. Acta Psychiatr Scand 76 (suppl):87–95, 1987

Liebowitz MR, Gorman JM, Fyer AJ, et al: Social phobia: review of a neglected anxiety disorder. Arch Gen Psychiatry 42:729–736, 1985

Lohr KN, Kamberg CJ, Keeler EB, et al: Chronic disease in a general adult population. West J Med 145:537–545, 1986

Majewska MD: Steroids and brain activity: essential dialogue between body and mind. Biochem Pharmacol 36:3781–3788, 1987

Marks IM: Fears, Phobias and Rituals, 2nd Edition. Oxford, Oxford University Press, 1987

Metz AM, Sichel DA, Goff DC: Postpartum panic disorder. J Clin Psychiatry 49:278–279, 1988

Miller JB, Stiver I: A relational approach to understanding women's lives and problems. Psychiatric Annals 23:424–431, 1993

Noshirvani HF, Kasvikis Y, Marks IM, et al: Gender-divergent aetiological factors in obsessive-compulsive disorder. Br J Psychiatry 158:260–263, 1991

Putnam FW, Gurroff JJ, Silberman EK, et al: The clinical phenomenology of multiple personality disorder: review of 100 recent cases. J Clin Psychiatry 47:285–293, 1986

Rasmussen SA, Tsuang MT: The epidemiology of obsessive compulsive disorder. J Clin Psychiatry 45:450–457, 1984

Robins LN, Helzer JE, Weissman MM, et al: Lifetime prevalence of specific disorders in three sites. Arch Gen Psychiatry 41:949–958, 1984

Ross CA, Anderson G: Phenomenological overlap of multiple personality disorder and obsessive-compulsive disorder. J Nerv Ment Dis 176:295–299, 1988

Saunders EA, Arnold F: Borderline personality disorder and childhood abuse: revisions in clinical thinking and treatment approach. Work in Progress 59. Wellesley, MA, Stone Center, 1991

Scheibe G, Albus M: Age at onset, precipitating events, sex distribution, and co-occurrence of anxiety disorders. Psychopathology 25:11–18, 1992

Schneier FR, Johnson J, Hornig CD, et al: Social phobia: comorbidity and morbidity in an epidemiological sample. Arch Gen Psychiatry 49:282–288, 1992

Shores MM, Glubin T, Cowley DS, et al: The relationship between anxiety and depression: a clinical comparison of generalized anxiety disorder, dysthymic disorder, panic disorder, and major depressive disorder. Compr Psychiatry 33:237–244, 1992

Soloff PH, Millward JW: Developmental histories of borderline patients. Compr Psychiatry 24:574–588, 1983

Stein MB, Schmidt PJ, Rubinow DR, et al: Panic disorder and the menstrual cycle: panic disorder patients, healthy control subjects, and patients with premenstrual syndrome. Am J Psychiatry 146:1299–1303, 1989

Swedo SE: Trichotillomania. Psychiatric Annals 23:402–407, 1993

Thyer BA, Tomlin P, Curtis GC, et al: Diagnostic and gender differences in the expressed fears of anxious patients. J Behav Ther Exp Psychiatry 16:111–115, 1985

Uhde TW, Tancer ME, Black B: Phenomenology and neurobiology of social phobia: comparison with panic disorder. J Clin Psychiatry 52 (suppl):31–40, 1991

van der Kolk BA, Greenberg M, Boyd H: Inescapable shock, neurotransmitters, and addiction to trauma: toward a psychobiology of post-traumatic stress. Biol Psychiatry 20:314–325, 1985

Welner A, Reich T, Robin E: Obsessive-compulsive neurosis record, follow-up and family studies, I: inpatient record study. Compr Psychiatry 17:577–589, 1976

Wolpe J, Lang P: A Fear Survey Schedule for use in behavior therapy. Behav Res Ther 2:27–30, 1964

Yonkers KA, Ellison JM: Anxiety disorders in women and their pharmacological treatment, in Psychopharmacology of Women: Sex, Gender, and Hormonal Consideration. Edited by Hamilton JA, Jensvold M, Halbreich U. Washington, DC, American Psychiatric Press (in press)

CHAPTER 7

Gender, Brain, and Schizophrenia

Anatomy of Differences/ Differences of Anatomy

Richard R. J. Lewine, Ph.D.
Mary V. Seeman, M.D., C.M., F.R.C.P.C.

T he point of origin for this chapter is the now well-established epidemiological fact that the age when men and women are at greatest risk for schizophrenia is significantly lower in men than in women (see Chapter 8). In this context, Lewine (1981) proposed two competing models of a putative timing difference: 1) a *trigger* model that hypothesizes a lowering of the threshold for schizophrenia among men and 2) a *suppressor* model that hypothesizes the presence of a protective, or delaying, factor among women, assuming a pool of individuals equally predisposed to the development of schizophrenia. That women lose this protective factor after menopause, as reflected in an increased late incidence of schizophrenia,

Preparation of this chapter was supported in part by grant 44151 (RL) from the National Institute of Mental Health. The authors wish to thank Susan Maxwell and Tammy LePage for their help with the bibliography.

suggests a possible hormonal mechanism. In either case—trigger or suppressor—we assume that gender differences in the brain play a significant role in schizophrenia.

Triggering and suppressing factors may be hypothesized as occurring at or immediately before onset of symptoms. They may also be viewed as long-standing or predisposing factors traceable to early life, indeed to prenatal life. Hormonal differentiation of the two sexes comes into play when testes are formed and begin to secrete testosterone. In human male embryos, this occurs at approximately week 20 of gestation. Testosterone, present to a significant degree in males only, enters the fetal brain and interacts with sex hormone receptors in various parts of the developing brain (mainly estrogen receptors, paradoxically) to speed or delay local neuronal growth. Although the process must be very complex and is still far from being understood, the simple picture is that male and female brains diverge from that point onward. Their brains are dimorphically organized during the prenatal period, although actual hormonal divergence does not occur until puberty (Seeman 1989a; Seeman and Lang 1990).

The original difference in organization can be conceptualized as involving both structural differences and differences in pace of development. Size differentials of brain nuclei imply greater or smaller requirements vis-à-vis blood supply and nutrients. This, in turn, has at least hypothetical implication for vulnerability to trauma, anoxia, or infection. Pace of development differentials has additional implications; quickly multiplying cells are perhaps more prone to transcription errors. Thus, prenatal hormonally induced differences in male and female brains establish different potentials for environmental interaction. How these sex differences might raise or lower the threshold for the action of putative schizophrenia genes is, of course, unknown. If the genes for schizophrenia act at the level of neurodevelopment, however (which seems more and more likely), it is plausible, and even probable, that sexual differentiation either enhances or attenuates whatever neuronal disarray the gene products induce.

At the later phase of central nervous system (CNS) activation, puberty ushers in a dramatically different hormonal environment for male and female brains. Not only are there marked differences in the levels of various gonadal steroids, but the rhythm of hormonal release is profoundly different in men and women. Men's brains are bathed in minor fluctuations occurring daily; women's brains are flooded with relatively major tides of various sex hormones in monthly cycles. This divergence between the sexes occurs during a period of active neuronal pruning that must, to some degree, be affected by the hormonal environment (Lewine 1992).

A host of other influences impacts on the brain during the developmental period of adolescence. Many of these are gender dimorphic. To name a few: immune functions reach maturity, males are preferentially exposed to physical and chemical injury, and social expectations of males and females in all cultures begin to diverge dramatically after puberty. Whereas for many mental illnesses discussed in other chapters females become *more* vulnerable than males after puberty, the reverse is true for schizophrenia; the changes of puberty appear to protect females for some time thereafter. For males, on the other hand, puberty (which occurs chronologically several years later than in females) is closely associated with the timing of the onset of schizophrenia.

A case can therefore be made for an interaction of male gender and predisposition to schizophrenia at the level of prenatal brain development as well as a subsequent, presumably related, interaction at the time of schizophrenia onset.

In this chapter, we first selectively review the current evidence that male and female brains show systematic, reproducible differences in schizophrenia. We then discuss the putative role of hormonal and immune factors and the theoretical implications of the available data.

Schizophrenia and the Brain

Lateral Ventricular Enlargement

The most consistently reported morphological gender difference in the brains of patients with schizophrenia is in the size of the lateral ventricles. The enlargement of this structure is usually taken as an indication of early, probably perinatal, brain insult (Castle and Murray 1991). Schizophrenic patients, as a group, have larger ventricle brain ratios (VBRs; the ratio of ventricle size to whole brain for a given brain imaging slice) than nonpsychiatric control subjects. A meta-analysis of published studies to date (Raz and Raz 1990) yielded a significant association between gender and VBR. This review concluded that the higher the proportion of men in a schizophrenia sample, the greater the schizophrenia/nonschizophrenia difference in VBRs.

At the same time, a somewhat less consistent picture was drawn by Flaum and colleagues (1990) in their review of about 50 controlled studies of schizophrenia that used computed tomography (CT) and approximately 12 studies that used magnetic resonance imaging (MRI). Of the only 13 studies reporting gender difference analyses, 5 found men to have a significantly larger VBR than women, 1 found women to have a significantly larger VBR than men, and 7 studies reported no gender effects. In the analyses of their own data, the investigators found that in 3 of their 4 independent samples, men with schizophrenia had significantly larger VBRs than male control subjects but that no significant differences existed between the women with schizophrenia and female control subjects.

Both quantitative and qualitative studies since 1990 tend to be consistent with the conclusion of Raz and Raz (1990). Lieberman and colleagues (1992) qualitatively analyzed MRI brain scans in first-episode and multiepisode patients with schizophrenia and found not only that both groups had a significantly higher rate of global abnormality ratings than a healthy contrast group (31%, 42%, and 5%, respectively), but also that rates of all abnormalities were higher in men with schizophrenia; only the difference in ventricular enlargement reached statistical significance. Comparable rates of qualitative anomalies by diagnosis and gender have been reported by Lewine and co-workers (in press) in a sample of 110 schizophrenic patients, 65 nonschizophrenic psychiatric patients, and 150 healthy control subjects. Ventricular enlargement and asymmetry, although rare overall (5 of 325, or 1.5%), were found exclusively in the male schizophrenia group.

Lateral ventricular volume increases were particularly prominent among young (< age 30 years) males (but not among females) with schizophrenia in an MRI study reported by O'Callaghan and associates (1992). This subgroup of patients with schizophrenia had an average increase of 91% over the control mean lateral ventricular volume, in contrast to an average increase of 33% across the entire schizophrenia sample. The ventriculomegaly found in these young schizophrenic male patients is particularly striking because the patients and control subjects were matched (by group) on age. In addition, the finding reflects the opposite trend to that expected as a function of age. That is, lateral ventricular volume is known to increase with age.

More complex interactions involving gender, age, and lateralization were reported by R. C. Gur and co-workers (1991) in an MRI study of aging and atrophy in healthy individuals. Aging was associated with a disproportionate degree of brain atrophy in men relative to women; this atrophy was, furthermore, particularly marked in the left hemisphere of men, whereas it was comparable in the two hemispheres of women. This study is at odds with that of O'Callaghan and colleagues, who reported that total ventricular volume increased significantly with age in both control subjects ($r = .46$) and schizophrenic patients ($r = .53$) but that the association between age and total ventricular volume was substantially stronger in female schizophrenic patients ($r = .75$) than in male schizophrenic patients ($r = .50$), female control subjects ($r = .57$), or male control subjects ($r = .35$). Age-gender interactions must be examined in all brain morphology investigations to help clarify this ambiguity.

Laterality and gender were found to interact in an MRI study of first-episode schizophrenic patients conducted by Bogerts and colleagues (1990). In a subsample of the patients reported by Lieberman and co-workers (1992), Bogerts and colleagues found that, relative to control subjects, both male and female patients with schizophrenia exhibited bilateral enlargement of the lateral ventricles, the temporal horn, or its anterior portion, whereas hippocampal tissue was significantly smaller only in the left brain hemisphere of male patients with schizophrenia.

Andreasen and associates (1990) rigorously examined the effects of gender, age, and stage of illness on ventricle enlargement in a large sample of patients with schizophrenia and healthy volunteers. Overall, patients with schizophrenia had a significantly higher mean VBR (6.49) than healthy control subjects (5.37). This difference was accounted for entirely by the significant difference in mean VBR between male control subjects (4.83) and male schizophrenic patients (6.64); the difference between female control subjects (5.87) and female schizophrenic patients (6.24) was not significant. When separate comparisons were conducted for age decades ranging from less than 20 to 60 years, it was found that, in each age period, the men with schizophrenia had higher mean VBRs than the control men, especially in the decade from age 30 to 40 years. (We note a similarity to the findings of O'Callaghan et al. [1992] in their young male schizophrenic patients.)

In contrast, among the women, the VBRs were either quite similar or in some instances slightly higher in the female control subjects than in the female schizophrenic patients. Finally, the distribution of abnormal VBRs, defined as one or two standard deviations above the control mean, showed a significant diagnosis by gender interaction. Specifically, 19% of the patients with schizophrenia were more than two standard deviations above the control mean, and 43% were more than one standard deviation above the control mean. Thirteen percent of the male schizophrenic patients were outside the control range. In contrast, only one (5.3%) of the healthy control subjects had a VBR more than two standard deviations above the mean, and two (10.6%) had values one standard deviation above the mean. The distributions for the female control subjects and schizophrenic patients overlapped almost completely.

Some investigators have, however, found more abnormalities among female schizophrenic patients. Nasrallah and colleagues (1990) reported that women with schizophrenia had smaller craniums and brains and larger lateral and third ventricles on MRI scans than did healthy control subjects. However, men with schizophrenia did not differ substantially from the male control subjects. Examination of the detailed data from this report reveals that this gender-by-diagnosis interaction may be largely attributable to somewhat anomalous values for the healthy female control group, raising questions about subject selection. For each of the five measures of lateral or third ventricular volume, the female control subjects had the smallest value. For example, on the VBR calculated from the midsagittal view, female control subjects had a mean VBR of 0.040, in contrast to female schizophrenic patients (0.061), male control subjects (0.056), and male schizophrenic patients (0.053). Although the female control

$(n = 20)$ group was somewhat younger and more educated than the female schizophrenia group, the differences were not statistically significant. A larger sample may yield different results.

In a recently published study, R. E. Gur and co-workers (1994) reported on measures of whole-brain volume in men and women with schizophrenia. MRIs of cranial, brain, ventricular, and sulcal volume were examined in 50 men, 31 women, and 81 demographically matched control subjects. The patients had smaller cranial and brain volumes than control subjects. They also had higher ventricular cerebrospinal fluid volumes and thus higher VBRs. Women with schizophrenia had significantly higher ratio elevations than men. The investigators had excluded subjects with histories of neurological difficulties, and because more of these are likely to have been men (Cannon et al. 1989), they believe they may have undersampled this neurodevelopmentally affected, predominantly male subpopulation of patients with schizophrenia. This could explain their findings.

The available data are by no means consistent. Degreef et al. (1992) reported a significant gender effect on lateral ventricle volume, with men (both those with schizophrenia and healthy control subjects) having larger ventricular volumes and temporal horn volumes than women. There were no significant gender-by-diagnosis interactions, suggesting that reports of larger lateral ventricles in male schizophrenic patients may not be specific to schizophrenia.

Distinctively negative results regarding gender differences in lateral ventricle size have been reported by DeLisi and associates (1991). Their morphometric analyses of first-episode "schizophrenic-like" patients revealed neither gender nor lateralization effects when controlling for total brain volume. However, the authors did report an association between enlargement of lateral ventricles and early onset. Because the first-episode patients were very broadly characterized as "schizophrenic-like," we can anticipate a change in the results as the diagnoses are clarified on follow-up.

Temporal Lobe and Corpus Callosum

Shenton and collaborators (1992) examined the relationship between temporal lobe volume and severity of thought disorder in a Veterans

Administration sample of men with schizophrenia. They found that there was a differential volume loss in the left (versus right) temporal lobe and that the magnitude of volume loss was significantly related to severity of thought disorder. Because women were not included in the study, we can only view this as presumptive evidence of gender differences, which, as shown later in this chapter, is supported by other studies. Differential left temporal volume loss in men with schizophrenia has been emphasized in a series of studies by Crow and his colleagues (Crow 1990a, 1990b; Crow et al. 1989a, 1989b), who, based on these findings, suggested a genetic theory of gender differences, which is presented later in this chapter.

Two independent and quite different brain studies have yielded data suggesting that schizophrenia is characterized by a reversal of a normal sexual dimorphism. Lewine and others (1990) found that only 12% of a healthy control male sample had corpora callosa less than 600 mm^2 in area; 45% of the healthy women had corpora callosa this small. Among the patients with schizophrenia, however, 56% of the men had corpora callosa less than 600 mm^2, whereas only 33% of the women with schizophrenia did. Not only did the male schizophrenic patients differ from the male control subjects (whereas the female control subjects and patients did not differ), but there was a reversal of the normal gender relationship in schizophrenia. That is, in the healthy sample, women more often than men were characterized as having "small" corpora callosa; in schizophrenia, the opposite was found.

Reversal of sexual dimorphism was also suggested in splenial shape. It has been reported, with some controversy, that the corpus callosum splenium (the posterior 20% of the corpus callosum) is rounder or more bulbous in women than in men (see Witelson 1986 for review). Lewine and colleagues (1991) replicated this finding in an MRI study of healthy control subjects. In their schizophrenia sample, however, women had the less bulbous splenia, the reverse of their normative sample. It is interesting that when the male schizophrenia sample was divided into those with bulbous ("female") splenia and those with elongated splenia ("male"), the two groups showed significant differences in severity of schizophrenia in the direction predicted by our knowledge of gender differences in schizophrenia expression. Male schizophrenic patients with "male" splenia had a significantly higher F and Sc elevation on the Minnesota Multiphasic Personality Inventory (Hathaway and McKinley 1943) (i.e., they were more ill) than male schizophrenic patients with "female" splenia.

Functional Brain Gender Differences

Josiassen and co-workers (1990) have reported global gender differences in cerebral event-related potentials (ERPs) recorded from the human scalp, as well as significant gender-by-diagnosis interactions that reflected a reversal in the pattern of intensity distributions of ERPs between genders in healthy control subjects and schizophrenic patients. Indeed, Josiassen and co-workers concluded that "the female schizophrenic patients follow a similar pattern and in many ways resemble the male control subjects" (p. 239).

The study of brain function, as reflected in regional cerebral blood flow (rCBF), has yielded consistent gender differences, both of a general nature and specific to schizophrenia (R. E. Gur and R. C. Gur 1990). In general, women exhibit greater rCBF than do men. It is interesting that this gender difference appears to be especially marked at younger ages (younger than 20) and almost disappears in patients older than age 30. In their study, Gur and Gur found that female schizophrenic patients' cerebral blood flow, in contrast to all other groups, was almost unaffected by task manipulation. Specifically, the female schizophrenic patients exhibited very little change in cerebral blood flow from resting state to verbal task to spatial task. The other groups exhibited rather large increases in cerebral blood flow over these same conditions.

In samples of healthy individuals, glucose metabolism rates have also been reported to be higher in women than in men (Baxter et al. 1987; Daniel et al. 1988). Of particular interest to researchers studying schizophrenia are reversals of sexual dimorphism under certain conditions, as reported in the study by Daniel and others. They found that rCBF increased with femininity (as measured by Bem's Sex Role Inventory [Bem 1974]), independent of biological sex. That is, both men and women who scored high on femininity had higher cerebral blood flow than did individuals scoring low on femininity. This is reminiscent of the findings of Lewine and colleagues (1991) regarding the association between corpus callosum splenium shape and gender differences in the clinical expression of schizophrenia.

In summary, although the picture remains inconsistent, when gender differences *are* found, there is usually greater brain morphological and functional divergence from control subjects in men with schizophrenia. These anomalies appear to be lateralized to the left hemisphere. It must be remembered, however, that most studies still do not report gender analysis results (Wahl and Hunter 1992).

Hormones

One way to understand these findings is to conceptualize a psychotic process as being superimposed on a somewhat anomalous brain, more often and more extensively anomalous in men than in women. The compromised brain can be hypothesized to result from faulty prenatal neurodevelopment and, perhaps, from additional CNS perturbations before onset of symptoms. The additional changes may be preprogrammed to emerge at a specific maturational stage or may result from crucially timed biological (trauma, infection, alcohol, drugs) or psychosocial (demands, conflicts, losses) challenges. Both at the prenatal and at the pubertal levels, female hormones, specifically estrogen, may serve an overall protective function. What is the evidence?

Speculation about the possible protective effects of estrogens must begin with a discussion of the known differences between female and male brains (Pilgrim and Reisert 1992). Reproductive behaviors, masterminded through hypothalamic centers in the medial preoptic region and the ventromedial nucleus (Pfaff 1980), are known to be sexually dimorphic in all species. Gonadotropin secretion, tonic in male animals and cyclic in female animals, is thought to be controlled by the synaptic interaction between gonadotropin-releasing hormone neurons in the preoptic area of the brain and dopamine neurons in the arcuate nucleus (Kordon 1988). These sex-specific brain functions point to sexually dimorphic neural circuits—dimorphic in cell numbers and sizes of individual neurons (Bleier et al. 1982; Hammer and

Jacobson 1984), in synaptic connectivity (Perez et al. 1990), and in neuronal firing patterns (Sakuma 1984). The brain distribution of neurons mediating specific neurotransmitters and their receptors is also sexually dimorphic. This is true in monoaminergic systems (Reisert and Pilgrim 1991), cholinergic systems (Luine and McEwen 1983), and neuropeptide systems (Alexander et al. 1991). Most important to the speculations advanced in this chapter, sex differences exist in the distribution, expression, and binding properties of estrogen and androgen receptors in the brain (Brown et al. 1988; Lauber et al. 1991; Roselli 1991). Potentially relevant to schizophrenia, these sex differences exist in the limbic system of the brain: in the amygdala (Malsbury and McKay 1989), the stria terminalis (Guillamon et al. 1988), and the hippocampus (Foy et al. 1984). The striatum is characterized by sex differences in both dopaminergic and γ-aminobutyric acid (GABA)ergic neurons (Ovtscharoff et al. 1992). Sex differences in the width of the corpus callosum and in hemispheric left-right asymmetry, referred to earlier in this chapter as controversial in human beings, are evidenced to some degree in all vertebrates and even in invertebrates (Hodgkin 1991).

What is the mechanism invoked for sexual differentiation of the male and female brain? Animal experiments have demonstrated that a critical organizational period exists, which, in different species, may occur prenatally, perinatally, or early in the postnatal period (Arnold and Gorski 1984). Testosterone, secreted by the fetal testes, enters the brain and is aromatized to estrogen (Lieberburg et al. 1978) in those brain areas where the enzyme aromatase exists.

Estrogen, via its effects on neuronal gene expression and neurite growth, results in the organization of specific neural circuits. The differentiation of the female brain was once thought to be a passive phenomenon, proceeding without enhancement by estrogens. This was considered probable because of the binding of circulating estrogen by α-fetoprotein in some species, not allowing the entry of estrogen into the brain. Androgens were thus thought to be the only gonadal steroids to enter the brain, there to be aromatized to estrogens. It is now thought (Toran-Allerand 1991) that the developing brain is exposed to both testicular androgens and ovarian secretions at critical periods and that, in both sexes, these hormones promote permanent differentiation of sex differences in a broad spectrum of behaviors, including cognitive functions. In primates of both sexes, the developing cerebral cortex contains large numbers of estrogen receptor–containing cells and high levels of estrogen receptors, but only transiently, during specific perinatal periods. Estrogens stimulate dendritic growth, synaptogenesis, and myelinogenesis, and they control programmed cell death (Murakami and Arai 1989). Gonadal steroids are not thought to act alone on neural organization but rather in concert with adrenal steroids, growth factors, and neurotransmitters. Reisert and Pilgrim (1991) conducted a series of experiments in rats; the results were interpreted to show that sex-linked differentiation of neurons proceeds, to a certain extent, independently of gonadal hormones. These investigators concluded that a sex-specific genetic program may explain the generation of neuronal sex differences, and the hormonal environment plays an epigenetic role.

Sex differences in humans are thought to be based on developmental mechanisms similar, if not identical, to those in other species (Kimura 1987). The distinct critical period for sexual differentiation of the human brain is not known, although it is thought to start in the early midtrimester of gestation (Dörner 1988). This is supported by the fact that testosterone production in the human male fetus starts 8 weeks after conception and peaks at week 20 (Reinisch and Sanders 1984). Lanthier and Padwardhan (1986) have suggested that there may be more than one time window of opportunity for organizational effects and that these critical periods may be both sex specific and neural circuit specific. It is also probable that feedback loops exist so that pathways that are used are further developed, whereas those that are not used atrophy, or as Carla Shatz (1992) described it, "cells that fire together, wire together" (p. 64). With respect to male-female differences, for instance, relative parental reinforcement of male motor activity in infancy versus relative restraint of female motor activity may accentuate or even create sex-specific brain circuitry differences. This has been demonstrated in rodents (Denenberg et al. 1991).

The interaction of sex and cortical development was popularized in the clinical literature by Geschwind and Galaburda (1987). They suggested that the slower pace of development of the left hemisphere in human male fetuses contributes to sexual dimorphism and plays a role in the various sex-specific prevalence rates of immune and neurological disorders. Specifically, they theorized that fetal testosterone effectively slows the development of the left hemisphere of the brain, thus rendering it more susceptible to compromise in males than in females. This observation is consistent with the apparently greater impairment of left over right hemisphere function in schizophrenia (see Walker and McGuire 1982). Geschwind and Galaburda also noted that fetal testosterone may play a sensitizing role in the expression of certain allergic phenomena such as atopic eczema, childhood asthma, and hay fever, disorders that are more common in boys than in girls.

Because allergic and infective etiologies have been invoked for schizophrenia, it is useful at this point to review sex differences in immune function.

Immune Function

An immunoreactive theory of increased male susceptibility to a variety of neurodevelopmental disorders was proposed in 1985 by Gualtieri and Hicks. Drawing on many sources of evidence, they hypothesized that there was "something about the male fetus that evokes an untoward uterine environment" (p. 431). They further speculated that maleness, represented by the presence of the H-Y antigen, induces maternal immunoreactivity, which then leads directly or indirectly to fetal damage. This interesting theory has not gained much support.

The observed seasonal variation in schizophrenia births, perhaps more marked in males (Torrey and Torrey 1980), could reflect impaired immunity to certain common viruses that are relatively prevalent in winter and early spring. King and associates (1985) found lower antibody titers to mumps, rubella, and measles in male psychiatric patients relative to females. The investigators concluded that this might reflect impairment of immune response, which would increase vulnerability to CNS infection or allow persistence of an acquired CNS virus over a longer time. Waltrip and co-workers (1990) elegantly developed the theory of viral reactivation as a possible cause of schizophrenia. Specifically, they postulated an abnormality of α-interferon, a cytokine mediator. They used the decrease in the inducibility of α-interferon production in females relative to males to support their theory.

Three relatively recent reviews (Grossman 1989; Sarvetnick and Fox 1990; Schuurs and Verheul 1990) record the many immune system differences between men and women:

Both humoral and cell-mediated immune responses are more active in women than in men. The mechanisms are, for the most part, unknown. Presumably, the immune responses arose to protect fetuses from external infection through effective immunological surveillance. The price that women pay for this relative protection from infective agents is their greater susceptibility to autoimmune disease—that is, overeffective immune surveillance. The system must be hormone responsive in some way to protect the fetus from being rejected as foreign tissue. The direct effects of raised levels of estrogens and progestins during pregnancy on lymphocyte activity have been well documented. Hormone-immune interactions function through steroid hormone receptors for estrogens, androgens, and progestins. These receptors are present in the thymus, spleen, and various classes of lymphocytes. Steroid-mediated events may be involved in lymphocytic development. It has been proposed that the greater immunostimulation present in females than in males results in part from the pattern of growth hormone (GH) release. The female pattern (induced by estrogens and progestins) is an elevated basal GH secretion accompanied by reduced pulsatile GH release. This pattern is reversed in males. Peak and trough levels of GH are known to influence other somatic mechanisms and may well help to create the sexual dimorphism that exists in the immune response.

Prolactin has also been shown to influence immune function in the expected direction. Estrogen stimulates prolactin secretion (as do neuroleptics) by downregulating the number of dopamine receptors in the anterior pituitary. Estrogen also regulates prolactin gene transcription (as it does for many other gene products; see Chapter 3). The sexual dimorphism in immune response predates puberty but becomes much more pronounced at that time.

There is no compelling evidence that antigen-antibody response has any bearing on the development of schizophrenia, but theories of neuronal disarray (Beckmann et al. 1987; Conrad and Scheibel 1987; Feinberg 1983; Gattaz et al. 1987; Haracz 1985; Weinberger 1987) can be accommodated both by known data about the effects of estrogen on synaptogenesis and by data on the enhancing effects of estrogen on the immune response and thus on protection from infective agents during pregnancy and the early postnatal period (see, however, Susser and Lin 1992; Takei et al. 1993, 1994).

Postpubertal Effects of Estrogens

Activational protective effects—that is, the antidopaminergic (or neuroleptic-like) action of estrogens postpuberty—are better known than estrogenic neurodevelopmental effects (Häfner et al. 1991a, 1991b; Seeman 1981, 1983). Premenstrual, postpartum, and postmenopausal exacerbations of schizophrenia, as well as the relative freedom from schizophrenic relapse experienced during pregnancy, are consistent with a protective effect of estrogens (Seeman and Lang 1990). Also consistent are the relatively late onset of schizophrenia in women and the second incidence peak at the time of menopause, a phenomenon that does not occur in men. In a study of 470,000 women experiencing psychiatric admission over a 12-year period, Kendell and colleagues (1987) reported a 3.4% increased risk of schizophrenia during the 90 days after childbirth. This, too, is consistent with increased risk as a result of the precipitous decline in estrogen levels.

Early reports linking exacerbation of psychosis to the premenstrual (low-estrogen) phase of the menstrual cycle had intimated a relationship between hormones and symptom intensity. Luggin and co-workers (1984) reported a statistically significant increase in psychiatric admissions during the menstrual period (also a low-estrogen phase) in 121 young women. No difference between psychotic and nonpsychotic women was found, suggesting a general phenomenon. Brockington and others (1988) and Gerada and Reveley (1988) provided more recent cases of premenstrual psychotic relapse. Lovestone (1992) described premenstrual psychosis associated with increased blink rate, a dopamine-mediated phenomenon.

Hallonquist and co-investigators (1993) followed five regularly menstruating women with a DSM-III-R diagnosis of schizophrenia through 2 consecutive menstrual cycles, obtaining daily symptom self-reports using the McNeil et al. (1989) Brief Symptom Checklist. They compared the symptom mean for 4 high-estrogen (midcycle) days with the mean of 4 low-estrogen days. They deliberately avoided the premenstrual and menstrual period and used the 4 days after menses as their low-estrogen phase. This was in order to disassociate it from the late luteal phase with its probable expectancy in the subjects' minds of increased psychopathology. Thus, subjects knew that the relationship between menstrual phase and symptom severity was being investigated, but they were blind to the specific time periods that were being scrutinized. All subjects were being treated with neuroleptic drugs. This dampened the symptomatology and might have dampened the amplitude of estrogen fluctuations, because neuroleptics are known to increase prolactin levels and to decrease estrogen secretion. The subjects had 2 consecutive, regular (less than 35 days) menstrual cycles and, thus, were assumed to be ovulating. They were outpatients and had only moderate levels of actively psychotic symptomatology. This meant they were in a stable phase of illness and were not progressively improving over the 2 months of the study, as an acutely ill sample might have done. Results supported the hypothesis. Mean global symptom severity (psychotic and nonpsychotic) was significantly higher in the low-estrogen phase than in the high-estrogen phase. The results were from the 10 cycles in the five women. Little can be concluded from the small sample size, although the investigators did attempt to obviate several sources of potential bias (e.g., subject attribution, confound with late luteal phase syndrome, progressive treatment effects).

Additional evidence for the estrogen protection hypothesis is that doses of antipsychotics prescribed to prevent relapses in women were lower than those prescribed to men (Seeman 1983, 1989b).

Androgens

There is no literature on the possible schizophrenia-enhancing role of androgens. From a brain organizational viewpoint, the neurodevelopmental disarray found in fetal development could be attributed to the effects of androgens that are aromatized to estrogens but act at receptors distributed differently in boys than in girls. Furthermore, interactions with the immune system may predispose boys to certain allergic phenomena, as hypothesized by Geschwind and Galaburda (1987), which may contribute to a viral influence on neurodevelopment (Scheibel and Conrad 1993).

At the activational level, androgens may exacerbate a dysfunction in axonal pruning that is thought to occur in schizophrenia (Lewine 1992). Axonal pruning is the process by which the excess interneuronal connections established during early neural development are reduced to adult numbers. Pruning occurs in association with general biological maturation. Puberty is hypothesized to "shut off" pruning. Saugstaad (1990) followed this line of reasoning in speculating that excessive pruning takes place when biological maturation is late, as in schizophrenia, whereas inadequate pruning occurs when maturation is early (e.g., in affective disorder).

Consequently, men, who mature more slowly than women (i.e., they have a later onset of puberty), would be exposed to more pruning and, therefore, less connectivity or axonal density. Saugstaad's view would thus predict a higher rate of schizophrenia among men, which is precisely the finding reported by Iacono and Beiser (1992). Consistent with this view, excessive pruning, resulting in greater than normal axon loss, has been found (in computer simulations) to result in cognitive loosening (Hoffman and Dobscha 1989).

In addition, androgens predispose to motor activity, impulsivity, and risk taking, which may provoke a series of biological or psychosocial sequelae that decrease the age at onset for schizophrenia and contribute to the relative severity of its course in men.

Critique

Provocative new findings on the specific effect of second trimester maternal influenza and malnutrition on the induction of schizophrenia in daughters (Susser and Lin 1992; Takei et al. 1993, 1994) call into question the protective role of female hormones and immune factors in neurodevelopment.

Contrary to expectation, second trimester environmental events appear to affect female fetuses more than male fetuses. Only if these events are lethal to male fetuses or newborns can these findings be brought in line with the evidence addressed in this chapter.

The study of the role of hormones in schizophrenia has been, and will continue to be, quite difficult. Antipsychotic medications affect the hypothalamic-pituitary-gonadal axis and interfere with the menstrual cycle, often resulting in amenorrhea. As yet, no estrogen studies have been done in women with schizophrenia who are not taking neuroleptic drugs, let alone who have never taken neuroleptic drugs; therefore, we are constrained in our interpretation of the existing data. Precise monitoring of the menstrual cycle is difficult, often placing considerable demands and responsibility on the individual women to help in the monitoring, for example, by taking basal temperatures before getting out of bed in the morning or by keeping detailed diaries. These tasks would be particularly difficult for the woman with schizophrenia. When the menstrual cycle is not affected by medication, water retention and consequent weight increase premenstrually may be sufficient in some women to cause dilution of medication concentrations, making studies of gender differences in medication dose and efficacy problematic (Yonkers et al. 1992). Finally, as is true for much of the gender differences database, sample sizes are often small, and studies are frequently conducted in the absence of specific gender hypotheses.

In summary, provocative findings are consistent with an important role for hormones in schizophrenia. The complex interactions among hormones, immune factors, medications, and biopsychosocial gender differences demand careful, highly focused research.

Theoretical Implications

Brain morphological and hormonal gender differences raise four broad theoretical questions with respect to schizophrenia.

1. *How do we best conceptualize schizophrenia as defined, in part, by gender differences?* One view is to return to Kraepelin's original notion of dementia praecox as an early-onset, male disorder. Castle and Murray (1991) have articulated this position in suggesting that "schizophrenia" is really two different disorders: 1) an early-onset neurodevelopmental disorder of men, and 2) a late-onset affective disorder of women.

   Another view is that schizophrenia is fundamentally the same disorder in men and women but that men's greater susceptibility to brain insult leads to an earlier triggering of schizophrenia in men than in women (Lewine 1981).

2. *Are men and women at equal genetic risk for schizophrenia?* The accepted answer, until recently, has been "yes." Within the last 5 years, however, a reevaluation of gender differences in genetic theory has taken place in two areas. Goldstein and her colleagues have reanalyzed the Iowa 500 data specifically to assess gender differences; they report that women are at significantly higher genetic risk for schizophrenia than men (see Chapter 9).

Even more controversial is Crow's X-linked pseudoautosomal hypothesis, which is based on the demonstration of asymmetric morphological anomalies, particularly those of the left temporal lobe, in schizophrenia. Crow and colleagues (1989a) reason that if schizophrenia is an anomaly of cerebral asymmetry (especially of the left "cognitive" hemisphere), then the genetic mechanism underlying it should also be related to the development of cerebral asymmetries. They propose Annett's "right shift factor" or the cerebral dominance gene as the locus of schizophrenia, which they furthermore assert may be transmitted in a Mendelian fashion. Pointing to data suggesting greater sibling concordance for schizophrenia by sex, Crow and colleagues hypothesize that the genetic factor for cerebral asymmetry may be located in the pseudoautosomal region of the sex chromosomes because pseudoautosomal transmission is characterized by sex concordance of siblings when the disease is paternally transmitted. Primarily of heuristic value, this hypothesis seems improbable at this stage, largely because the empirical bases for the primary assumptions of asymmetry of morphological abnormality and sibling concordance of illness by sex are so meager. Other genetic mechanisms that may underlie gender differences are discussed in Chapter 3.

3. *Is schizophrenia a progressive disorder characterized by brain atrophy, or is it a neurodevelopmental anomaly best characterized by dysplasia?* Early efforts to document the progressive deterioration presumed to underlie schizophrenia have yielded to a neurodevelopmental model (see Lewine 1992). Longitudinal studies of brain morphology reveal surprisingly little morphological deterioration in individuals with schizophrenia, despite often considerable clinical and behavioral deterioration. Although the deterioration model may not apply to schizophrenia in general,

a review of gender differences suggests it may be applicable to a small subgroup of men with schizophrenia.

A considerably more controversial hypothesis is the possibility that brain structures or functions may exhibit sexual dimorphisms that are linked to gender-related behaviors, independent of biological sex (Daniel et al. 1988; Lewine et al. 1990). Thus, although higher cerebral blood flow may be linked to gender, the relationship may be mediated by femininity, independent of biological sex (Daniel et al. 1988). Likewise, Lewine and colleagues found that the "female" corpus callosum, regardless of the sex it occurred in, was associated with a clinical symptom picture more typical of schizophrenia in women than in men. These studies point to potentially complex relationships between brain and psychopathology mediated by "psychological gender." The prepotency of "brain gender" over gender-relevant behavior is manifestly true for nonhuman species. In humans, however, one can never overestimate the role of learning and experience and the feedback that is subsequently exerted on neural circuitry (see Shatz 1992).

4. *What does the study of gender differences tell us about the etiology of schizophrenia?* To date, we must conclude that there are very few, if any, gender differences in schizophrenia that are not also true in general for men versus women. On the other hand, if these differences exist in men and women regardless of illness, why is the sex distribution of schizophrenia so different from that of other psychiatric disorders?

In contrast to the etiological puzzle, factors that affect the course—onset, duration, and response to treatment—seem more ready to yield to gender-related explanations, as detailed in this chapter. At any rate, we must remind ourselves that no explanation is likely to apply to all of the schizophrenias.

Caveats

As reiterated by Wahl and Hunter (1992), gender differences in the study of schizophrenia continue to be considered only sporadically, despite considerable growing interest in the field. Often it is impossible to determine whether gender effects were analyzed, found to be negligible, and hence not reported, or whether they were not examined at all. Understanding of gender differences will continue to be constrained, therefore, until this issue receives more widespread attention.

Even when gender effects are examined, patient sampling continues to be problematic (Hambrecht et al. 1992). Some of the discrepant gender difference findings may be attributable to sampling characteristics, such as inpatient versus outpatient treatment, acute versus chronic illness, and public versus private institutions, and whether patients (usually men) are participating in a concurrent medication study. Walker and Lewine (1993), for example, have suggested that the particular nature of the patient population from which schizophrenic patients are sampled may have an important impact on the severity of illness by gender. Specifically, samples derived from more severely ill, committed inpatients may overrepresent severely ill women, whereas outpatient samples may overrepresent severely ill men (Lewine et al. 1981).

Furthermore, the database from which we make gender difference inferences is almost exclusively cross-sectional. Neurodevelopmental processes must ultimately be addressed with longitudinal studies. Finally, small sample sizes and medication effects will continue to hamper our efforts, especially in the study of hormones. Despite the obstacles, however, the investigation of schizophrenia gender differences promises to yield valuable information about brain-behavior relationships across the spectrum of normal and abnormal behavior.

In the end, we may learn little about schizophrenia per se but, rather, a considerable amount about neurodevelopmental gender differences and behavioral organization. Brain morphology and hormones are not independent. Gonadal hormones have considerable impact on neural organization, and our understanding of morphological differences may lead ultimately to elucidation of hormonal mechanisms (Geschwind and Galaburda 1987). In any event, we are well beyond the stage of descriptive summaries (Lewine 1981) and must now turn our attention to reasoned theories, informed by a general knowledge of brain and behavior development in women and men.

References

Alexander MJ, Kiraly ZJ, Leeman SE: Sexually dimorphic distribution of neurotensin/neuromedin N mRNS in the rat preoptic area. J Comp Neurol 311:84–96, 1991

Andreasen N, Swayze V, Flaum M: Ventricular enlargement in schizophrenia evaluated with computed tomographic scanning. Arch Gen Psychiatry 47:1008–1015, 1990

Arnold AP, Gorski A: Gonadal steroid induction of structural sex differences in the central nervous system. Annu Rev Neurosci 7:413–442, 1984

Baxter L, Mazziotta J, Phelps M, et al: Cerebral glucose metabolic rates in normal human females versus normal males. Psychiatry Res 21:237–245, 1987

Beckmann H, Gattaz WF, Jakob H: Biochemical and neuropathological indices for the aetiology of schizophrenia, in Search for the Causes of Schizophrenia. Edited by Häfner H, Gattaz WF, Janzarik W. New York, Springer-Verlag, 1987, pp 241–249

Bem SL: The measurement of psychological androgeny. J Consult Clin Psychol 42:155–162, 1974

Bleier R, Byne W, Siggelkow I: Cytoarchitectonic sexual dimorphisms of the medial preoptic and anterior hypothalamic areas in guinea pig, rat, hamster, and mouse. J Comp Neurol 212:118–130, 1982

Bogerts B, Ashtari M, Degreef G, et al: Reduced temporal limbic structure volumes on magnetic resonance images in first episode schizophrenia. Psychiatry Res Neuroimaging 35:1–13, 1990

Brockington IF, Kelly A, Hall P, et al: Premenstrual relapse of puerperal psychosis. J Affect Disord 14:287–292, 1988

Brown TJ, Hochberg RB, Zielinski JE, et al: Regional sex differences in cell nuclear estrogen-binding capacity in the rat hypothalamus and preoptic area. Endocrinology 123:1761–1770, 1988

Cannon TD, Mednick SA, Parnas J: Genetic and perinatal determinants of structural brain deficits in schizophrenia. Arch Gen Psychiatry 46:883–889, 1989

Castle D, Murray R: The neurodevelopmental basis of sex differences in schizophrenia (editorial). Psychol Med 21:565–575, 1991

Conrad AJ, Scheibel AB: Schizophrenia and the hippocampus: the embryological hypothesis extended. Schizophr Bull 13:577–587, 1987

Crow TJ: The continuum of psychosis and its genetic origins. Br J Psychiatry 156:788–797, 1990a

Crow TJ: Nature of the genetic contribution to psychotic illness—a continuum viewpoint. Acta Psychiatr Scand 81:401–408, 1990b

Crow T, Ball J, Bloom S, et al: Schizophrenia as an anomaly of development of cerebral asymmetry: a postmortem study and a proposal concerning the genetic basis of the disease. Arch Gen Psychiatry 46:1145–1150, 1989a

Crow T, Colter N, Frith C, et al: Developmental arrest of cerebral asymmetries in early onset schizophrenia. Psychiatry Res 29:247–253, 1989b

Daniel D, Mathew R, Wilson W: Sex roles and regional cerebral blood flow. Psychiatry Res 27:55–64, 1988

Degreef G, Ashtari M, Bogerts B, et al: Volumes of ventricular system subdivisions measured from magnetic resonance images in first episode schizophrenic patients. Arch Gen Psychiatry 49:531–537, 1992

DeLisi L, Hoff A, Schwartz J, et al: Brain morphology in first-episode schizophrenic-like psychotic patients: a quantitative magnetic resonance imaging study. Biol Psychiatry 29:159–175, 1991

Denenberg VH, Fitch RH, Schrott LM, et al: Corpus callosum: interactive effects of testosterone and handling in the rat. Behav Neurosci 105:562–566, 1991

Dörner G: Sexual endocrinology and terminology in sexology. Exp Clin Endocrinol 91:129–134, 1988

Feinberg I: Schizophrenia: caused by a fault in programmed synaptic elimination during adolescence? J Psychiatr Res 17:319–334, 1983

Flaum M, Arndt S, Andreasen N: The role of gender in studies of ventricle enlargement in schizophrenia: a predominantly male effect. Am J Psychiatry 147:1327–1332, 1990

Foy MR, Chiaia NL, Teyler TJ: Reversal of hippocampal sexual dimorphism by gonadal steroid manipulation. Brain Res 321:311–314, 1984

Gattaz WF, Kohlmeyer K, Gasser T: Structural brain abnormalities in schizophrenia, in Search for the Causes of Schizophrenia. Edited by Häfner H, Gattaz WF, Janzarik W. New York, Springer-Verlag, 1987, pp 250–259

Gerada C, Reveley A: Schizophreniform psychosis recurring in association with the menstrual cycle. Br J Psychiatry 152:700–702, 1988

Geschwind N, Galaburda A: Cerebral Lateralization: Biological Mechanisms, Associations and Pathology. Cambridge, MA, MIT Press, 1987

Grossman C: Possible underlying mechanisms of sexual dimorphisms in the immune response, fact and hypothesis. J Steroid Biochem Mol Biol 34:241–251, 1989

Gualtieri T, Hicks RE: An immunoreactive theory of selective male affliction. Behavioral and Brain Sciences 8:427–441, 1985

Guillamon A, Segovia S, del Abril A: Early effects of gonadal steroids on the neuron number in the medial posterior region and the lateral division of the bed nucleus of the stria terminalis in the rat. Brain Res Dev Brain Res 44:281–290, 1988

Gur RC, Mozley PD, Resnick SM, et al: Gender differences in age effect on brain atrophy measured by magnetic resonance imaging. Proc Natl Acad Sci U S A 88:2845–2849, 1991

Gur RE, Gur RC: Gender differences in regional cerebral blood flow. Schizophr Bull 16:247–254, 1990

Gur RE, Mozley PD, Shtasel DL, et al: Clinical subtypes of schizophrenia: differences in brain and CSF volume. Am J Psychiatry 151:343–350, 1994

Häfner H, Behrens S, De Vry J, et al: An animal model for the effects of estradiol on dopamine-mediated behavior: implications for sex differences in schizophrenia. Psychiatry Res 38:125–134, 1991a

Häfner H, Behrens S, De Vry J, et al: Oestradiol enhances the vulnerability threshold for schizophrenia in women by an early effect on dopaminergic neurotransmission. Eur Arch Psychiatry Clin Neurosci 241:65–68, 1991b

Hallonquist JD, Seeman MV, Lang M, et al: Variation in symptom severity over the menstrual cycle in schizophrenics. Biol Psychiatry 33:207–209, 1993

Hambrecht M, Maurer K, Häfner H: Evidence for a gender bias in epidemiological studies of schizophrenia. Schizophr Res 8:223–231, 1992

Hammer RP Jr, Jacobson CD: Sex difference in dendritic development of the sexually dimorphic nucleus of the preoptic area in the rat. Int J Dev Neurosci 2:77–85, 1984

Haracz JL: Neural plasticity in schizophrenia. Schizophr Bull 11:191–229, 1985

Hathaway SR, McKinley JC: Minnesota Multiphasic Personality Inventory. Minneapolis, University of Minnesota, 1943

Hodgkin J: Sex determination and the generation of sexually dimorphic nervous system. Neuron 6:177–185, 1991

Hoffman R, Dobscha S: Cortical pruning and the development of schizophrenia: a computer model. Schizophr Bull 15:477–489, 1989

Iacono W, Beiser M: Are males more likely than females to develop schizophrenia? Am J Psychiatry 149:1070–1074, 1992

Josiassen R, Roemer R, Johnson M, et al: Are gender differences in schizophrenia reflected in brain event-related potentials? Schizophr Bull 16:229–246, 1990

Kendell RE, Chalmers JC, Platz C: Epidemiology of puerperal psychoses. Br J Psychiatry 150:662–673, 1987

Kimura D: Are men's and women's brains really different? Can J Psychol 28:133–147, 1987

King DJ, Cooper SJ, Earle JAP, et al: A survey of serum antibodies to eight common viruses in psychiatric patients. Br J Psychiatry 147:137–144, 1985

Kordon C: Hypothalamic-hypophyseal mechanisms involved in the regulation of hormones and behaviour, in New Concepts in Depression. Edited by Briley M, Fillion G. Basingstoke, England, Macmillan, 1988, pp 235–246

Lanthier A, Padwardhan VV: Sex steroids and 5-en-3B-hydroxysteroids in specific regions of the human brain and cranial nerves. J Steroid Biochem Mol Biol 25:445–449, 1986

Lauber AH, Mobbs CV, Muramatsu M, et al: Estrogen receptor messenger RNA expression in rat hypothalamus as a function of genetic sex and estrogen dose. Endocrinology 129:3180–3186, 1991

Lewine RJ: Sex differences in schizophrenia: timing or subtypes. Psychol Bull 30:432–444, 1981

Lewine RJ: Brain morphology in schizophrenia. Current Opinion in Psychiatry 5:92–97, 1992

Lewine RJ, Watt N, Grubb T: High-risk-for-schizophrenia: sampling bias and its implications. Schizophr Bull 7:273–280, 1981

Lewine RJ, Gulley LR, Risch SC, et al: Sexual dimorphism, brain morphology, and schizophrenia. Schizophr Bull 16:193–203, 1990

Lewine RJ, Flashman L, Gulley L, et al: Sexual dimorphism in corpus callosum and schizophrenia. Schizophr Res 4:63–64, 1991

Lewine RJ, Hudgins P, Brown F, et al: Gender differences in qualitative brain morphology findings in schizophrenia, major depression, bipolar disorder and normal volunteers. Schizophr Res (in press)

Lieberburg I, MacLusky NJ, Roy EJ, et al: Sex steroid receptors in the perinatal rat brain. American Zoologist 18:539–544, 1978

Lieberman J, Bogerts B, Degreef G, et al: Qualitative assessment of brain morphology in acute and chronic schizophrenia. Am J Psychiatry 149:784–794, 1992

Lovestone S: Periodic psychosis associated with the menstrual cycle and increased blink rate. Br J Psychiatry 161:402–404, 1992

Luggin R, Bernsted L, Petersson B, et al: Acute psychiatric admission-related to the menstrual cycle. Acta Psychiatr Scand 69:461–465, 1984

Luine VN, McEwen BS: Sex differences in cholinergic enzymes of diagonal band nuclei in the rat preoptic area. Neuroendocrinology 36:475–482, 1983

Malsbury CW, McKay K: Sex difference in the substance P-immunoreactive innervation of the medial nucleus of the amygdala. Brain Res Bull 23:561–567, 1989

McNeil DE, Greenfield TK, Attkisson CC, et al: Factor structure of a brief symptom checklist for acute psychiatric inpatients. J Clin Psychol 45:66–72, 1989

Murakami S, Arai Y: Neuronal death in the developing sexually dimorphic periventricular nucleus of the preoptic area in the female rat: effect of neonatal androgen treatment. Neurosci Lett 102:185–190, 1989

Nasrallah H, Schwarzkopf B, Olson S, et al: Gender differences in schizophrenia on MRI brain scans. Schizophr Bull 16:205–210, 1990

O'Callaghan E, Redmond O, Ennis J, et al: Abnormalities of cerebral structure in schizophrenia on magnetic resonance imaging: interpretation in relation to the neurodevelopmental hypothesis. J R Soc Med 85:227–231, 1992

Ovtscharoff W, Reisert I, Pilgrim C: Sexual dimorphisms of dopaminergic input and GABAergic targets in the developing rat striatum (abstract). Anat Anz 174 (suppl):18, 1992

Perez J, Naftolin F, Carcia-Segura LM: Sexual differentiation of synaptic connectivity and neuronal plasma membrane in the arcuate nucleus of the rat hypothalamus. Brain Res 527:116–122, 1990

Pfaff DW: Estrogens and Brain Function: Neural Analysis of a Hormone-Controlled Mammalian Reproductive Behavior. New York, Springer-Verlag, 1980

Pilgrim C, Reisert I: Differences between male and female brains—developmental mechanisms and implications. Horm Metab Res 24:353–359, 1992

Raz S, Raz N: Structural brain abnormalities in the major psychoses: a quantitative review of the evidence from computerized imaging. Psychol Bull 108:93–108, 1990

Reinisch JM, Sanders SA: Prenatal gonadal steroidal influences on gender-related behavior. Prog Brain Res 61:407–416, 1984

Reisert I, Pilgrim C: Sexual differentiation of monoaminergic neurons—genetic and epigenetic? Trends Neurosci 14:468–472, 1991

Roselli CE: Sex differences in androgen receptors and aromatase activity in microdissected regions of the rat brain. Endocrinology 128:1310–1316, 1991

Sakuma Y: Influences of neonatal gonadectomy or androgen exposure on the sexual differentiation of the rat ventromedial hypothalamus. J Physiol (Lond) 349:273–286, 1984

Sarvetnick N, Fox HS: Interferon-gamma and the sexual dimorphism of autoimmunity. Molecular Biological Medicine 7:323–331, 1990

Saugstaad L: Social class, marriage and fertility in schizophrenia: the author replies. Schizophr Bull 16:175–178, 1990

Scheibel AB, Conrad AS: Hippocampal dysgenesis in mutant mouse and schizophrenic man: is there a relationship? Schizophr Bull 19:21–33, 1993

Schuurs AHWM, Verheul HAM: Effects of gender and sex steroids on the immune response. J Steroid Biochem Mol Biol 35:157–172, 1990

Seeman MV: Gender and the onset of schizophrenia: neurohumoral influences. Psychiatric Journal of the University of Ottawa 6:136–138, 1981

Seeman MV: Interaction of sex, age, and neuroleptic dose. Compr Psychiatry 24:125–128, 1983

Seeman MV: Prenatal gonadal steroids and schizophrenia. Psychiatric Journal of the University of Ottawa 14:473–475, 1989a

Seeman MV: Prescribing neuroleptics for men and women. Journal of Social Pharmacology 3:219–236, 1989b

Seeman MV, Lang M: The role of estrogens in schizophrenia gender differences. Schizophr Bull 16:185–194, 1990

Shatz CJ: The developing brain. Sci Am 267:60–67, 1992

Shenton M, Kikinis R, Jolesz F, et al: Abnormalities of the left temporal lobe and thought disorder in schizophrenia. N Engl J Med 327:604–612, 1992

Susser E, Lin S: Schizophrenia after prenatal exposure to the Dutch hunter winter of 1944–1945. Arch Gen Psychiatry 49:983–988, 1992

Takei N, O'Callaghan E, Sham PC, et al: Does prenatal influenza divert susceptible females from later affective psychosis to schizophrenia? Acta Psychiatr Scand 88:328–336, 1993

Takei N, Sham PC, O'Callaghan E, et al: Prenatal exposure to influenza and the development of schizophrenia: is the effect confined to females? Am J Psychiatry 151:117–119, 1994

Toran-Allerand CD: Organotypic culture of the developing cerebral cortex and hypothalamus: relevance to sexual differentiation. Psychoneuroendocrinology 16:7–24, 1991

Torrey EF, Torrey BB: Sex differences in the seasonality of schizophrenic births. Br J Psychiatry 137:101–104, 1980

Wahl O, Hunter J: Are gender effects being neglected in schizophrenia research? Schizophr Bull 18:313–318, 1992

Walker EF, Lewine RJ: Sampling biases in studies of gender and schizophrenia. Schizophr Bull 19:1–14, 1993

Walker E, McGuire M: Intra- and interhemispheric information processing in schizophrenia. Psychol Bull 92:701–715, 1982

Waltrip RW II, Carrigan DR, Carpenter WT: Immunopathology and viral reactivation: a general theory of schizophrenia. J Nerv Ment Dis 178:729–738, 1990

Weinberger DR: Implications of normal brain development for the pathogenesis of schizophrenia. Arch Gen Psychiatry 44:660–669, 1987

Witelson S: Wires of the mind: anatomical variation in the corpus callosum in relation to hemispheric specialization and integration, in Two Hemispheres–One Brain: Function of the Corpus Callosum. Edited by Lepore F, Ptito M, Jasper M. New York, Alan R Liss, 1986, pp 117–138

Yonkers K, Kando J, Cole J, et al: Gender differences in pharmacokinetics and pharmacodynamics of psychotropic medication. Am J Psychiatry 149:587–595, 1992

CHAPTER 8

The Impact of Gender on Understanding the Epidemiology of Schizophrenia

Jill M. Goldstein, Ph.D.

K raepelin first described dementia praecox as a disorder of early onset and downward course, a disorder that featured neurological abnormalities, physical anomalies, and deterioration of the intellect. He observed that men were three times more likely than women to show these particular features (Kraepelin 1893). Despite Kraepelin's work, very little research had *specifically* focused on identifying the role of gender in the etiology and course of schizophrenia until the last 10 years. Gender had seemed relatively unimportant to researchers because it did not impact on what had always been considered an equal incidence and prevalence of schizophrenia among women and men, an assumption that is being challenged by recent work. Also being investigated are differences in onset age, in

Preparation of this chapter was supported in part by a National Institute of Mental Health Scientist Development Award MH00976. The author wishes to thank Julie Goodman, M.A., for her help in tabling the incidence and prevalence studies.

premorbid history, in expression of illness, and in its course.

In this chapter, I question whether gender influences the distribution of schizophrenia in a given population and, if so, how this helps in understanding the nature of the disorder. Methodological issues are a primary concern because I believe that discrepancies across studies are frequently a result of differences in methodology.

Age at Onset

Because there have been two recent exhaustive reviews on gender differences in age at onset of schizophrenia (Angermeyer and Kuhn 1988; Lewine 1988), I only refer here to the more recent work (Goldstein et al. 1989; Häfner et al. 1989) and discuss possible explanations of the findings. The consensus is that men have an earlier onset age, which is not merely an artifact of admission practices. It has been found to be specific to schizophrenia (Angermeyer and Kuhn 1988).

It is unknown whether the age at onset discrepancy is confined to a particular time or place. In a substantial review of the literature, it has been reported that the magnitude of the difference in age at first *admission* varies according to geographic region (Angermeyer and Kuhn 1988). The World Health Organization's (WHO) cross-cultural study of first-episode patients with schizophrenia reported that women with schizophrenia had a higher mean age at onset than men in both developing and developed countries (Hambrecht et al. 1992). The difference was smaller in developing countries because very few onsets occurred after age 40 years, presumably a result of earlier mortality in developing countries (Hambrecht et al. 1992).

Differences in age at first admission, as distinct from age at onset, may be caused by cultural differences in the elapsed time before parents bring children into treatment. This may differ depending on sex role (Angermeyer and Kuhn 1988; Lewine 1981). To illustrate this phenomenon, a study demonstrated that the risk of a hospital admission after a first episode was similar in unmarried men and women but differed for married people (Häfner et al. 1989). However, when age at true onset is examined, studies consistently show a significant gender difference, similar across cultures (Sartorius et al. 1986).

The peak period of onset for men is age 18–25 years and for women is age 25 years to mid-30s (Angermeyer et al. 1989; Goldstein et al. 1989; Häfner et al. 1989). The actual size of the age difference depends on the strictness of the criteria for defining a case (Angermeyer and Kuhn 1988; Häfner et al. 1989). In early adolescence, the onset ratio of men to women is generally 2:1; at age 50 and older, two new female cases are admitted for every male (Goldstein et al. 1989; Häfner et al. 1989). Approximately 3%–10% of women have an age at onset greater than 45 years versus few, if any, male cases (Angermeyer et al. 1989; Goldstein et al. 1989; Häfner et al. 1989).

Sampling Bias in
Age at Onset Studies

The age at onset in patients is biased by the underlying age distribution of the population studied (W. J. Chen et al. 1992; Heimbuch et al. 1980). If men and women in a given population have different age distributions, observed gender differences in age at onset of a specific illness may be a reflection of that difference. Because women in the general population tend to live longer than men, they are more likely to have a later age at onset. Specific gender differences in mortality among patients with schizophrenia may exacerbate the problem (W. J. Chen et al. 1993; Goldstein et al. 1992).

A recent study by Faraone and colleagues (1994) reexamined gender differences in age at onset by applying methods of statistical correction. The study used retrospective cohorts—the Iowa 500 and non-500 (Morrison et al. 1972; Tsuang and Winokur 1975). Of 332 patients with a DSM-III (American Psychiatric Association 1980) diagnosis of schizophrenia, 319 had reliable age at onset information. They were approximately equally divided by sex. The DSM-III criterion limiting age at onset to 45 years was not adhered to in this study. To correct the observed age at onset distributions, a nonparametric method proposed by Baron and colleagues (1983) was used, in addition to modifications adjusting for increased mortality after onset. The observed age at onset distribution of schizophrenia was found to be biased toward younger ages. The observed ages at onset were greater than 35 years for 5.6% of the men and 18.5% of the women, which, after correction, increased to 11.8% and 30.1%, respectively. This distribution was replicated in simulation studies (W. J. Chen et al. 1993). The study also showed that the gender difference in age at onset was real. In other words, women with schizophrenia still had a significantly higher mean age at onset, controlling both for the age composition of the population of origin and for the differential excess mortality among men and women with schizophrenia (Faraone et al. 1994).

Explanations

Numerous post-hoc explanations exist for the gender differences in age at onset. Explanatory perspectives range from biology to social role–social stress (Angermeyer and Kuhn 1988; Castle and Murray 1991; Seeman 1982). Because of estrogen's antidopaminergic effect, it has been suggested that estrogens may play a protective role for women with schizophrenia and prolong their premorbid period (Häfner et al. 1991; Lewine 1981; Seeman 1981, 1982; Seeman and Lang 1990). It has also been suggested that late adolescence may be a more socially demanding developmental period for boys than for girls because of social expectations for them to be working independently and actively courting girls (Al-Issa 1982; Angermeyer and Kuhn 1988; Bleuler 1978; Lewine 1981; Seeman 1982).

In an elegant study testing the hypothesis that estrogens may explain the age at onset differences between men and women, Häfner and co-workers (1991) studied the effects of estrogen implants on behavior induced by a dopamine (DA) agonist and a DA antagonist in ovariectomized neonatal and adult rats. They concluded that estrogen exposure caused a downward regulation of D_2 receptor numbers, which was most noticeable in the youngest brains. The experimental laboratory animal data seemed to confirm the clinically derived explanations for the later age at onset in women with schizophrenia.

An alternative hypothesis is that androgens trigger earlier onset in adolescent males (Lewine 1981, 1988). Finally, it has been suggested that gender differences in age at onset may be related to gender differences in the familial risk for schizophrenia (Goldstein et al. 1992; Pulver et al. 1992; see Chapter 9).

Premorbid History

Because women, on average, have a later age at onset, they can, on average, be expected to function better premorbidly. This has been consistently demonstrated across time periods (Farina et al. 1962; Gittelman-Klein and Klein 1969; Salokangas 1983). Not only were women with schizophrenia more often married (Ciompi 1980; Salokangas 1983), but they also tended to have had better early childhood histories, in terms of school achievement and sociability (Gittelman-Klein and Klein 1969). Studies of children at high risk for schizophrenia have consistently suggested that males are at higher risk than females for early neurobehavioral deficits that lead to poor premorbid functioning. In addition, male children with schizophrenia have been found to have more physical anomalies (Green et al. 1989; Waddington et al. 1990) and to have been exposed to more obstetric complications than girls with schizophrenia (Foerster et al. 1991a; Lewis and Murray 1987). Thus, it has been proposed that males are at higher risk for a neurodevelopmental form of schizophrenia (Castle and Murray 1991; Castle et al. 1993; Goldstein et al. 1990; Murray et al. 1992).

Recent work reporting gender differences in premorbid functioning examined the specificity of the effect for schizophrenia compared with affective psychoses (Foerster et al. 1991a, 1991b). The sample included a series of consecutive admissions over a 1-year period to a psychiatric ward in a general hospital and a psychiatric hospital in London. All subjects met DSM-III criteria for schizophrenia or affective disorders with psychotic features ($n = 73$). Mothers were interviewed blindly to better evaluate the patients' premorbid schizoid and schizotypal characteristics and premorbid social functioning. Mothers of schizophrenic males reported significantly higher levels of schizoid and schizotypal traits compared with mothers of schizophrenic females and mothers of patients with affective psychoses. In addition, schizophrenic males had a history of significantly worse premorbid social functioning. Importantly, the investigators demonstrated that age at first admission, as an indicator of age at onset, did not explain the gender effect for premorbid history (Foerster et al. 1991b). The investigators further analyzed these data and showed that mothers of schizophrenic males had had significantly more obstetric complications than mothers of the other groups (Foerster et al. 1991a). In addition, patients with schizophrenia had significantly lower birth weight than patients with affective psychosis; this was associated with increased later expression of schizoid and schizotypal traits and poor social adjustment. This relationship was particularly true for males.

Findings by Foerster and colleagues (1991a, 1991b) were consistent with previous literature, even though the sample of patients with schizophrenia, especially the women ($n = 10$ women and $n = 35$ men), was quite small. However, because the sample was a hospitalized group of severely ill patients with schizophrenia (an average of approximately four admissions), one would expect gender differences to have been attenuated (Goldstein 1993). That is, females with a better prognosis were not represented.

Marital status, as a signpost of premorbid adjustment, is confounded with age at onset. Women with schizophrenia have consistently been shown to marry and procreate more often than men with schizophrenia (e.g., Häfner et al. 1989; Watt and Szulecka 1979; Wattie and Kedward 1985). It is, however, unclear whether women are more often married because they have a later age at onset or, perhaps, because it confers protection. There is some evidence for the first assumption, based on the recent work on the effects of estrogens in explaining later age at onset among women (Häfner et al. 1991; Riecher-Rössler and Häfner 1993; Seeman and Lang 1990). However, this would not exclude an effect for marital status as an additional protective factor.

Gender and Symptomatology
in Schizophrenia

Most studies that have reported findings on symptomatology in schizophrenia do not directly test for gender differences (Wahl and

Hunter 1992). Early literature, however, suggested that there may be gender differences in the symptom expression of schizophrenia. Men with schizophrenia were described generally as more socially organized, controlled, constrained, quiet, clean, and compliant, but less exhibitionistic, than women with schizophrenia. Women with schizophrenia were observed to be more explosive, violent, sexually acting out, exhibitionistic, hostile, seductive, and agitated than men with schizophrenia.

In a microanalysis of the interactions of parents with schizophrenia and their offspring, Cheek (1964) found that women with schizophrenia exhibited more active and dominating behavior in family interactions and in their attitudes on questionnaires compared with men with schizophrenia and a control group of healthy women. Men with schizophrenia were more withdrawn and passive and showed lower rates of hostility and disagreements with family members compared with women with schizophrenia and a control group of healthy men. Lorr and Klett (1965) also found that female patients with psychosis, mostly schizophrenic, exhibited more belligerence, hostility, resistance, and excitability than male patients with psychosis. Finally, compared with men with schizophrenia, women with schizophrenia were found to exhibit significantly more sexual delusions (Kraepelin 1893), to express more affective symptoms in general (Flor-Henry 1983; Lewine 1981; Walker et al. 1985), and to have fewer schizoid traits and negative symptoms (Lewine 1981).

Taken individually, the early studies had a number of methodological problems, such as sampling biases and measurement inadequacies. There were intriguing consistencies, however. Women with schizophrenia were described as exhibiting more affective symptoms, as well as more explosivity, hostility, sociopathy, and sexual deviance. Men with schizophrenia tended to be more quiet, withdrawn, passive, and schizoid.

One might argue that the gender differences in these early studies were simply a result of diagnostic inaccuracy. That is, perhaps there were more manic disorders among the group of women with schizophrenia. The symptom pattern found for women would be consistent with both disorders, and there is evidence that more schizophrenic women than men are rediagnosed as having affective disorders when current diagnostic criteria are used (Lewine et al. 1984).

In a study specifically designed to test this hypothesis, Goldstein and Link (1988) analyzed the symptomatology of 169 patients with a DSM-III diagnosis of schizophrenia (104 men/65 women) who were in the early stages of the disorder. Restricted maximum likelihood factor analysis, as programmed in Linear Structural Relationships by the Method of Maximum Likelihood (LISREL; Joreskog and Sorbom 1981), was used to test for gender differences in the expression of the disorder. Schizophrenic men and women differed significantly in terms of the severity of certain symptoms and the organization of the symptom patterns. The expression of paranoia, impulsivity, and depressive symptomatology was more characteristic of women with schizophrenia, and the expression of negative symptomatology was more characteristic of men. Findings were not attributable to diagnostic misclassification, differential diagnosis of schizoaffective disorder, or differences in the chronicity of the illness between men and women (Goldstein and Link 1988).

Before the study by Goldstein and Link, Lewine and Meltzer (1984) conducted a study that found that men with schizophrenia had a significantly higher overall negative symptom rating than women with schizophrenia. However, in the Lewine and Meltzer study, the negative symptom rating included several depression items, such as loss of interest, depressed appearance, fatigue, and retardation, as well as a few positive symptoms, such as formal thought disorder (loose associations and incoherence) and inappropriate affect. Thus, one was unable to evaluate whether the depressive items lowered the negative symptom score for men.

Several recent studies have specifically examined gender differences in symptom expression (Goldstein et al. 1990; Haas et al. 1988, 1990; Hambrecht et al. 1992; Harris et al. 1991; McGlashan and Bardenstein 1990; Rector and Seeman 1992; Ring et al. 1991; Shtasel et al. 1992). A number of these studies support the finding that men with schizophrenia express more negative symptoms (Carpenter et al. 1988; Goldstein et al. 1990; Haas et al. 1988; Hambrecht et al. 1992; Harris et al. 1991; Ring et al. 1991; Shtasel et al. 1992) and less affective symptomatology than women with schizophrenia (Copolov et al. 1990; Goldstein et al. 1990; Hambrecht et al. 1992; McGlashan and Bardenstein 1990; Ring et al. 1991; Shtasel et al. 1992). Note that the studies by Goldstein and associates (1990) and Shtasel and colleagues

(1992) used symptom assessments of *unmedicated* patients.

Most of these studies reported no significant gender differences in overall positive symptomatology scores (Haas et al. 1990; Hambrecht et al. 1992; McGlashan and Bardenstein 1990; Ring et al. 1991; Shtasel et al. 1992). Studies that have tested hypotheses regarding specific positive symptoms, however, *have* reported significant effects. Goldstein and Link (1988) did *not* report significant gender differences for positive symptoms in general but, specifically, for persecutory delusions. In another study using a much larger and different sample, Goldstein and colleagues (1990) replicated the finding that women with schizophrenia expressed more persecutory delusions (and dysphoria). Hambrecht and colleagues (1992) also reported significantly higher rates of fantastic and persecutory delusions in women with schizophrenia than in men in the multinational WHO Determinants of Outcome Study of patients being treated for the first time (Sartorius et al. 1986). Rector and Seeman (1992) reported significantly higher rates of auditory hallucinations in women with schizophrenia than in men. Other hallucinatory modalities were not significantly different, although the trend was for women to express more olfactory hallucinations than men. This difference was noted earlier in the U.S. Epidemiologic Catchment Area study (Tien 1991) and the WHO cross-national study of patients who were admitted to the hospital for the first time (Marneros 1984).

Only a few investigators have addressed the question of whether the gender differences in symptom expression are specific to schizophrenia. Flor-Henry (1983) has argued that gender differences are not specific to schizophrenia. Similar male symptom patterns are found in autism, psychopathy, sexual deviations, and early-onset obsessive-compulsive states, perhaps because of gender differences in the cerebral organization of the brain. For instance, studies of schizophrenia have shown that men with schizophrenia exhibit significantly more antisocial character pathology than women with schizophrenia (Haas et al. 1990; Hambrecht et al. 1992; Test et al. 1990). Higher rates of antisocial behavior have been found among healthy men compared with women, thus suggesting that this is not specific to schizophrenia.

In a recent well-designed study using a large *nonclinical* sample of undergraduates, Raine (1992) used the Student's *t* test to determine mean gender differences in the symptom expression of schizotypal features. He found that women scored significantly higher than men on cognitive-perceptual items, in specific, ideas of reference and odd beliefs and magical thinking. Furthermore, there was some evidence that women had more unusual perceptual experiences and odd speech or behavior. Men scored significantly higher than women on constricted affect and having no close friends. These findings are highly reminiscent of the studies (reported above) showing more persecutory or other delusions and auditory hallucinations in women with schizophrenia and more flat affect and social withdrawal among men with schizophrenia. Although the mean symptom differences between men and women in the Raine study were small, they suggested that gender differences in symptom expression in schizophrenia may reflect an exaggeration of normal gender differences. Thus, both Raine's and Flor-Henry's work suggests that gender differences in the expression of schizophrenia reflect sex differences in cerebral organization.

Gender and the Course of Schizophrenia

I reviewed the literature on course of illness and treatment outcome (see Angermeyer et al. 1989, 1990 and Chapter 10). Factors that seem to account for the variability across studies are diagnostic inconsistency, sample selection, differences in lengths of follow-up, and differences in operationalizing dimensions of outcome. The main problems with sample selection are 1) the need to differentiate between first admissions and multiple admissions and 2) the adequacy of the sample size, which influences the statistical power of the test of differences. It is important to study first admissions because those women who *do* experience a better course to their disorder and recover after one episode would no longer be represented in a sample of patients with multiple hospitalizations. Thus, gender differences in a multiply hospitalized group would be attenuated. This was argued in a previous review in which we demonstrated that studies of first-admission patients consistently tended to show significant gender differences in rehospitalization and length of hospital stays, with women having better outcomes, whereas studies that used multiply hospitalized patients were more variable (Angermeyer et al. 1989).

Recent work has suggested that gender differences in rehospitalization and lengths of hospital stay may be partially a result of the protective effects of estrogens, as discussed in the above section "Age at Onset." It has been observed that the longer the observation period, the less marked the treatment outcome difference between the sexes (Angermeyer et al. 1990; Eaton et al. 1992; Goldstein 1988). This difference may be partially caused by estrogen potentiation of the antipsychotic effect of neuroleptic drugs (Riecher-Rössler et al. 1994; Seeman 1983; Seeman and Lang 1990). As women age and reach menopause, gender differences in the course of treatment become attenuated. In contrast, studies of short- and long-term follow-up of social adjustment consistently have shown that women with schizophrenia function better than men (McGlashan and Bardenstein 1990; Scottish Schizophrenia Research Group 1992; Test et al. 1990). These findings are not likely to be accounted for by any one factor but, rather, by a combination of illness-related variables, treatment-related variables, and sex-role expectations (Angermeyer et al. 1989; Goldstein and Kreisman 1988; Haas et al. 1990; Test et al. 1990).

Incidence and Prevalence

Historically, it has been reported that the annual incidence of schizophrenia ranges from approximately 0.5 to 2.0 per 10,000 population, and the prevalence ranges from 1% to 12% in different regions of the world. It has generally been accepted that the incidence and prevalence do not vary according to gender (Neugebauer et al. 1980; Wyatt et al. 1988). However, there is a current challenge to this assumption (Cooper et al. 1987; Iacono and Beiser 1992b). The challenge can, in part, be explained by the possibility that the diagnostic criteria used in the earlier studies differentially included more female affective psychoses and thus attenuated the gender effect for schizophrenia. However, no one has systematically reviewed the more current literature. Therefore, in this section of the chapter, I examine the evidence for an effect of gender on the incidence and/or prevalence of schizophrenia in studies from 1980 to the present.

A MEDLINE search resulted in 35 studies from a range of countries during this observation period, 31 of which reported data by gender. The studies differ with respect to their case finding strategies, diagnostic inclusion criteria, and adjustment for the age structure and gender distribution of the population at risk (Tables 8–1 and 8–2). These factors influence the rate estimates for men and women. The studies can be considered separately according to their case finding strategy (i.e., psychiatric case registries, population-based sampling, and hospital-based [first-admission] sources). Regarding the admissibility of treatment statistics, a number of studies have shown that the use of treated rates is a good approximation to the true rates (Dilling and Weyerer 1984; Folnegovic et al. 1990; Link and Dohrenwend 1980; Ring et al. 1991; Stromgren 1987) because, for schizophrenia, most affected individuals eventually receive treatment. However, to contrast the sexes, treated-rate estimates must include all types of treatment services because women with schizophrenia are more often found in outpatient services, compared with men with schizophrenia who are more often found in the hospital (Angermeyer et al. 1989). Thus, the use of case registries is a more comprehensive sampling frame than hospital-based statistics.

Incidence

The case registry studies came from Denmark, England, Ireland, Scotland, Germany, and Croatia. These registries included patients who were seen in inpatient facilities, psychiatric departments in general hospitals, and outpatient and day-treatment services. Some registries included community visits by mental health professionals and social services and services provided to those patients living in group homes or hostels (Bamrah et al. 1991). The Danish studies used the design of sampling census days from different years (Munk-Jorgensen et al. 1986; Stromgren 1987). The investigators counted the number of first admissions or first contact with day treatment. They adjusted the rates for the age structure of the population at risk and then presented sex-specific rates.

In case registry studies using ICD-8 criteria for schizophrenia alone, the male-to-female risk ratio was 1.32:1.79 (World Health Or-

Table 8–1. Studies (1980–present) of male/female incidence rates of schizophrenia and related disorders

Study	Sample	Diagnostic criteria	Age/Sex adjusted	Annual incidence per 100,000 population				Male-to-female risk ratio	Significance tests
Population-based									
Sartorius et al. 1986	First contact with any "helping agency" for psychosis in eight sites, over 2-year period	[a,b]	Y/Y	Broad (schizophrenia) and related disorders	M 18–37	F 12–48		0.77–1.87	No formal tests; in 6/8, males higher
				Restrictive (CATEGO S+)*	8–17	5–14		0.73–1.8	
Iacono and Beiser 1992b	First-episode cases of psychosis making contact with any psychiatry service, group contact, or community care in Vancouver, over 2.5 years	[a,c,d,e,f]	Y/Y		M	F	% M		All significant
				ICD-9	10.90	4.12	75	2.64	
				12-point	6.81	2.55	76	2.67	
				RDC	7.59	2.55	75	2.98	
				DSM-III	6.81	1.96	76	3.47	
				Feighner	5.64	1.72	73	3.20	
Case register									
Gam 1980	All patients first admitted to psychiatric institutions in Denmark, 1970–1977	[g,h]	Y/Y	Sex-specific rates, not presented				Reported higher among men, but no figures presented	
Munk-Jorgensen et al. 1986	First admissions to Danish psychiatric facilities (inpatient, outpatient, day treatment); a day census in 1972	[h] (295.0–.9)	Y/Y	Total population	M 19.3	F 10.8		1.79	Significant
				Adjusted for M/F population	15.0	8.7		1.72	

(continued)

Table 8-1. Studies (1980–present) of male/female incidence rates of schizophrenia and related disorders *(continued)*

Study	Sample	Diagnostic criteria	Age/Sex adjusted	Annual incidence per 100,000 population			Male-to-female risk ratio	Significance tests
				M	F	Total		
Cooper et al. 1987	First contacts with Mapperly Psychiatric Hospitals, Nottingham, England, 8/1/78–7/31/80	a,e	Y/Y	DSM-III	–	–	8.0		No formal tests
				DSM-III retro. 17.0	7.0	13.0	2.43	
				ICD-9 restrct. (295) –	–	20.0		
				ICD-9 broad 28.0	14.0	22.0	2.00	
McGovern and Cope 1987	First admissions to Birmingham Psychiatric Hospital, England, 1/1/80–12/31/83	i	Y/Y	M	F			No tests
				Afro-Caribbean				
				(16–29 years) 138.0	98.0		1.41	
				(30–64 years) 45.3	52.8		0.86	
				White (16–29 years) 20.5	7.0		2.93	
				(30–64 years) 9.8	13.3		0.74	
NiNullain et al. 1987	First contact, case register in three countries, Ireland (1973–1974), ages 15–65	b,h	Y/Y	M	F			Not significant
				CATEGO 295/297 47.3	24.9		1.90	
				CATEGO 295 37.0	20.4		1.81	
				CATEGO 295 20.6	15.8		1.30	
				CATEGO S+ 20.6	13.8		1.51	
Häfner et al. 1989	All Danish citizens (1976) and inhabitants of Mannheim, West Germany (1978–1980), first hospitalized for schizophrenia, ages 12–59	h	Y/Y	*For schizophrenia only:* M	F			Significant for Denmark
				Denmark 10.7	8.1		1.32	
				Mannheim 32.1	32.3		1.00	

Study	Description	Y/Y	Location/details	M	F	Ratio	Tests
Folnegovic et al. 1990	First admissions to psychiatric institutions in Croatia, 1965–1984 [a,h,j]	Y/Y	1965–1969 1970–1974 1975–1979 1980–1984	28 30 28 29	26 28 27 26	1.08 1.07 1.04 1.12	No tests
Orbell et al. 1990	First versus all admissions to psychiatric hospitals and units in London, Edinburgh, and Belfast in 1981 (national statistics) [a]	Y/Y	England Scotland Ireland	10 3 14	7 9 9	1.43 1.44 1.56	No tests
E. Y. H. Chen et al. 1991	Subsample of the Cooper study; test reported; defined catchment area of Nottingham; 40 Afro-Caribbeans; 40 matched control subjects [h]	Not reported	All Afro-Carribbeans with first episode; 60% ($n = 24$) were male; no rates reported				No tests
Castle et al. 1993	All nonorganic nonaffective psychotic patients from the Camberwell Cumulative Psychiatric Case Register who had first contact with psychiatric services, 1965–1984 [a,d,e,f,k]	Y/Y	For DSM-III-R schizophrenia alone: ≤45 >45 All ages	11.1 5.2 9.0	5.2 9.0 6.7	2.14 0.58 1.34	All significant

(continued)

Table 8–1. Studies (1980–present) of male/female incidence rates of schizophrenia and related disorders *(continued)*

Study	Sample	Diagnostic criteria	Age/Sex adjusted	Annual incidence per 100,000 population	Male-to-female risk ratio	Significance tests
Hospital-based						
Schwarz et al. 1980	All first-admitted inpatients and outpatients of three psychiatric hospitals in Mannheim, from 1/78–9/78 (*n* = 70)	h,l	N/Y	No rates reported	Males = 58.6% Females = 41.4%	The distribution of men and women with schizophrenia significantly different from the sex distribution in the general population
Bland and Orn 1984	First admissions to psychiatric institutions in Canada, 1978 (national statistics)	h	Y/Y	M F 31.0 22.0	1.41	No tests
Häfner et al. 1991	Representative sample of consecutive first admissions, from defined catchment area (Mannheim) over 2-year period; ages 12–59	a	Y/Y	M F 13.2 13.14	1.0	Not significant

Ring et al. 1991	First admissions for psychosis, ages 16–49 years, to National Health Service Psychiatric Units, south and central Manchester, England, 1987–1988	[d] (personal interviews)	Y/Y	Definite schizophrenia	M 19	F 14	1.36	Not significant

Note. retro. = retrospective, restrct. = restrictive

*CATEGO is an automated diagnostic computer program developed to make diagnoses from the Present State Examination developed in the U.K. (Wing et al. 1974).

[a] ICD-9 = *International Classification of Diseases, 9th Revision* (World Health Organization 1989).

[b] CATEGO (personal interviews).

[c] 12-point.

[d] (personal interviews)

[e] RDC = Research Diagnostic Criteria (Spitzer et al. 1978).

[e] DSM-III = *Diagnostic and Statistical Manual of Mental Disorders, 3rd Edition* (American Psychiatric Association 1980).

[f] Feighner's criteria (personal interviews) (Feighner et al. 1972).

[g] Most of the sample (65%) were rediagnosed using available record information.

[h] ICD-8 = *International Classification of Diseases, 8th Revision* (World Health Organization 1968).

[i] Criteria not stated (schizophrenia and paranoid psychoses).

[j] ICD-7 = *International Classification of Diseases, 7th Revision* (World Health Organization 1955).

[k] DSM-III-R = *Diagnostic and Statistical Manual of Mental Disorders, 3rd Edition, Revised* (American Psychiatric Association 1987).

[l] 63% were rediagnosed with personal interview (included schizophrenia and related psychotic disorders).

ganization 1968). The difference was significant for two Danish studies
(Häfner et al. 1989; Munk-Jorgensen et al. 1986) and not significant
for a German study (1.00) (Häfner et al. 1989) and an Irish study (1.3)
(NiNullain et al. 1987). No formal tests were reported for the studies
conducted in England (E. Y. H. Chen et al. 1991; Cooper et al. 1987;
Orbell et al. 1990). In several instances, ICD-8 schizophrenia was
combined with paranoid disorders (Häfner et al. 1989; McGovern
and Cope 1987; NiNullain et al. 1987). A lower male-to-female risk
ratio was reported when paranoid disorders were included.

In only two case registry studies, research psychiatrists interviewed patients and rediagnosed their disorders (Cooper et al. 1987;
NiNullain et al. 1987). In one study, research psychiatrists rediagnosed
patients' disorders based on medical records (Castle et al. 1991). This
issue is an important one. Clinical diagnoses are less stringent than
research diagnoses, and, as I discuss later in this chapter, the stringency of the diagnosis has a differential effect on the rates among men
and women.

Cooper and colleagues (1987) conducted a very thorough study
in Nottingham over a 2-year period (1978–1980) as part of the WHO
Collaborative Study on the Determinants of Outcome and Severe
Mental Disorders (Sartorius et al. 1986). They used case registry information and structured clinical interviews by psychiatrists. They
made consensus diagnoses based on all available material. Although
the investigators did not conduct any formal statistical tests for the
effect of gender, the male-to-female risk ratio was 2:2.4, a higher risk
ratio than other case registry studies in which only clinical diagnoses
were used. NiNullain and co-workers (1987), who also rediagnosed
disorders based on structured interviews with patients and record
material, reported a higher relative risk among men with schizophrenia than women, although the differences were not significant. Unfortunately, there was low statistical power in this study to test for
gender differences because the sample included only 27 patients with
schizophrenia (34 patients when paranoid disorders were included).

Castle and colleagues (1993), using the Camberwell Psychiatric
Case Registry, rediagnosed the conditions of 470 patients who were
first admitted between 1965 and 1984. They applied several diagnostic classification systems to estimate sex-specific rates. This is the only
study in the literature reporting sex-specific rates in patients with a

Table 8–2. Studies (1980–present) of male/female prevalence of schizophrenia and related disorders

Study	Sampling design	Diagnostic criteria	Age/Sex adjusted	Point, period, and/or lifetime prevalence	Male-to-female prevalence ratio	Significance tests
Case register						
Dilling and Weyerer 1984	Representative random sample from resident registries of three communities in Upper Bavaria (Germany), 1975–1977	a	?/Y	1-week prevalence/ 1,000 (note: only six cases of schizophrenia identified) — M 4.0 F 4.0	1.00	No tests (only six cases)
Munk-Jorgensen et al. 1986	Comparison of 2 census days; all patients in Danish psychiatric institutions (inpatient, outpatient, and day treatment), on 7/28/77 and 9/29/82	a	Y/Y	Point prevalence/ 10,000 — 1977 M 8.3 F 6.9; 1982 M 7.8 F 6.6	1.20 / 1.18	No tests
Freeman and Alport 1987	Salford Psychiatric case register; includes psychiatry and social service use; no group-only data, 1973–1974	b,c	Y/Y	1-year prevalence/ 1,000 — M 7.02 F 6.61	1.06	No formal tests, but likely not significant
Stromgren 1987	All residents of Bornholm on census days, 1935 and 1983	a	Y/Y	Point prevalence/ unstated unit (total population 50,000) — 1935 M 0.37 F 0.41; 1983 M 0.32 F 0.25	0.90 / 1.28	Significant decrease

(continued)

Table 8–2. Studies (1980–present) of male/female prevalence of schizophrenia and related disorders *(continued)*

Study	Sampling design	Diagnostic criteria	Age/Sex adjusted	Point, period, and/or lifetime prevalence			Male-to-female prevalence ratio	Significance tests
Case register *(continued)*								
Bamrah et al. 1991	All residents of Salford, England, who made contact with psychiatric services during 1984	d	Y/Y	*1-year prevalence/ 1,000* Main and borderline schizophrenia	M 7.68	F 7.35	Total 7.51	1.04	No tests
Population-based								
Nandi et al. 1980	Epidemiological survey of two rural villages in West Bengal; key informants used	e	Unclear, re: age in some cases, sex adjusted	*Point prevalence/ 1,000 for schizophrenia* Brahmin Scheduled caste Tribes	M 3.5 1.7 0.8	F 11.0 1.8 1.7		0.32 0.94 0.47	No tests
Kauders et al. 1982	All known schizophrenic persons in the Palau Islands (Micronesia), 1972–1980	f	N/N	*Percentages among 15,000 population* All schizophrenic persons (n = 73) Age < 35 years Age 35+	M 79 85 15	F 21 42 58		No rates calculated	No tests

Study		Description		Measure						
Halldin 1984	[a]	Representative selection, stratified by age and sex of population of Stockholm County, 1970–1971; 2-stage case finding strategy; ages 18–65	Y/Y	*1-year prevalence/ 1,000*	M 7.0	F 6.0	1.17			Not significant
Robins et al. 1984	[g]	One selected member, age 18+, of each selected household in New Haven, 1981–1982	Y/Y	*Lifetime prevalence/ 1,000*						Significant for New Haven

Robins et al. 1984:

	M	F	ratio
New Haven	12	26	0.46
Baltimore	12	19	0.63
St. Louis	10	11	0.91

Study		Description		Measure						
Sikanarty and Eaton 1984	[a]	Epidemiological study of all facilities and services treating psychiatric disorders, plus sample from traditional healers and homeless persons; point prevalence, 2-week period in 1978	Y/Y	*For Ghana: 2-week point prevalence/ 1,000 For Monroe Co.: annual incidence/ 1,000 for nonwhites*						No tests

Sikanarty and Eaton 1984:

	M		F		ratio	
Ages	Ghana	Monroe	Ghana	Monroe	Ghana	Monroe
15–24	0.57	8.60	0.34	3.00	1.7	2.87
25–44	1.68	14.44	0.26	11.96	6.46	1.20
45–64	0.98	12.41	1.42	12.69	0.69	0.98
≥ 65	0	3.03	1.08	1.27	0	2.39
Total (n)	19		9		2.1	

Study		Description		Measure						
Bland et al. 1988	[g]	Community survey of Edmonton, Canada, 1983–1986; only household residents reported here, age 18+	Y/Y	*Lifetime prevalence/ 1,000*	M 5.0	F 7.0	0.71			Not significant

(continued)

Table 8–2. Studies (1980–present) of male/female prevalence of schizophrenia and related disorders (continued)

Study	Sampling design	Diagnostic criteria	Age/Sex adjusted	Point, period, and/or lifetime prevalence			Male-to-female ratio	Significance tests
Population-based (continued)								
C. K. Lee et al. 1990	All family members, ages 18–65, of randomly selected households in Seoul, Korea	g	Y/Y	*Lifetime prevalence/ 1,000* Schizophrenia Schizophrenia, schizophreniform disorder	M 4.1 4.8	F 2.4 2.4	 1.71 2.0	Not significant
Youseff et al. 1991	All existing cases of schizophrenia in the eastern half of the rural county Cavan, Ireland, on 11/2/87 and 11/2/88	h	Y/Y	*1-year prevalence/ 1,000* ≤ 15 years 15–44 years Total population	M 5.1 7.0 3.6	F 4.1 5.7 2.9	 1.23 1.24	Difference not significant
Hospital-based								
Bland and Orn 1984	Admissions for psychiatric disorders in Canada, 1978 (national statistics)	a	Y/Y	*1-year prevalence/ 1,000*	M 10.36	F 6.76	1.5	No tests
Wattie and Kedward 1985	All schizophrenic persons, ages 17–63, treated in four Canadian provinces 18 months to 10 years before the index interview	i	N/N	*Percentage of patients* (No rates or population figures reported) < 30 years > 50 years	M (n = 109) 54 7.3	F (n = 73) 28.8 23.3		Significant relationship between sex and age

[a] ICD-8 = *International Classification of Diseases, 8th Revision* (World Health Organization 1968) (personal interviews by psychiatrists).

[b] Structured Symptom checklist subjected to records.

[c] CATEGO (schizophrenia, schizoaffective, and paranoid disorders).

[d] ICD-9 = *International Classification of Diseases, 9th Revision* (World Health Organization 1989).

[e] Clinical criteria; loosely defined schizophrenia (personal interviews by psychiatrists and case records).

[f] Clinical diagnoses; 50% personally interviewed and rediagnosed by DSM-III (*Diagnostic and Statistical Manual of Mental Disorders, 3rd Edition* [American Psychiatric Association 1980]).

[g] DSM-III (personal interviews, Diagnostic Interview Schedule [DIS; Robins et al. 1981]).

[h] DSM-III-R = *Diagnostic and Statistical Manual of Mental Disorders, 3rd Edition, Revised* (American Psychiatric Association 1987) (personal interviews).

[i] RDC = Research Diagnostic Criteria (Spitzer et al. 1978).

DSM-III-R (American Psychiatric Association 1987) diagnosis of schizophrenia. Findings showed that the more stringent the diagnostic criteria, the higher the male-to-female risk ratio. Males younger than age 45 years had the highest incidence of schizophrenia, a significant difference from females. Women older than age 45 years had a significantly higher incidence of schizophrenia than men older than age 45. However, the higher incidence among older women did not offset the higher incidence among younger males. That is, for all ages combined, males still had a significantly higher incidence of DSM-III-R schizophrenia than females. The risk ratio was 1.34 (Castle et al. 1991, 1993).

This study is particularly important because it has been argued that only in youth do males differ from females and that studies reporting significant gender differences in incidence have not included later-onset females (Hambrecht et al. 1992). However, the study by Castle and associates included older-onset females and did not limit the age at onset to 45 years. Although the investigators did find a significantly higher incidence of schizophrenia among older females than among older males, this did not completely offset the relatively higher incidence among young males.

Two incidence studies could be considered population based, but they were not true community studies (Iacono and Beiser 1992a; Sartorius et al. 1986). The WHO Collaborative Study on Determinants of Outcome of Severe Mental Disorders was an important contribution to assessing rates cross-culturally (Jablensky et al. 1980; Sartorius et al. 1986). One of the purposes of this study was to assess the occurrence rates of schizophrenia across age groups, the two sexes, geographically diverse areas, and cultures. The study was an attempt to improve on the sampling strategy in the WHO International Pilot Study of Schizophrenia (Jablensky et al. 1980), which obtained consecutive first admissions of "potential" schizophrenic patients to psychiatric services. The improved case finding network was extended to all potential schizophrenic patients over a 2-year period, with a first lifetime contact to a variety of institutional and community care services, including traditional healers and religious agencies. Structured clinical interviews were used to obtain symptom and diagnostic information. Although the study did not report statistical tests of gender differences in rates, using a case definition of schizophrenia and schizoaffective disorders, there was a higher than parity male-to-female risk ratio in six out of eight countries in which incidence was calculated. The risk ratio ranged from 1.22 to 1.8 (Sartorius et al. 1986).

In a recent study that used a similar sampling strategy to the WHO Collaborative Study, Iacono and Beiser (1992b) found a significantly higher incidence for men than for women. As with the WHO study, this sampling strategy comes closest to estimating "true incidence," short of a community survey. Consensus diagnoses were made, based on structured clinical interviews and all other record and clinical information. Rates of disorder were presented under various diagnostic systems. The study was exemplary in its effort to find "true" first-episode cases, in that anyone who had ever taken antipsychotic, antimanic, or antidepressive medications was excluded. Although this exclusion criterion may have differentially barred from inclusion in the study more women than men, the investigators argued that relative incidence was not changed when subjects with a history of treatment were included (Iacono and Beiser 1992b). The male-to-female risk ratio ranged from 2.65 to 3.47, a significant difference regardless of the diagnostic system applied to the data. It is noteworthy that, in comparing diagnostic systems, ICD-9 (World Health Organization 1989), the system used by European studies, resulted in the lowest male-to-female risk ratio. This will be discussed in more detail later in this chapter.

One reason that Iacono and Beiser found a greater risk ratio than other studies may be the low proportion of older-onset women in their sample (i.e., women older than age 40). (Few men have onset of schizophrenia at these ages [Angermeyer and Kuhn 1988; Goldstein et al. 1989].) It is unclear from the data presented how many women from this age group were in their sample. It may be that older women were not presenting for treatment or that they were overrepresented in those who were taking medications on an outpatient basis before their first episode and were thus excluded from the study. An analysis of subjects of this age from the screened-out group might help to clarify this important issue. The Iacono and Beiser study is one of only three in which patients were personally interviewed, and their disorders were rigorously rediagnosed by research criteria. As discussed below, this methodology may differentially affect risk estimates for men and women.

Finally, there were two hospital-based incidence studies (Bland and Orn 1984; Ring et al. 1991). Bland and Orn's cross-national Canadian study of first admissions in 1978 reported a male-to-female risk ratio of 1.41, although statistical tests were not applied. Diagnoses were obtained from clinical records based on ICD-8 criteria. In the English study by Ring and colleagues, Research Diagnostic Criteria (Spitzer et al. 1978) were applied, resulting in a male-to-female risk ratio of 1.36 for definite schizophrenia (which was not significant). Rates for atypical psychosis were significantly higher for women than for men (Ring et al. 1991).

Discussion of Incidence Studies

The incidence rates for men and women appear to depend, in part, on the diagnostic inclusion criteria. The majority of studies that used broader inclusion criteria reported little difference in incidence between men and women. For example, studies on schizophrenia and paranoid disorders (e.g., Häfner et al. 1989) reported less difference between the sexes than studies that reported rates for schizophrenia alone (e.g., Munk-Jorgensen et al. 1986). In fact, Häfner et al. (1989) presented rates for schizophrenia alone and schizophrenia plus paranoid disorders, which demonstrated that, in Denmark, the male-to-female risk difference was attenuated when paranoid disorders were included.

Orbell and colleagues (1990) presented data that clearly demonstrate this finding as well. For schizophrenia alone, the male-to-female relative risk ratios were 1.43, 1.44, and 1.56 for England, Scotland, and Ireland, respectively. However, for paranoid disorders, the risk was reversed. *Females* showed a greater relative risk than males—that is, 2.5, 1.8, and 3.0 female-to-male risk ratios for England, Scotland, and Ireland, respectively. This reversal was also true for other nonaffective psychoses (Orbell et al. 1990).

Thus, incidence studies that report a combined rate for schizophrenia, paranoid disorders, and other nonaffective psychoses may be attenuating the effect of gender on the incidence of schizophrenia. Because it is still unclear which disorders should be included in the genetic spectrum of schizophrenia, it would be helpful if incidence

studies reported rates for schizophrenia and schizophreniform disorder separately rather than in combination. This is particularly important with regard to assessing gender differences in incidence because,
in some studies, women have been found to express higher rates of
schizoaffective and paranoid disorders than men (e.g., Orbell et al.
1990; Ring et al. 1991). Furthermore, a certain proportion of patients
with a diagnosis of schizophreniform disorder acquire diagnoses of
affective psychoses when rediagnosed 6 months to 1 year later (Pulver
et al. 1992). Studies that used ICD-8 criteria or Research Diagnostic
Criteria reported less of a difference, especially when the diagnosis
included disorders other than schizophrenia alone. Iacono and Beiser
(1992a) clearly demonstrated that the more stringent the criteria for
diagnosing schizophrenia, the greater the gender difference in incidence. Feighner's criteria (Feighner et al. 1972) and DSM-III criteria
were the most stringent and showed the greatest male-to-female relative risk ratios. This was also supported by a case registry study
(Cooper et al. 1987).

It has been argued that gender differences in incidence using
DSM-III criteria are artifactually inflated. DSM-III may exclude
more women than men because of the age at onset under 45 years
criterion (Hambrecht et al. 1992). Furthermore, Feighner's criteria
may increase the estimate for men, because "poor premorbid history"
and "being single" are criteria for the diagnosis, features that are more
characteristic of men with schizophrenia than women. Thus, the male-
to-female risk ratio for DSM-III and Feighner's criteria may be artifactually inflated.

A key factor that may explain discrepancies across studies is the
difference in the percentage of older-onset women in different samples (e.g., see Castle et al. 1993).

Finally, the method of calculation may differentially affect the
rates for men and women. In many studies, the number of cases is
divided by the total population at risk during a specified time. It would
be helpful to see age-specific rates stratified by gender because, after
onset, a subject is eliminated from the population at risk that is used
to estimate rates for the subsequent age groups. That is, the denominator for calculating incidence (the population at risk) decreases for
older age groups because those who have become ill are eliminated
from the at-risk population. Because, relative to men, women have

an older age at onset, the population at risk (the denominator) differs between men and women at different ages. A smaller denominator increases the risk estimate. To control for this, the subjects in a sample must come from the population that is used as the denominator. Analytic techniques, such as survival analysis, can be used to control for variable ages at onset and differential mortality (E. T. Lee 1980).

In summary, incidence studies conducted from 1980 to the present have, in general, reported a higher incidence of schizophrenia among men than women. The statistical significance of the difference in effect sizes is, in part, dependent on the stringency of the diagnostic criteria, the inclusivity or exclusivity of the definition of a "case," the methods for sampling and diagnosing cases (personal interviews versus clinical records), and statistical techniques applied to calculate rates. It would be helpful if studies would separate rates for schizophrenia and/or schizophreniform disorder from rates of other nonaffective psychoses because it has been shown that gender affects the expression of some of the other nonaffective psychoses. Studies currently under way investigating first-episode psychoses will provide incidence estimates for DSM-III-R schizophrenia and related disorders (e.g., Bromet et al. 1992).

Prevalence

Fifteen prevalence studies were conducted from 1980 to the present that analyzed data by gender. Five case registry studies were from England (Bamrah et al. 1991; Freeman and Alport 1987), Denmark (Munk-Jorgensen et al. 1986; Stromgren 1987), and Germany (Dilling and Weyerer 1984); eight population-based studies were from Africa (Sikanarty and Eaton 1984), Ireland (Youseff et al. 1991), Korea (C. K. Lee et al. 1990), the United States (Robins et al. 1984), the Palau Islands (Kauders et al. 1982), Sweden (Halldin 1984), India (Nandi et al. 1980), and Canada (Bland et al. 1988); and two hospital-based studies were from Canada (Bland and Orn 1984; Wattie and Kedward 1985).

Prevalence studies are somewhat more difficult to compare than incidence studies because the estimate of prevalence is reported in different ways: *point* prevalence, which refers to a day's census; *period* prevalence, which refers to a time anywhere from 1 week to 1 year; and *lifetime* prevalence. In addition, it has been argued that there is a large difference in prevalence across geographical areas and cultures (Sartorius et al. 1986; Torrey 1987). In general, prevalence studies show that the male-to-female risk ratio ranges from 1.0 to 2.1. In the only three studies in which statistical tests were applied, the differences were nonsignificant. In three other studies, the prevalence among females was higher than among males (C. K. Lee et al. 1990; Nandi et al. 1980; Robins et al. 1984); this is discussed in detail below. As with incidence studies, the difference in the rate ratios was, in part, a result of differences in diagnostic criteria and sampling frame.

In general, the use of clinical diagnoses produced a small difference in prevalence rates between men and women (Bamrah et al. 1991; Freeman and Alport 1987; Munk-Jorgensen et al. 1986), with men showing slightly higher rates. One epidemiological study of two rural villages in India that used clinical criteria for diagnosis showed higher rates among women (Nandi et al. 1980). However, this study used a very broad definition of schizophrenia, and rates were not adjusted for the age or sex distribution of the population. The only study that used clinical diagnoses and showed a possibly significantly higher male-to-female ratio (1.5) was the hospital-based study by Bland and Orn (1984). The use of hospital statistics alone, however, may underestimate the rate for females.

Discrepancies illustrate the importance of the sampling frame when assessing the validity of reported prevalence rates. In fact, one would anticipate higher rates among *females* if the population source were the community. A higher prevalence among females was indeed reported in the two studies that used lay interviewers and reported community rates alone, excluding institutionalized cases (Bland et al. 1988; Robins et al. 1984). The reliability and validity of diagnostic assessments done by lay interviewers using close-ended questionnaires have been called into question. For example, the reliability of diagnosing schizophrenia in the Robins and colleagues study (1984) produced a Kappa of 0.19 (very low interrater reliability) when comparing lay interviewers' with psychiatrists' assessments (Anthony et al. 1985). The United States study reported higher prevalence rates of schizophrenia than other studies in the literature and may, perhaps, reflect the inclusion of affective psychoses in the diagnosis of schizophrenia, an artifact of the clinical inexperience of lay interviewers.

A study done in Korea (C. K. Lee et al. 1990), which was very similar to the United States study by Robins and colleagues (1984), reported a male-to-female risk ratio of 1.7–2.0 (nonsignificant). The actual prevalence (0.34%) was very low, suggesting an underestimation by lay interviewers; an underreporting by household members because of cultural stigma; or, alternatively, a very low prevalence for urban Korea. (Low prevalence also makes it difficult to rely on statistical tests of the effect of gender because of low statistical power.) To complicate the picture further, another issue for the United States and Korean studies was the use of DSM-III criteria, which exclude cases that have an age at onset after 45 years. As discussed previously, this may differentially exclude more women, and thus prevalence rates for women in these studies may be underestimated.

A population-based study that used DSM-III-R criteria found a male-to-female ratio of approximately 1.2, which was not significant (Youseff et al. 1991). The purpose of this exemplary study was to identify all cases of schizophrenia over a 1-year period in a defined rural area of Ireland. Patients from a case registry were personally interviewed, and sophisticated statistical methods were used to calculate and compare rates. The prevalence rate among men was 7.0 and among women was 5.7 for ages 15–44. There were only 48 male and 35 female schizophrenic patients; thus, the statistical power to test for gender differences may have been low. Youseff and colleagues reported rates for schizophrenia alone. Additional data on prevalence rates for other disorders that are considered part of the schizophrenia spectrum would further contribute to understanding the effect of gender on the expression of different forms of schizophrenia.

In two additional studies that used comprehensive sampling strategies (Halldin 1984; Sikanarty and Eaton 1984), gender differences in prevalence rates varied. Sikanarty and Eaton (1984) reported rates from a representative sample of cases of schizophrenia in Ghana, from all psychiatric facilities and community services caring for individuals with psychiatric disorders, in addition to a sample from traditional healers and homeless persons. Halldin (1984) conducted a study of a representative selection of the population of Stockholm County in Sweden. In both studies, ICD-8 criteria were used based on personal interviews and case records. Halldin (1984) reported a small male-to-female rate difference (1.7), and Sikanarty and Eaton (1984) reported an approximate 2:1 difference. However, Halldin reported rates for schizophrenia combined with other psychoses, and Sikanarty and Eaton reported rates for schizophrenia alone. Combining rates for all psychoses may attenuate gender differences. Alternatively, valid gender discrepancies may exist in these two cultures.

Finally, an attempt was made to identify all known cases of schizophrenia in the Palau Islands (Micronesia) over an 8-year period (Kauders et al. 1982). Medical records and key informants were used to identify cases. Approximately 50% were personally interviewed and rediagnosed by DSM-III criteria. Kauders and associates reported a very large male-to-female difference—approximately 4:1. Fifty-eight men and 15 women were identified. However, no adjustment for the age structure of the population was applied. In addition, 73 cases over an 8-year period for a population of 15,000 is an extremely low prevalence. It is unclear whether this is a true reflection of the prevalence on this island or whether methodological artifacts are affecting the estimates. The methods were poorly described in the Kauders and colleagues report (1982).

Discussion of Prevalence Studies

In general, prevalence studies report a lower male-to-female rate ratio than the incidence studies. Prevalence studies are vulnerable to the same methodological issues that were discussed in the above section, "Incidence." In a prevalence study that addressed many of these issues, the male-to-female rate ratio for schizophrenia was only 1.23 (Youseff et al. 1991).

If one is convinced that the incidence is truly higher in men, then the duration of the illness in women would have to be longer for the prevalence in men and women to be similar (e.g., more males committing suicide) (Test et al. 1990). It is important for future studies on incidence and prevalence to report the data in such a way as to address the diagnostic issues raised in this chapter because they differentially affect the estimate of rates for men and women. In addition, the 6-month duration of symptoms criterion of DSM-III, DSM-III-R, and DSM-IV (American Psychiatric Association 1994) might differentially affect the rates for men and women (e.g., women may show more brief reactive psychoses).

Furthermore, it is important to present age-specific rates to determine whether higher rates of schizophrenia among men apply only to younger ages and whether women "catch up" after menopause, as has been argued for the incidence data (Hambrecht et al. 1992). Finally, some studies have argued that, preferentially for women, the prevalence of schizophrenia has decreased over the last 50 years (Stromgren 1987). It is unknown whether this represents a true decrease or whether, in previous years, the diagnosis of schizophrenia included what are now called affective psychoses. Because affective psychosis is more prevalent in women than in men, changes in diagnostic criteria might account for the apparent decrease of schizophrenia among women.

Summary of Findings

Evidence from several large bodies of literature reviewed in this chapter supports the hypothesis that men and women with schizophrenia express the illness differently. Men with schizophrenia have a significantly earlier age at onset than women, controlling for the age composition of the population of origin and differential excess mortality among men and women with schizophrenia. This difference has been found across cultures and historical periods. Some evidence suggests that the antidopaminergic effect of estrogens may contribute to this difference in age at onset.

Men with schizophrenia also experience a poorer premorbid history than women with schizophrenia. Women are older at onset and therefore have a longer developmental period before illness and a higher likelihood of marriage. Women have also been found to have better early childhood histories, in terms of school achievement and social functioning. High-risk studies have shown that, compared with female children of schizophrenic women, male children exhibit more frequent early neurobehavioral deficits, such as neuromotor and attentional dysfunction, more aggression, lower IQs, more schizoid or schizotypal traits, lower birth weight, and more obstetric complications, all of which may lead to premorbid deficits. Findings regarding poorer premorbid histories among men with schizophrenia have been found to be specific to schizophrenia when compared with affective psychosis.

Men and women with schizophrenia also have been found to show some symptom differences. Women with schizophrenia express more affective symptoms, paranoia, and auditory hallucinations. Men with schizophrenia have more negative symptoms, in particular, flat or constricted affect, loss of drive or will, and social withdrawal. Some evidence suggests that gender differences in symptom expression may not be specific to schizophrenia but, rather, may reflect general gender differences in the development and organization of the brain. This may result in gender dimorphism in the expression of several neurodevelopmental disorders.

Factors that explain gender differences in age at onset, symptomatology, and premorbid history also, in part, may explain gender differences in the course of schizophrenia. Women tend to have better treatment outcomes (i.e., less frequent rehospitalization, shorter lengths of hospital stay, less psychopathology during remission, and superior social adjustment). As with age at onset, differences in treatment outcomes may be, in part, a result of hormones. This is supported by the finding that the influence of gender on treatment outcomes is attenuated as women age and reach menopause. Although estrogens may help to explain gender differences in treatment outcomes, they do not readily explain better social adjustment among women. Perhaps the better premorbid development among women allows for better social adjustment after illness onset. Social role expectations differ for men and women, and these factors have also been found to influence social outcomes.

Thus, men and women with schizophrenia tend to express the illness differently. Do these differences translate into gender differences in incidence or prevalence of schizophrenia? In general, recent studies have shown that the incidence is higher among men than among women, especially when stringent diagnostic criteria for schizophrenia are applied. The statistical significance of the gender effect size is, in part, dependent on the definition of a case, methods for sampling and diagnosing cases, and statistical techniques applied to the data.

The variability in the results across studies underscores the need to separate schizophrenia from other diagnostic groups, such as paranoid disorders and schizoaffective disorders, because women have been found to have relatively higher rates of the latter disorders. Therefore, combining all of these disorders in the estimate of rates for schizophrenia attenuates the gender effect. Because it is still unclear what to include in the genetic spectrum, it would be helpful to estimate separate sex-specific rates for different diagnostic entities, as well as to show combined rates. This will contribute to understanding the boundaries of the definition of schizophrenia and related disorders and how gender affects the expression of these disorders.

Prevalence studies have reported a lower male-to-female rate ratio than incidence studies. The prevalence studies are vulnerable to the same methodological problems as the incidence studies (e.g., diagnostic issues). In general, the studies report a higher prevalence among young men and a higher prevalence among older women postmenopause, resulting in an attenuated overall gender effect on prevalence. However, it remains unclear whether the higher prevalence among older women offsets the higher rate among young men. Thus, it is important to present age-specific rates by gender to answer this question. Estimating the effect of gender on prevalence is important for many reasons, including the incorporation of accurate prevalence parameters into genetic modeling studies.

References

Al-Issa I (ed): Gender and Schizophrenia, Gender and Psychopathology. New York, Academic Press, 1982

American Psychiatric Association: Diagnostic and Statistical Manual of Mental Disorders, 3rd Edition. Washington, DC, American Psychiatric Association, 1980

American Psychiatric Association: Diagnostic and Statistical Manual of Mental Disorders, 3rd Edition, Revised. Washington, DC, American Psychiatric Association, 1987

American Psychiatric Association: Diagnostic and Statistical Manual of Mental Disorders, 4th Edition. Washington, DC, American Psychiatric Association, 1994

Angermeyer MC, Kuhn L: Gender differences in age at onset of schizophrenia: an overview. Eur Arch Psychiatry Neurol Sci 237:351–364, 1988

Angermeyer MC, Goldstein JM, Kuhn L: Gender differences in schizophrenia: rehospitalizaiton and community survival. Psychol Med 19:365–382, 1989

Angermeyer MC, Kuhn L, Goldstein JM: Gender and the course of schizophrenia: differences in treated outcomes. Schizophr Bull 16:293–307, 1990

Anthony JC, Folstein M, Romanoski AJ, et al: Comparison of the lay Diagnostic Interview Schedule and a standardized psychiatric diagnosis: experience in eastern Baltimore. Arch Gen Psychiatry 42:667–675, 1985

Bamrah JS, Freeman HL, Goldberg DP: Epidemiology of schizophrenia in Salford, 1974-84: changes in an urban community over ten years. Br J Psychiatry 159:802–810, 1991

Baron M, Gruen R, Asnis L, et al: Age-of-onset in schizophrenia and schizotypal disorders. Neuropsychobiology 10:199–204, 1983

Bland RC, Orn H: Long term mental illness in Canada: an epidemiological perspective on schizophrenia and affective disorders. Can J Psychiatry 29:242–246, 1984

Bland RC, Orn H, Newman SC: Lifetime prevalence of psychiatric disorders in Edmonton. Acta Psychiatr Scand 77:24–32, 1988

Bleuler M: The Schizophrenic Disorders: Long-Term Patient and Family Studies. Translated by Clemens S. New Haven, CT, Yale University Press, 1978

Bromet EJ, Schwartz JE, Fennig S, et al: The epidemiology of psychosis: the Suffolk County Mental Health Project. Schizophr Bull 18:243–255, 1992

Carpenter WT Jr, Heinrichs DW, Wagman AMI: Deficit and nondeficit forms of schizophrenia: the concept. Am J Psychiatry 145:578–583, 1988

Castle DJ, Murray RM: The neurodevelopmental basis of sex differences in schizophrenia. Psychol Med 21:565–575, 1991

Castle DJ, Wessely S, Der G, et al: The incidence of operationally defined schizophrenia in Camberwell 1965-1984. Br J Psychiatry 159:790–794, 1991

Castle DJ, Wessely S, Murray RM: Sex and schizophrenia: effects of diagnostic stringency, and associations with premorbid variables. Br J Psychiatry 162:658–664, 1993

Cheek F: A serendipitous finding: sex roles and schizophrenia. Journal of Abnormal Social Psychology 69:393–400, 1964

Chen EYH, Harrison G, Standen PJ: Management of first episode psychotic illness in Afro-Caribbean patients. Br J Psychiatry 158:517–522, 1991

Chen WJ, Faraone SV, Tsuang MT: Estimating age at onset distributions: a review of methods and issues. Psychiatric Genetics 2:219–238, 1992

Chen WJ, Faraone SV, Orav EJ, et al: Estimating age at onset distributions: the bias from prevalent cases and its impact on risk estimation. Genet Epidemiol 10:43–59, 1993

Ciompi L: The natural history of schizophrenia in the long-term. Br J Psychiatry 136:413–420, 1980

Cooper JE, Goodhead D, Craig T, et al: The incidence of schizophrenia in Nottingham. Br J Psychiatry 151:619–626, 1987

Copolov DL, McGorry PD, Singh BS, et al: The influence of gender on the classification of psychotic disorders—a multidiagnostic approach. Acta Psychiatr Scand 82:8–13, 1990

Dilling H, Weyerer S: Prevalence of mental disorders in the small-town, rural region of Traunstein (Upper Bavaria). Acta Psychiatr Scand 69:60–79, 1984

Eaton WW, Mortensen PB, Hermann H, et al: Long term course of hospitalization for schizophrenia, part I: risk for rehospitalization. Schizophr Bull 18:217–228, 1992

Faraone SV, Chen WJ, Goldstein JM, et al: Gender differences in age at onset of schizophrenia. Br J Psychiatry 164:625–629, 1994

Farina A, Garmezy N, Zalvsky N, et al: Premorbid behavior and prognosis in female schizophrenic patients. J Consult Clin Psychol 26:56–60, 1962

Feighner JP, Robins E, Guze SB, et al: Diagnostic criteria for use in psychiatric research. Arch Gen Psychiatry 26:57–63, 1972

Flor-Henry P: The influence of gender on psychopathology: animal experiments, in Cerebral Basis of Psychopathology. Edited by Flor-Henry P. Boston/Bristol/London, John Wright, PSG, 1983, pp 97–116

Foerster A, Lewis SW, Owen MJ, et al: Low birth weight and a family history of schizophrenia predict poor premorbid functioning in psychosis. Schizophr Res 5:13–20, 1991a

Foerster A, Lewis SW, Owen MJ, et al: Pre-morbid adjustment and personality in psychosis: effects of sex and diagnosis. Br J Psychiatry 158:171–176, 1991b

Folnegovic Z, Folnegovic-Smalc V, Kulcar Z: The incidence of schizophrenia in Croatia. Br J Psychiatry 156:363–365, 1990

Freeman HL, Alport M: Prevalence of schizophrenia in an urban population. Br J Psychiatry 149:603–611, 1987

Gam J: A 5-year retrospective investigation of all first admitted schizophrenics to Danish psychiatric institutions in the fiscal year from April 1st, 1970, to April 1st, 1971, in Epidemiological Research as Basis for the Organization of Extramural Psychiatry. Edited by Stromgren E, Dupont A, Nielsen J. Acta Psychiatr Scand Suppl 62 (285):332–336, 1980

Gittelman-Klein R, Klein DF: Premorbid asocial adjustment and prognosis in schizophrenia. J Psychiatr Res 7:35–53, 1969

Goldstein JM: Gender differences in the course of schizophrenia. Am J Psychiatry 145:684–689, 1988

Goldstein JM: Sampling biases in studies on gender and schizophrenia: a reply. Schizophr Bull 19:9–14, 1993

Goldstein JM, Kreisman D: Gender, family environment, and schizophrenia. Psychol Med 18:861–872, 1988

Goldstein JM, Link BG: Gender and the expression of schizophrenia. J Psychiatr Res 22:141–155, 1988

Goldstein JM, Tsuang MT, Faraone SV: Gender and schizophrenia: implications for understanding the nature of the disorder. Psychiatry Res 28:243–253, 1989

Goldstein JM, Santangelo SL, Simpson JC, et al: The role of gender in identifying subtypes of schizophrenia: a latent class analytic approach. Schizophr Bull 16:263–275, 1990

Goldstein JM, Faraone SV, Chen WJ, et al: Gender and the familial transmission of schizophrenia: disentangling confounding factors. Schizophr Res 7:135–140, 1992

Green MF, Satz P, Gaier DJ, et al: Minor physical anomalies in schizophrenia. Schizophr Bull 15:91–99, 1989

Haas GL, Glick ID, Clarkin JF, et al: Inpatient family intervention: a randomized clinical trial, II: results at hospital discharge. Arch Gen Psychiatry 45:217–224, 1988

Haas GL, Glick ID, Clarkin JF, et al: Gender and schizophrenia outcome: a clinical trial of an inpatient family intervention. Schizophr Bull 16:277–292, 1990

Häfner H, Riecher A, Maurer K, et al: How does gender influence age at first hospitalization for schizophrenia? A transnational case register study. Psychol Med 19:903–918, 1989

Häfner H, Behrens S, DeVry J, et al: An animal model for the effects of estradiol on dopamine mediated behavior: implications for sex differences in schizophrenia. Psychiatry Res 38:125–134, 1991

Halldin J: Prevalence of mental disorder in an urban population in central Sweden. Acta Psychiatr Scand 69:503–518, 1984

Hambrecht M, Maurer K, Sartorius N, et al: Transnational stability of gender differences in schizophrenia? An analysis based on the WHO study on determinants of outcome of severe mental disorders. Eur Arch Psychiatry Clin Neurosci 242:6–12, 1992

Harris MJ, Jeste DV, Krull A, et al: Deficit syndrome in older schizophrenic patients. Psychiatry Res 39:285–292, 1991

Heimbuch RC, Matthysse S, Kidd KK: Estimating age of onset distributions for disorders with variable onset. Am J Hum Genet 32:564–574, 1980

Iacono WG, Beiser M: Are males more likely than females to develop schizophrenia? Am J Psychiatry 149:1070–1074, 1992a

Iacono WG, Beiser M: Where are the women in first-episode studies of schizophrenia? Schizophr Bull 18:471–480, 1992b

Jablensky A, Schwarz R, Tomov T: The WHO collaborative study on impairments and disabilities associated with schizophrenic disorders. A preliminary communication: objectives and methods. Acta Psychiatr Scand 62:152–163, 1980

Joreskog KG, Sorbom D: An Analysis of Linear Structural Relationships by the Method of Maximum Likelihood. User's Guide, Version V. Uppsala, Sweden, University of Uppsala, 1981

Kauders FR, MacMurray JP, Hammond KW: Male predominance among Palauan schizophrenics. Int J Soc Psychiatry 28:97–103, 1982

Kraepelin E: Psychiatrie, 4th Edition. Leipzig, Germany, Barth, 1893

Lee CK, Kwak YS, Yamamoto J, et al: Psychiatric epidemiology in Korea, part I: gender and age differences in Seoul. J Nerv Ment Dis 178:242–246, 1990

Lee ET: Statistical Methods for Survival Data Analysis. Belmont, CA, Lifetime Learning Publications, 1980

Lewine RRJ: Sex differences in schizophrenia: timing or subtypes? Psychol Bull 90:432–444, 1981

Lewine RRJ: Gender and schizophrenia, in Handbook of Schizophrenia, Vol 3. Edited by Tsuang MT, Simpson JC. Amsterdam, Elsevier, 1988, pp 379–397

Lewine RRJ, Meltzer HY: Negative symptoms and platelet monoamine oxidase activity in male schizophrenics. Psychiatry Res 12:99–109, 1984

Lewine RRJ, Burbach D, Meltzer HY: Effect of diagnostic criteria on the ratio of male to female schizophrenic patients. Am J Psychiatry 141:84–87, 1984

Lewis SW, Murray RM: Obstetric complications, neurodevelopmental deviance, and risk of schizophrenia. J Psychiatr Res 21:413–421, 1987

Link B, Dohrenwend BP: Formulation of hypotheses about the ratio of untreated to treated cases in true prevalence studies of functional psychiatric disorders in adults in the United States, in Mental Illness in the United States: Epidemiological Estimates. Edited by Dohrenwend BP, Dohrenwend BS, Gould M, et al. New York, Praeger, 1980, pp 133–149

Lorr M, Klett CJ: Constancy of psychotic syndromes in men and women. J Consult Clin Psychol 29:309–313, 1965

Marneros A: Frequency of occurrence of Schneider's first rank symptoms in schizophrenia. Eur Arch Psychiatry Neurol Sci 234:78–82, 1984

McGlashan TH, Bardenstein KK: Gender differences in affective, schizoaffective, and schizophrenic disorders. Schizophr Bull 16:319–329, 1990

McGovern D, Cope RV: First psychiatric admission rates of first and second generation Afro Caribbeans. Social Psychiatry 22:139–149, 1987

Morrison J, Clancy J, Crowe R, et al: The Iowa 500, I: diagnostic validity in mania, depression, and schizophrenia. Arch Gen Psychiatry 27:457–461, 1972

Munk-Jorgensen P, Weeke A, Jensen EB, et al: Changes in utilization of Danish psychiatric institutions, II: census studies 1977 and 1982. Compr Psychiatry 27:416–429, 1986

Murray RM, O'Callaghan E, Castle DJ, et al: A neurodevelopmental approach to the classification of schizophrenia. Schizophr Bull 18:319–332, 1992

Nandi DN, Mukherjee SP, Boral GC, et al: Socio-economic status and mental morbidity in certain tribes and castes in India: a cross-cultural study. Br J Psychiatry 136:73–85, 1980

Neugebauer R, Dohrenwend PR, Dohrenwend BS: Formulation of hypotheses about the true prevalence of functional psychiatric disorders among adults in the U.S., in Mental Illness in the United States: Epidemiological Estimates. Edited by Dohrenwend BP, Dohrenwend BS, Gould M, et al. New York, Praeger, 1980, pp 45–94

NiNullain M, O'Hare A, Walsh D: Incidence of schizophrenia in Ireland. Psychol Med 17:943–948, 1987

Orbell S, Trew K, McWhirter L: Mental illness in Northern Ireland: a comparison with Scotland and England. Soc Psychiatry Psychiatr Epidemiol 25:165–169, 1990

Pulver AE, Liang KY, Brown CH, et al: Risk factors in schizophrenia: season of birth, gender, and familial risk. Br J Psychiatry 160:65–71, 1992

Raine A: Sex differences in schizotypal personality in a nonclinical population. J Abnorm Psychol 101:361–364, 1992

Rector NA, Seeman MV: Auditory hallucinations in women and men. Schizophr Res 7:233–236, 1992

Riecher-Rössler A, Häfner H: Schizophrenia and oestrogens—is there an association? Eur Arch Psychiatry Clin Neurosci 242:323–328, 1993

Riecher-Rössler A, Häfner H, Stumbaum M, et al: Can estradiol modulate schiozphrenic symptomatology? Schizophr Bull 20:203–214, 1994

Ring N, Tantam D, Montague L, et al: Gender differences in the incidence of definite schizophrenia and atypical psychosis—focus on negative symptoms of schizophrenia. Acta Psychiatr Scand 84:489–496, 1991

Robins LN, Helzer JE, Croughan J, et al: National Institute of Mental Health Diagnostic Interview Schedule: its history, characteristics, and validity. Arch Gen Psychiatry 38:381–389, 1981

Robins LN, Helzer JE, Weissman MM, et al: Lifetime prevalence of specific psychiatric disorders in three sites. Arch Gen Psychiatry 41:949–958, 1984

Salokangas RKR: Prognostic implications of the sex of schizophrenic patients. Br J Psychiatry 142:145–151, 1983

Sartorius N, Jablensky A, Korten A, et al: Early manifestations and first-contact incidence of schizophrenia in different cultures. Psychol Med 16:909–928, 1986

Schwarz R, Biehl H, Krumm B, et al: Case-finding and characteristics of schizophrenic patients of recent onset in Mannheim: a report from the WHO collaborative study on the assessment of disability associated with schizophrenic disorders. Acta Psychiatr Scand 62:212–219, 1980

Scottish Schizophrenia Research Group: The Scottish first episode schizophrenia study, five-year follow-up: clinical and psychosocial findings. The Scottish Schizophrenia Research Group. Br J Psychiatry 161:496–500, 1992

Seeman MV: Gender and the onset of schizophrenia: neuro-humoral influences. Psychiatric Journal of the University of Ottawa 6:136–138, 1981

Seeman MV: Gender differences in schizophrenia. Can J Psychiatry 27:107–111, 1982

Seeman MV: Interaction of sex, age, and neuroleptic dose. Compr Psychiatry 24:125–128, 1983

Seeman MV, Lang M: The role of estrogens in schizophrenia gender differences. Schizophr Bull 16:185–194, 1990

Shtasel DL, Gur RE, Gallacher F, et al: Gender differences in the clinical expression of schizophrenia. Schizophr Res 7:225–231, 1992

Sikanarty T, Eaton WW: Prevalence of schizophrenia in the Labadi District of Ghana. Acta Psychiatr Scand 69:156–161, 1984

Spitzer RL, Endicott J, Robins E: Research Diagnostic Criteria: rationale and reliability. Arch Gen Psychiatry 35:773–782, 1978

Stromgren E: Changes in the incidence of schizophrenia? Br J Psychiatry 150:1–7, 1987

Test MA, Burke SS, Wallisch LS: Gender differences of young adults with schizophrenic disorders in community care. Schizophr Bull 16:331–344, 1990

Tien AY: Distribution of hallucinations in the population. Soc Psychiatry Psychiatr Epidemiol 26:287–292, 1991

Torrey EF: Prevalence studies in schizophrenia. Br J Psychiatry 150:598–608, 1987

Tsuang MT, Winokur G: The Iowa-500: field work in a 35-year follow-up of depression, mania, and schizophrenia. Canadian Psychiatric Association Journal 20:359–365, 1975

Waddington JL, O'Callaghan E, Larkin C: Physical anomalies and neurodevelopmental abnormality in schizophrenia: new clinical correlates (abstract). Schizophr Res 3:90, 1990

Wahl OF, Hunter J: Are gender effects being neglected in schizophrenia research? Schizophr Bull 18:313–318, 1992

Walker E, Bettes BA, Kain EL, et al: Relationship of gender and marital status with symptomatology in psychotic patients. J Abnorm Psychol 94:42–50, 1985

Watt DC, Szulecka TK: The effect of sex, marriage and at first admission on the hospitalization of schizophrenics during two years following discharge. Psychol Med 9:529–539, 1979

Wattie BJS, Kedward HB: Gender differences in living conditions found among male and female schizophrenic patients on a follow-up study. Int J Soc Psychiatry 31:205–216, 1985

Wing JK, Cooper JE, Sartorius N: Measurement and Classification of Psychiatric Symptoms: An Instruction Manual for the PSE and CATEGO Program. New York, Cambridge University Press, 1974

World Health Organization: International Classification of Diseases, 7th Revision. Geneva, World Health Organization, 1955

World Health Organization: International Classification of Diseases, 8th Revision. Geneva, World Health Organization, 1968

World Health Organization: International Classification of Diseases, 9th Revision. Geneva, World Health Organization, 1989

Wyatt RJ, Alexander R, Egan M, et al: Schizophrenia, just the facts: what we know, how well do we know it? Schizophr Res 1:3–18, 1988

Youseff HA, Kinsella A, Waddington JL: Evidence for geographical variations in the prevalence of schizophrenia in rural Ireland. Arch Gen Psychiatry 48:254–258, 1991

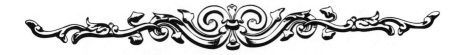

CHAPTER 9

Gender and the Familial Transmission of Schizophrenia

Jill M. Goldstein, Ph.D.

T he familial nature of schizophrenia is well established in the literature. The prevalence of schizophrenia is elevated among first-degree relatives of schizophrenic probands, with morbidity risk estimates ranging from 3% to 15% (Gottesman and Shields 1982; Kendler et al. 1985). However, neither the precise mode of inheritance nor the gene locus has been identified for schizophrenia. It has been generally accepted that the elevated risk among relatives of patients with schizophrenia does not vary by sociodemographic characteristics of the proband. However, some literature suggests that the risk may differ by the proband's gender (Bellodi et al. 1986; Goldstein et al. 1990; Pulver et al. 1990; Shimizu et al. 1987).

Yet, after an extensive review of the literature from the late 1920s through the present, we found that most studies did not examine the

Preparation of this chapter was supported by a National Institute of Mental Health Scientist Development Award K21 MH00976. The author wishes to thank Susan Santangelo, Sc.D., for her help with an earlier draft of this chapter.

impact of gender on the transmission of schizophrenia. Of the 100 studies investigating the familial transmission of schizophrenia that were reviewed for this chapter, only 26 had conducted gender-specific analyses or had reported the data in such a way as to make it possible to do so. Most reports neglected to present the gender distribution of the sample.

This is the first systematic review of the literature regarding the issue of gender and familial transmission of schizophrenia. The studies reviewed in detail below have made at least a cursory attempt to examine the impact of gender on the transmission of schizophrenia. They may be categorized as either concordance studies or family transmission studies. Concordance studies date from the late 1920s. Family transmission studies range from the 1939 paper by Pollock and colleagues to the present. In this chapter, I note methodological weaknesses and strengths of these studies. Research methodology and diagnostic practices have changed markedly over this time span.

Concordance Studies

Twin Concordance Studies

Most of the early twin studies found that concordance rates among female monozygotic (MZ) and dizygotic (DZ) twins were higher than among male MZ or DZ twins (Luxenberger 1928, 1934; Rosanoff et al. 1934; Rosenthal 1962; Slater 1958). Only Kallman (1946) claimed that there were no significant differences in twin concordance rates by gender. He failed to report the distribution of his data by gender, however, so it is difficult to evaluate his results. The three post–World War II studies that included twins of both sexes did not find significant differences in concordance rates by gender (Fischer 1973; Gottesman and Shields 1972; Kringlen 1968).

Other investigators have written about the methodological differences between the early and late twin studies that might account for the discrepant findings regarding gender differences in concordance rates (Gottesman and Shields 1972, 1982; Lewine 1979; Samuels 1979).

Most cite the differences in sampling methods between pre– and post–World War II studies. For example, much has been made of the fact that almost all of the pre–World War II studies sampled chronic resident populations from mental institutions in which women were overrepresented. One exception was the study by Rosanoff and colleagues (1934), which used a sample of convenience from different areas of the United States and Canada. In contrast, samples in the post–World War II twin studies were obtained by matching psychiatric case registries with twin birth registries and taking consecutive admissions. It has been suggested that excessive female pair concordance among pre–World War II studies was an artifact of oversampling females from severe, chronic institutionalized populations (Gottesman and Shields 1982). However, as I argue below, it is still unclear whether the early findings were an artifact.

The other major difference between the early and later twin studies is that diagnostic criteria and procedures changed. Earlier criteria (e.g., clinical diagnoses, DSM-I, or DSM-II [American Psychiatric Association 1952, 1968]) tended to be quite broad and included substantial proportions of patients with what are now considered affective disorders, which are known to be more prevalent among women (Goldstein and Link 1988; Lewine et al. 1984). The argument against the validity of the early sex-concordance findings was that oversampling women from severe, chronic populations differentially increased the probability of finding concordance among women, based on the assumption that greater severity implied greater genetic risk (Gottesman and Shields 1982). On the other hand, one could argue that using broad criteria for schizophrenia, as did the early studies, created greater phenotypical variability among the oversampled females (e.g., broad criteria meant greater heterogeneity including nongenetic, environmentally caused psychoses). Thus, *lower* concordance may have been found among females. Alternatively, greater phenotypical variability may have resulted in the inclusion of more affective psychoses among the females, which may have artificially inflated the concordance among these so-called female schizophrenic patients, because affective psychosis has been found to have greater genetic penetrance than schizophrenia.

The post–World War II studies examined concordance among twins using a range of definitions for "being affected." In fact, higher concordance rates were found for female MZ pairs by Kringlen (1968) and Fischer (1973) for narrower definitions of schizophrenia, although the rate differences were not maintained for the broader definitions (i.e., the schizophrenia spectrum disorders). Kringlen (1968), Fischer (1973), and Stromgren (1987) (i.e., his analysis of data from Luxenburger) all reported higher twin concordance in males when broad criteria were used and higher concordance in females when narrow criteria were used. Thus, the use of broad criteria in males did not introduce genetic variability but, in females, it did.

Gottesman and Shields (1972) have argued that the variation in male and female twin concordance rates based on the inclusivity/exclusivity of the criteria can be interpreted as evidence for "greater phenotypic variability in the male" (pp. 307–308). That is, they suggest that even when narrow criteria are used, there is more phenotypical variability in male probands and thus lower concordance among male twins.

I would argue that the evidence does not support greater phenotypical variability among men with schizophrenia compared with women. That is, there is evidence that *women* have a greater phenotypical variability when broad criteria are used, given that there are more female affective disorders included in a broad diagnostic approach (Lewine et al. 1984). In addition, as demonstrated in incidence studies, females tend to express more atypical psychoses (e.g., Ring et al. 1991) and paranoid psychoses (Orbell et al. 1990), again supporting the argument that the use of broad diagnostic criteria results in relatively more variability among female schizophrenic patients. Thus, depending on whether the spectrum diagnosis is itself highly heritable, females might have *lower* twin concordance rates. More recently, others have argued that the deciding factor in sex concordance is whether the illness is inherited from the mother or the father (see below).

In fact, all of the twin concordance studies were conducted before the development of criteria such as DSM-III, DSM-III-R, or DSM-IV (American Psychiatric Association 1980, 1987, 1994) for schizophrenia. By current diagnostic criteria, men with schizophrenia are more frequently hospitalized (and at younger ages) than women with schizophrenia (Angermeyer et al. 1990; Goldstein 1988; Salokangas 1983). Thus, Gottesman and Shield's argument that sampling consecutive admissions is a better approach to answering the question of differential sex-concordance rates may not hold true because consecutive admissions may oversample men if current diagnostic standards are used (Goldstein 1993; Wahl and Hunter 1992).

Studies of Concordance Among Sibling Pairs: The Pseudoautosomal Locus Theory

Some investigators have proposed a genetic susceptibility locus for schizophrenia in the pseudoautosomal region of the sex chromosomes (Collinge et al. 1991; Crow 1988; Crow et al. 1989; DeLisi and Crow 1989; see Chapters 3 and 7). Based on this theory, one would expect that among patients with schizophrenia, there would be concordance by sex among siblings when the gene is paternally inherited.

Early investigations of affected siblings have reported same-sex concordance, particularly among female siblings (Mott 1910; Myerson 1925; Penrose 1945; Schulz 1932; Tsuang 1967). These studies have been criticized on methodological grounds (Sturt and Shur 1985). The arguments are similar to those raised against same-sex concordance among twins. Sturt and Shur (1985) argue that reports of same-sex concordance among affected sibling pairs are a result of 1) differential diagnostic heterogeneity among male and female schizophrenic patients, 2) biased ascertainment of cases (e.g., preferential reporting of same-sex pairs when both are affected, the use of hospital reports to identify cases that might lead to incomplete ascertainment, or an excess of one sex or another among the probands), 3) lack of control for the expected sex and age distribution of schizophrenia, 4) lack of control for family size among male versus female proband families, and 5) lack of adjustment for differential age at onset among male versus female schizophrenic patients.

In a study intended to avoid these methodological problems, Sturt and Shur (1985) found no significant association between the sex of the proband and the sex of the affected first-degree relative. However, informative sibships (i.e., sibling groupings in which an individual with schizophrenia had a sibling with schizophrenia, whether a sister or a brother) were available for only six male proband and seven female proband families. Thus, finding significant same-sex concordance *among siblings* was unlikely. In addition, none of the relatives were interviewed. Diagnosis in relatives was based on family reports to the clinician. The diagnosis in probands was clinically derived and broadly defined using ICD-8 (World Health Organization 1968) criteria. These factors, as stated by Sturt and Shur themselves, can lead to unreliability and, therefore, less likelihood to discover significant differences.

Crow et al. (1989) employed three different methods to categorize illness as either paternally or maternally inherited (or both) and found that in 120 families having at least one sibling pair with schizophrenia, affected members were significantly more likely to be of the same sex when the illness was inherited paternally. The study has been criticized methodologically (Curtis and Gurling 1990) regarding biased ascertainment of cases resulting in an excess of male probands, inappropriate data analysis methods, lack of blind diagnostic assessment of relatives, and incomplete ascertainment of relatives. Crow and colleagues (1990) reanalyzed their data to address some of these criticisms, and same-sex sibling concordance in paternally transmitted schizophrenia remained significant.

However, an additional unaddressed problem was the inclusion of affective disorders in family members as evidence of the "schizophrenia" disease process. The question of whether the genetic transmission of schizophrenia is the same as that of more global psychosis remains unanswered. The effect of including affective disorders or psychosis not otherwise specified (NOS) should be tested separately to clarify the issue of specificity.

A study that used some patients from Crow et al.'s (1989) study and from other United Kingdom families (Collinge et al. 1991) used the affected sibling-pair method of linkage analysis to test the pseudoautosomal hypothesis. This study defined illness in family members as Research Diagnostic Criteria (RDC; Spitzer et al. 1978) schizophrenia or schizoaffective disorder. A deoxyribonucleic acid (DNA) probe was chosen to identify the telomeric end of the pseudoautosomal region (locus: DXYS14). The identity by descent (IBD) score method of Green and Woodrow (1977) was used to analyze data from 83 sibships in which there was an excess of same-sex (mostly male-male) siblings. The authors were able to reject the null hypothesis of independent assortment of alleles. They suggested that their findings were consistent with a locus for schizophrenia on the distal short arms of the X and Y chromosomes (Collinge et al. 1991). However, the finding of apparent nonindependent assortment of alleles does not prove linkage. Linkage may be the most plausible explanation, but other possibilities, including genomic imprinting, were not considered (see Chapter 3).

Three recent reports (Asherson et al. 1992; D'Amato et al. 1992; Gorwood et al. 1992) attempted to replicate the findings of Crow and colleagues (1989) and Collinge and co-workers (1991). In Wales, Asherson and colleagues conducted a linkage analysis of schizophrenia using DXYS14, the same marker that Collinge and colleagues used in their affected sibling-pair analysis. Asherson's group also conducted a sibling-pair analysis to examine sex concordance among siblings. Six large families were studied using the lod score method to detect linkage, and 22 independent sibling pairs were used for sibling-pair analysis. RDC and other diagnostic criteria (unspecified in the paper) were used to diagnose relatives. Under eight different genetic model assumptions, based on penetrance parameters and gene frequencies, the two-point lod scores indicated no positive linkage with the pseudoautosomal region. The affected sibling-pair method also suggested no linkage. The study reported a significant same-sex concordance among siblings, but there was no significant effect of paternal versus maternal inheritance. The authors suggested that same-sex concordance requires an explanation other than pseudoautosomal gene location.

In contrast, a French group of investigators found positive linkage between the DXYS14 locus and schizophrenia (D'Amato et al. 1992) and significant same-sex concordance with paternal inheritance (Gorwood et al. 1992). DSM-III diagnoses were used (including schizophrenia, schizophreniform, schizoaffective disorder, and schizotypal personality disorder [SPD]). The method for affected sibling-pair analysis was used, replicating that of Collinge and colleagues' study. Thirty-three sibling pairs were analyzed, and findings were consistent with nonrandom segregation of alleles at the DXYS14 locus among affected siblings. In addition, results suggested that this marker was not linked with the sex-determining locus. In a further analysis of these data, Gorwood and colleagues (1992) demonstrated significant same-sex concordance among affected siblings in paternally derived pairs compared with maternally derived pairs. The same method used by Crow and colleagues (1989, 1990 [in reply]) was employed, with methodological changes suggested by Curtis and Gurling (1990).

As with other linkage studies of schizophrenia, support for a pseudoautosomal locus has been inconsistent. Contradictory results from studies that used the affected sibling-pair method may have been caused by differences in sample sizes (resulting in differences in statistical power), differences in the definition of the phenotype, and differences in the genetic assumptions regarding penetrance parameters and gene frequencies. For example, the studies using the sibling-pair method that reported positive results had larger samples than did Asherson and colleagues (1992), who reported negative results. Gorwood and associates (1992) reported significant same-sex concordance among paternally derived pairs (sample total, 39 pairs); D'Amato and co-workers (1992), using 33 pairs from the same sample, reported nonsignificant same-sex concordance. This illustrates that a difference of 6 sibling pairs can affect the level of significance of the findings.

In addition, the linkage studies differed as to whether they included other psychoses in the definition of the phenotype, such as unspecified functional psychosis or affective psychosis. It is imperative that investigators present their data analyses in such a way as to clarify whether their significant findings relate to schizophrenia alone, schizophrenia and the traditional psychotic spectrum (i.e., schizophreniform and schizoaffective disorder), schizophrenia and the full spectrum (i.e., including SPD), or schizophrenia and other types of psychoses. This would allow the reader to judge whether the possibility of a pseudoautosomal locus might apply to schizophrenia alone, to spectrum disorders, or to psychosis in general. Finally, as was done by Asherson and colleagues, it would be useful in these initial studies that attempt to replicate the study by Crow et al. (1989) to present linkage findings using different genetic assumptions because the parameters for schizophrenia are unclear. Although this may increase Type I error (Risch 1991), it would allow for the possibility of replication of the findings in a subsequent study.

Family Transmission Studies

Early Studies

The earliest report that compared the inheritance of psychotic disorders in families of male versus female probands was by Pollock and colleagues (1939). This study attempted to assess the morbidity risk to first- and second-degree relatives of 175 patients (53% male) diagnosed with dementia praecox. The sample was obtained from consecutive admissions, more than 91% of whom were first admissions, to a New York State hospital during 1928–1930. Diagnoses in the 2,515 relatives were assessed by the family history method. Results showed a slightly higher risk for psychosis in relatives of male probands. Statistical tests comparing the risk in relatives of male probands with that in relatives of female probands were not conducted.

A study by Reed and associates (1973) examined the morbidity risk to first-degree relatives of 89 probands (64% female) with a diagnosis of "functional psychosis" admitted to a Pennsylvania state hospital before 1917. The sample was not consecutive and contained a disproportionate number of females. The study findings included the following:

- Approximately 20% of the mothers of probands had psychosis versus 14.5% of the fathers of probands.
- When the mother of the proband had psychosis, 39% of the proband's siblings had psychosis; when the father had psychosis, 17% of the proband's siblings had psychosis.
- When the proband was a mother with psychosis, 21% of her children had psychosis; when the proband was a father, 13% of his children had psychosis.
- Seventy-eight percent of the offspring with psychosis had a mother who was a proband; 15% of the offspring with psychosis had a father who was a proband.

In general, the study concluded that mothers with psychosis produced about twice as many offspring with psychosis as did fathers with psychosis.

The report failed to specify the ascertainment scheme, diagnostic criteria, and methods for assessing and categorizing relatives. In addition, there was no age correction, although the relatives were primarily in their 50s and older, thus past the period of risk. However, the study's most serious methodological flaw was its failure to control for differential fertility effects in male and female probands. It is well known that impairment of fertility is greater in male than in female schizophrenic patients (Vogel 1979). Thus, the higher rate of psychosis among offspring of ill mothers could simply be a result of differential family size of male and female probands.

Modern Studies

The only modern study conducted before 1980 was a segregation analysis of Kallman's (1946) twin/family data (Elston et al. 1978). This analysis was a minor manipulation of the data rather than an actual investigation of sex differences in transmission. The investigators applied a number of one-locus segregation models to Kallman's data and, in one instance, allowed the means and variances of the age at onset distributions to be sex specific in order to improve the fit of the model. However, all tested models were ultimately rejected, including the one that included the sex-specific age at onset distribution.

Modern studies can be characterized by their use of current diagnostic criteria and sophisticated quantitative methods. Some have used the family history method, in which information on relatives is obtained either from the proband, from an informant, from the proband's medical record, or from the proband's clinician. Others have used the family study method, in which relatives are personally interviewed to obtain diagnostic information. The use of the family history versus family study method is important to consider when interpreting results from studies because family history studies underestimate illness in relatives. This is particularly true of schizophrenia spectrum disorders such as SPD. If SPD prevalence were unequal in the two sexes, the underestimation of SPD in families might exert a profound effect on the results of sex-specific family transmission studies of schizophrenia.

Family history method. Most family transmission studies that have directly tested for the effect of gender have used the family history method to obtain information on relatives. I discuss the family history studies in chronological order. Until the mid-1980s, there were very few reports in the literature on the effect of gender on the transmission of schizophrenia, in part because of Gottesman and Shields' (1972, 1982) strong critique of the early studies that purported to show an effect. However, in 1986 and 1987, two groups from different countries—Italy (Bellodi et al. 1986) and Japan (Shimizu et al. 1987)—independently reported a higher morbidity risk to relatives of schizophrenic female patients versus male patients.

Bellodi and colleagues (1986) studied a consecutive series of 229 inpatients with schizophrenia (62% male) and their 457 parents and 588 siblings, all diagnosed using DSM-III criteria. Although the patient sample and selection methods were not well described, patients were diagnosed using a well-known semistructured interview. The family history method was used to collect clinical data on relatives. Relatives were classified as affected if they met criteria for the schizophrenia spectrum disorders (schizophrenia, atypical psychosis, paranoid disorder, or SPD). The data were age corrected, using different age at onset distributions for men and women. By logistic regression analysis, Bellodi and colleagues showed that the risk to relatives of female probands with schizophrenia (9.48%) was significantly higher than the risk to relatives of male probands with schizophrenia (5.13%). The study also reported a difference in the risk for spectrum disorders among male versus female relatives. Although this finding did not reach significance, male relatives seemed to be at lower risk for spectrum disorders than female relatives.

The study by Bellodi and colleagues was thoughtfully conducted and methodologically sophisticated. However, it is unclear whether their findings relate to a gender effect on spectrum disorders or to schizophrenia alone. They used the family history method, which underestimates the less severe disorders in the spectrum such as SPD. SPD may be an important expression of the schizophrenia genotype, especially among relatives of male probands, as I discuss later in this chapter. In addition, SPD itself may be more prevalent among men because men tend to express more of the negative symptoms of schizophrenia (e.g., Foerster et al. 1991; Goldstein and Link 1988; Lewine 1981), some of which are reflected in the criteria for SPD. Men also show more early childhood schizoid and schizotypal traits (Foerster et al. 1991). Therefore, an underestimation of SPD has a differential effect on any investigation into sex-linked schizophrenia transmission. The sex effect reported by Bellodi and colleagues may therefore be interpreted as pertaining to the psychotic spectrum disorders because these disorders are more reliably assessed using the family history method.

The study by Shimizu and others (1987) examined rates of schizophrenia in 3,350 parents and 4,935 siblings of 1,691 patients with schizophrenia (60% male). The patients were all younger than age 50 years. DSM-III criteria were used to diagnose subjects based on medical records, family history data, and/or clinical interviews. The parents of female probands had a significantly higher rate of schizophrenia (5.7%) than did the parents of male probands (2.8%). In addition, female probands were significantly more likely than male probands to have been members of multiply affected families. Thus, the density of illness within female families was greater than among male families. No significant differences were found for the rates of schizophrenia in siblings of male versus female probands. However, the sibling rates may have been underestimated because it is unclear how many siblings had passed through the period of risk.

A study by Nimgaonkar and associates (1988) was designed to assess prospectively the relationship among family history of schizophrenia, obstetric complications, and computed tomography (CT) scan findings in a consecutive series of 48 hospitalized patients with schizophrenia. A semistructured clinical interview and hospital records were used to diagnose probands based on RDC. The 242 first-degree and 535 second-degree relatives were classified by raters who were blind to patient status; they used family history RDC based on an informant and hospital records. Correction for variable ages at onset was not reported. The designation "familial" was given to patients with a history of psychotic illness, including affective psychoses, among their first-degree relatives. I undertook a post-hoc comparison of familiality in male ($n = 32$) and female ($n = 16$) probands, which showed that there was a slight excess of familial females (44% of female probands versus 34% of male probands), although the difference was not significant (odds ratio for familiality given female gender = 1.48). It is possible that the small sample size, ascertainment bias (fewer first-degree relatives were ascertained among the nonfamilial than among the familial patients), or the overinclusive definition of "affected" may have attenuated the effect size for gender.

In fact, in another family history study that examined the relationship among perinatal and childhood factors, gender, family history, and clinical symptoms, relatives of female schizophrenic patients were found to have a significantly greater risk for chronic psychosis than relatives of male patients (Nasrallah and Wilcox 1989). This was a retrospective study of 199 patients (102 men and 97 women) from the Iowa 500 study. Feighner's criteria (Feighner et al. 1972) were used to diagnose patients, based solely on chart review. Chart review alone was also used to determine history of psychiatric illness in family members, as evidenced by the institutionalization of the family member. Age correction was not done. However, even in the face of these methodological problems, a significant sex of proband effect was reported. This finding is particularly interesting because Feighner's criteria include single status and poor premorbid history—factors that are more characteristic of men with schizophrenia than women—which are biased toward including more men. A higher risk for relatives of men would have been expected if men were overrepresented in the proband sample.

Of the studies that used the family history method, a series of papers published by Pulver and colleagues at Johns Hopkins University (Pulver and Liang 1991; Pulver et al. 1990; Wolyniec et al. 1992) was the most methodologically sophisticated. Patients were sampled from consecutive admissions to 15 hospitals in the greater Baltimore area. They were given a best estimate research diagnosis based on DSM-III criteria using several sources of information, including a semistructured interview, hospital records, and global functioning at 6 months' follow-up. Family history RDC were used to classify the relatives, based on family history information collected (blindly) from two informants. The 1,853 first-degree relatives of 374 (73% male) schizophrenic probands were identified. Correction for variable age at onset was incorporated into the method of analysis. Pulver and Liang (1991) used a multivariate survival model (Liang 1991) that was superior to the Cox Proportional Hazards (PH) model used in the earlier study (Pulver et al. 1990) in that it accounted for correlated ages at onset among the relatives. The association between proband age at onset and risk to relatives was examined separately for male and female probands. The risk to relatives of male probands whose age at onset was less than 17 was found to be significantly higher than that to relatives of male probands whose onset was later. No association was found between age at onset of female probands and risk to their first-degree relatives. The failure to detect an association between age at onset and risk to relatives among the families of female probands may have been the result of low statistical power ($n = 101$, or 27%).

Female probands were found to have come from multiply affected families significantly more often than male probands. In addition, risk to relatives was found to be significantly correlated among the relatives of female probands but not among relatives of male probands.

Further work by this group (Wolyniec et al. 1992) investigated the relationships between season of birth, gender, and familial risk. The sample was the same as that in the previous report, with the addition of 2 male and 5 female probands, for a total of 381 probands and 1,931 first-degree relatives. Methods were the same as in the previous paper. Risk was modeled separately by proband gender using Cox PH models, controlling for the relative's age, season of birth, gender, and number of first-degree relatives. Among the relatives of female probands, the morbid risk for schizophrenia was highest for those born between February and May. Among the families of male probands, morbid risk was also highest for those born from February to May but only in relatives younger than age 30 years. The exact meaning of these findings is unclear.

Wolyniec et al. (1992) reanalyzed their data including relatives diagnosed with both schizophrenia and unspecified functional psychosis (collectively referred to as nonaffective psychosis) as affected. Cox PH models were used, adjusting for duration of illness of the proband and gender of the relative and incorporating an interaction term for proband gender and gender of family member. The first-degree relatives of female probands were found to have a significantly higher rate of nonaffective psychosis than the first-degree relatives of male probands. The increased risk to relatives of female probands was found to be consistent for parents, siblings, and children and for both male and female relatives. The fact that the relatives of the two proband groups did not differ with respect to either psychotic or nonpsychotic affective disorders lends support to the validity of the findings. The investigators acknowledge that their use of the Cox PH model assumes that morbid risks, as measured by onset times, were uncorrelated among family members and that this assumption may be wrong. However, failure to adjust for correlation of onsets among family members would tend to inflate the risk estimates but should not bias them for one or the other gender.

Family study method. Only three reports have used the family study method of collecting clinical information. They used the data from the Iowa 500 and non-500 studies (Morrison et al. 1972; Tsuang and Winokur 1975). Probands with a chart diagnosis of schizophrenia were obtained from 510 consecutive admissions to a tertiary psychiatric hospital in Iowa between 1934 and 1945. Patients were interviewed in the 1970s and blindly rediagnosed by DSM-III criteria in the mid-1980s using all available information (Kendler et al. 1985). Age at onset, however, was not restricted to 45 years. Family members were diagnosed using DSM-III criteria by investigators who were blind to proband status.

The first study examined the rates of atypical versus typical schizophrenia in male and female relatives of probands (Loyd et al. 1985). Nine hundred eighty-four first-degree relatives of 417 probands (typical and atypical) were assessed. "Atypical" was defined as DSM-III paranoid disorder, schizoaffective disorder, atypical psychosis, schizophreniform disorder, and SPD. "Typical" was defined as DSM-III schizophrenia. Stromgren's abridged method of age correction was used (Stromgren 1987). The authors reported no significant differences in the risk for atypical versus typical schizophrenia in male versus female relatives among atypical or typical schizophrenic proband families. One must keep in mind that their definition of atypical included a number of diagnoses that have not been shown to have a differential distribution by sex. Only schizoaffective disorders and paranoid disorder have been found to occur at higher rates among females (Goldstein and Link 1988; Lewine 1981; Orbell et al. 1990; Ring et al. 1991). Thus, the effect of gender may have been attenuated by including the other diagnoses. In fact, in a recent study by Goldstein and colleagues (1993) using the same data set as Loyd and colleagues, the effect of gender on the transmission of schizoaffective disorder was investigated. Goldstein and colleagues reported a significantly higher rate of schizophrenia and schizophreniform and schizoaffective disorders in the relatives of female schizoaffective probands compared with relatives of male probands. The finding held when probands were divided into "mainly schizophrenic" and "mainly affective" and when divided into "schizoaffective, depressed" versus "schizoaffective, manic."

Goldstein and co-workers (1990) also examined the effect of probands' and relatives' gender on the transmission of schizophrenia using Kaplan-Meier estimates obtained from survival analysis (Lee 1980). Seven hundred fourteen relatives of 332 (51.5% male) DSM-III schizophrenic patients were studied. The analyses were controlled for age and fertility effects. Goldstein and co-workers reported a significantly higher risk for schizophrenia in relatives of female versus male probands (5.2%, SE 1.1, for relatives of female probands versus 2.2%, SE 0.8, for relatives of male probands). The finding was consistent among parents, siblings, and children, although there was low statistical power to test for effects among separate classes of relatives. There were no significant differences between relatives of female versus male probands for rates of anxiety, affective, or alcohol disorders. Furthermore, females were more likely to be from families in which more than one person was affected, and *only* female probands were from families in which two or more members were affected. Thus, not only were there more relatives affected among female proband families, but the density of illness within female proband families was greater.

When the definition of illness in relatives was expanded to include schizophreniform and schizoaffective disorders, gender differences remained. However, when the definition of illness in relatives was expanded to include the full spectrum (schizophrenia, schizoaffective disorder, schizophreniform, paranoid, atypical psychosis, and SPD), gender differences in familial risk were attenuated (9.4%, SE 1.5) versus (8.7%, SE 1.7). This was due to the inclusion of SPD, for which relatives of male probands had a significantly higher risk than relatives of female probands. Thus, the results of this study showed that relatives of female probands were at higher risk for the *psychotic* forms of the illness spectrum (schizophrenia and schizophreniform and schizoaffective disorders), whereas relatives of male probands were at higher risk for the *nonpsychotic* form (SPD).

When the data were analyzed by sex of the relative, no significant differences were found for any definition of illness or for sex concordance among siblings who were both ill. However, few same-sex siblings were both ill, so this study could not truly test for concordance. It is unfortunate that the study could not test whether same-sex concordance was related to paternal versus maternal inheritance.

The strength of the study by Goldstein and colleagues (1990) was the use of family member diagnostic data obtained primarily by personal interviews (i.e., the family study method). The study has been criticized for obtaining relatively few personal interviews with parents (only 7% of the interviewed relatives were parents because most had died before the time of the interview). This may have underestimated illness and changed the denominator (those at risk) used in the survival analyses, which, in turn, may have led to an overestimation of the significance of effects (Wolyniec et al. 1992). To increase the sensitivity of the estimates of illness, diagnoses were made from the medical records of all dead relatives who were hospitalized, which may have increased morbidity estimates. However, comparisons of patterns of illness that both included and excluded these cases showed similar results (Kendler et al. 1985). In addition, it has been shown that parents are less likely to be ill than siblings or children of the proband because fertility is decreased in schizophrenia (Vogel 1979). Because the significant effect of the proband's gender was restricted to siblings alone, the validity of the findings is supported. Furthermore, the effect seemed to apply to children of probands, but the results were not significant because of the small number of children. Finally, the Iowa study reported a 3% prevalence rate of schizophrenia among the relatives of schizophrenic persons (Kendler et al. 1985), which, although it was at the lower end of the reports in the literature at the time, is supported by more recent studies.

In contrast to studies using the family history method, Goldstein and colleagues (1990) reported a significant difference in the rate of SPD among relatives of male probands compared with relatives of female probands. Family history studies cannot examine SPD because it is highly underestimated or unestimated. Thus, the significant findings in the family history studies (reported above) regarding higher rates of illness among female proband families relate to the psychotic spectrum disorders rather than to the full schizophrenia spectrum. On the other hand, when the data were collected for the Iowa study, criteria for SPD were not operationalized. Thus, SPD is most likely also underestimated in the Iowa study, but it is unlikely to be differentially underestimated among female families. Replication is necessary using the family study method with large samples.

Goldstein and colleagues (1990) reported no significant differences in the rates of illness for male versus female relatives. However, there were relatively few affected relatives (27 with schizophrenia and 33 with other spectrum disorders); thus, the statistical power to detect significant differences by sex of the relative may have been low.

In a further set of analyses, Goldstein and colleagues (1993) examined whether the effects of season of birth, age at onset, premorbid history, and symptomatology (flat affect, depression, and paranoia) could help to explain the elevated rates of schizophrenia in relatives of female probands. These variables were chosen because they have been shown to be differentially expressed among men and women. Findings showed no significant effects of these factors to help explain the gender transmission effect. There was adequate power to test these factors, so negative results are meaningful. There also were no significant interactions of these factors with gender. Dividing the probands into groups of age at onset below and above 17 years as was done by Pulver's group did not elicit interactive effects. However, few patients had an age at onset of less than 17 years; thus, there was low statistical power to test for an interaction. Variables used in this analysis may not have been those key to explaining the higher rates of illness among female proband families. For example, premorbid history was used as an indicator of neurodevelopmental factors and season of birth as an indicator of neonatal viral factors, both of which may be important for understanding differential effects of gender (O'Callaghan et al. 1991). However, these indicators are crude. More precise indicators of the explanatory factors of interest are needed.

Goldstein and colleagues (1993) suggest that gender differences in transmission may, in part, be a function of pleiotropy. That is, the schizophrenia gene may be differentially expressed in relatives of male versus female probands. These investigators have recently found that if flat affect in otherwise healthy relatives is included in the definition of a case, gender differences in transmission are attenuated. Relatives of male probands were found to have a significantly higher rate of flat affect than relatives of female probands. (The relatives with observed flat or blunted affect were free of any psychiatric disorder.) This finding suggests that the expression of the abnormal gene or genes involved in schizophrenia may be differentially affected by gender. If pleiotropy were operating, one should see differences in schizophrenia prevalence between male and female relatives of probands of both sexes. This has not been demonstrated. However, prevalence rates depend on the definition of a case. If the genetic spectrum of schizophrenia includes flat affect in the definition of the phenotype, as argued for in a recent study (Tsuang et al. 1991), one might see a greater gender difference in prevalence.

Summary

In this chapter, I addressed whether gender had an effect on the familial transmission of schizophrenia and related spectrum disorders. Taken together, the evidence from twin and sibling concordance studies and family transmission studies suggests that there is an important effect of gender that needs to be understood. The pre– and post–World War II twin studies examining same-sex concordance were inconsistent. It was suggested that this inconsistency was caused by ascertainment bias. Because more chronically ill women were hospitalized than men, it was argued that one would expect to find more female same-sex concordance among twins. However, same-sex concordance in these studies was dependent on the strictness of the diagnostic criteria that were used. That is, using narrow criteria, female twins were found to show more same-sex concordance than male twins. Using broad criteria, male twins were more concordant. It has been shown that, compared with males, more female schizophrenic patients, diagnosed using criteria before DSM-III, have been rediagnosed as having affective disorders based on current criteria. Thus, a sample of female patients with schizophrenia diagnosed before DSM-III was more likely than a male sample to include affective psychosis.

More recent studies that have hypothesized a pseudoautosomal locus for schizophrenia have argued that same-sex concordance would occur primarily if the abnormal gene(s) was paternally inherited. Thus, inconsistency in previous studies may have been a result of the lack of control for paternal or maternal transmission. As I have argued, interstudy inconsistency is most likely caused by differences in the definition of the phenotype, statistical power, and genetic assumptions based on penetrance parameters and gene frequency estimates.

The pseudoautosomal hypothesis has been revised recently by the same investigators who proposed it (Crow et al. 1994; DeLisi et al. 1994). They suggest that the inconsistent results from linkage studies of the telomeric, pseudoautosomal region implicated a schizophrenia gene in a nearby sex-specific region of the X and Y chromosomes. Their results showed some support for a dominant X-Y model of transmission in which homologous genes on X and Y contributed to the genetic susceptibility to schizophrenia. Although further work is needed before one can make definitive statements about X-Y transmission in schizophrenia, the model provides a mechanism for gender differences in the expression and transmission of schizophrenia. Because homologous genes are not identical, their effects on pathophysiology and phenotypic expression are not necessarily identical. Given that women cannot transmit the Y form of the homologous gene, the model also allows for differences in affected relatives based on the sex of the proband, which has been the main finding from family transmission studies of sex and schizophrenia. That is, family history and family study methods have provided evidence from different countries and different areas of the United States that relatives of female probands with schizophrenia are at significantly higher risk for schizophrenia and the psychotic forms of the spectrum than relatives of male probands. Furthermore, the density of the illness within families is greater for female proband families than male proband families. It is unclear whether this effect extends to the full spectrum (i.e., when SPD is included in the affected phenotype). Only one study was able to test this theory because the other studies used the family history method and thus could not reliably diagnose SPD.

Family transmission studies have, in general, also reported a nonsignificant effect of the relative's gender on the expression of schizophrenia and spectrum disorders. However, all of the studies had a relatively small number of affected relatives, resulting in low statistical power to test the effect of the relative's gender. Therefore, it is important to replicate these studies using the family study method to estimate the size and significance of this effect; an effect of the relative's gender on transmissibility would imply that there is a significant gender difference in the prevalence of the disorder. Because gender differences in the prevalence of currently diagnosed schizophrenia and/or spectrum disorders are still undetermined in the literature, a family study would be one useful approach.

Furthermore, it has been suggested that the effect of gender on the transmission of schizophrenia may be related to age at onset and season of birth. For example, in one family history study, male probands who had an age at onset below 17 had a higher rate of affected relatives than those who became ill after age 17, whereas age at onset was not related to risk in the relatives of female probands. This was not replicated by a family study. However, the effect of onset age should be examined further because both studies had few early-onset probands and, thus, low statistical power to test for a gender effect.

In addition, season of birth may be an indicator of environmental factors that are differentially influenced by gender (O'Callaghan et al. 1991). Several studies have reported significant gender differences in season of birth. One study reported a significant relationship between viral infection prenatally and subsequent onset of schizophrenia among women but not men (O'Callaghan et al. 1991). Environmental factors, such as prenatal exposure to viral infection (O'Callaghan et al. 1991), may have a different impact on the development of the brain in male and female fetuses. This may interact with genetic factors to produce a differential expression of the gene(s) for schizophrenia in men and women. Further work in this area is needed.

Recent work has also suggested that pleiotropy may contribute to explaining the gender effect on transmission. That is, the schizophrenia gene(s) may be somewhat differently expressed in men and women. For instance, flat affect has been found significantly more often in otherwise healthy relatives of male probands compared with healthy relatives of female probands.

Chapter 3 in this volume contains a discussion of other mechanisms that may account for differences between men and women in the heritability of schizophrenia.

References

American Psychiatric Association: Diagnostic and Statistical Manual: Mental Disorders. Washington, DC, American Psychiatric Association, 1952

American Psychiatric Association: Diagnostic and Statistical Manual of Mental Disorders, 2nd Edition. Washington, DC, American Psychiatric Association, 1968

American Psychiatric Association: Diagnostic and Statistical Manual of Mental Disorders, 3rd Edition. Washington, DC, American Psychiatric Association, 1980

American Psychiatric Association: Diagnostic and Statistical Manual of Mental Disorders, 3rd Edition, Revised. Washington, DC, American Psychiatric Association, 1987

American Psychiatric Association: Diagnostic and Statistical Manual of Mental Disorders, 4th Edition. Washington, DC, American Psychiatric Association, 1994

Angermeyer MC, Kuhn L, Goldstein JM: Gender and the course of schizophrenia: differences in treated outcomes. Schizophr Bull 16:293–307, 1990

Asherson P, Parfitt E, Sargeant M, et al: No evidence for a pseudoautosomal locus for schizophrenia: linkage analysis of multiply affected families. Br J Psychiatry 161:63–68, 1992

Bellodi L, Bussoleni C, Scorza-Smeraldi R, et al: Family study of schizophrenia: exploratory analysis for relevant factors. Schizophr Bull 12:120–128, 1986

Collinge J, DeLisi LE, Boccio A, et al: Evidence for a pseudoautosomal locus for schizophrenia using the method of affected sibling pairs. Br J Psychiatry 158:624–629, 1991

Crow TJ: Sex chromosomes and psychosis: the case for a pseudoautosomal locus. Br J Psychiatry 153:675–683, 1988

Crow TJ, DeLisi LE, Johnstone EC: Concordance by sex in sibling pairs with schizophrenia is paternally inherited: evidence for a pseudoautosomal locus. Br J Psychiatry 155:92–97, 1989

Crow TJ, DeLisi LE, Johnstone EC: In reply . . . a locus closer to the telomere? Br J Psychiatry 156:416–420, 1990

Crow TJ, DeLisi LE, Lofthouse R, et al: An examination of linkage of schizophrenia and schizoaffective disorder to the pseudoautosomal region (Xp22.3). Br J Psychiatry 164:159–164, 1994

Curtis D, Gurling H: Unsound methodology in investigating a pseudoautosomal locus in schizophrenia. Br J Psychiatry 156:415–416, 1990

D'Amato T, Campion D, Gorwood PH, et al: Evidence for a pseudoautosomal locus for schizophrenia, II: replication of a non-random segregation of alleles at the DXYS14 locus. Br J Psychiatry 161:59–62, 1992

DeLisi LE, Crow TJ: Evidence for a sex chromosome locus for schizophrenia. Schizophr Bull 15:431–440, 1989

DeLisi LE, Devoto M, Lofthouse R, et al: Search for linkage to schizophrenia on the X and Y chromosomes. Am J Med Genet 54:113–121, 1994

Elston RC, Namboodiri KK, Spence MA, et al: A genetic study of schizophrenia pedigrees, II: one locus hypotheses. Neuropsychobiology 4:193–206, 1978

Feighner JP, Robins E, Guze SB, et al: Diagnostic criteria for use in psychiatric research. Arch Gen Psychiatry 26:57–63, 1972

Fischer M: Genetic and environmental factors in schizophrenia. Acta Psychiatr Scand 238 (suppl):61–72, 1973

Foerster A, Lewis SW, Owen MJ, et al: Pre-morbid adjustment and personality in psychosis: effects of sex and diagnosis. Br J Psychiatry 158:171–176, 1991

Goldstein JM: Gender differences in the course of schizophrenia. Am J Psychiatry 145:684–689, 1988

Goldstein JM: Impact of sampling biases in explaining discrepancies in studies on gender and schizophrenia: a reply. Schizophr Bull 19:9–14, 1993

Goldstein JM, Link BG: Gender and the expression of schizophrenia. J Psychiatr Res 22:141–155, 1988

Goldstein JM, Faraone SV, Chen WJ, et al: Sex differences in the familial transmission of schizophrenia. Br J Psychiatry 156:819–826, 1990

Goldstein JM, Faraone SV, Chen WJ, et al: The role of gender in understanding the transmission of schizoaffective disorder. Br J Psychiatry 163:763–768, 1993

Gorwood PH, Leboyer M, D'Amato T, et al: Evidence for a pseudoautosomal locus for schizophrenia, I: a replication study using phenotype analysis. Br J Psychiatry 161:55–58, 1992

Gottesman II, Shields J: Schizophrenia and Genetics: A Twin Study Vantage Point. New York, Academic Press, 1972

Gottesman II, Shields J: Schizophrenia: The Epigenetic Puzzle. Cambridge, MA, Cambridge University Press, 1982

Green JR, Woodrow JC: Sibling method for detecting HLA linked genes in diseases. Tissue Antigens 9:31–35, 1977

Kallman FJ: The genetic theory of schizophrenia: an analysis of 691 schizophrenic twin index families. Am J Psychiatry 103:309–322, 1946

Kendler KS, Gruenberg AM, Tsuang MT: Psychiatric illness in first-degree relatives of schizophrenic and surgical control patients. Arch Gen Psychiatry 42:770–779, 1985

Kringlen E: An epidemiological-clinical twin study on schizophrenia, in The Transmission of Schizophrenia. Edited by Rosenthal D, Kety S. Oxford, Pergamon, 1968, pp 49–63

Lee ET: Statistical Methods for Survival Data Analysis. Belmont, CA, Lifetime Learning Publications, 1980

Lewine RRJ: Sex differences in schizophrenia: a commentary. Schizophr Bull 5:4–7, 1979

Lewine RRJ: Sex differences in schizophrenia: timing or subtypes? Psychol Bull 90:432–444, 1981

Lewine RRJ, Burbach D, Meltzer HY: Effect of diagnostic criteria on the ratio of male to female schizophrenic patients. Am J Psychiatry 141:84–87, 1984

Liang KY: Estimating effects of probands' characteristics on familial risk, I: adjustment for censoring and correlated ages at onset. Genet Epidemiol 8:329–338, 1991

Loyd DW, Simpson JC, Tsuang MT: A family study of sex differences in the diagnosis of atypical schizophrenia. Am J Psychiatry 142:1366–1368, 1985

Luxenberger H: Vorlaufiger Bericht uber psychiatrische Serienuntersuchungen an Zwillingen [First report of a series of psychiatric twins]. Zeitschrift fur die gesamte Neurologie und Psychiatrie [Journal of Neurology and Psychiatry] 116:297–326, 1928

Luxenberger H: Die Manifestationswahrscheinlichkeit der Schizophrenie im Lichte der Zwillingsforschung [The expression of schizophrenia in twins]. Zeitschrift fur Psychische Hygiene [Journal of Psychiatric Hygiene] 7:174–184, 1934

Morrison J, Clancy J, Crowe R, et al: The Iowa 500, I: diagnostic validity in mania, depression, and schizophrenia. Arch Gen Psychiatry 27:457–461, 1972

Mott FW: Hereditary aspects of nervous and mental diseases. BMJ 2:1013–1020, 1910

Myerson A: Inheritance of Mental Disease. Baltimore, MD, Williams & Wilkins, 1925

Nasrallah HA, Wilcox JA: Gender differences in the etiology and symptoms of schizophrenia: genetic vs brain injury effects. Annals of Clinical Psychiatry 1:51–53, 1989

Nimgaonkar VL, Wessley S, Murray RM: Prevalence of familiality, obstetric complications, and structural brain damage in schizophrenic patients. Br J Psychiatry 153:191–197, 1988

O'Callaghan E, Sham P, Takei N, et al: Schizophrenia after prenatal exposure to 1957 A2 influenza epidemic. Lancet 337:1248–1250, 1991

Orbell S, Trew K, McWhirter L: Mental illness in Northern Ireland: a comparison with Scotland and England. Soc Psychiatry Psychiatr Epidemiol 25:165–169, 1990

Penrose LS: Survey of cases of familial mental illness. Mimeographed document prepared for the Division of Psychiatric Research, Ontario Department of Health, abstracted in Digest of Neurology and Psychiatry 13:644, 1945

Pollock HM, Malzberg B, Fuller RG: Hereditary and Environmental Factors in the Causation of Manic-Depressive Psychoses and Dementia Praecox. Utica, NY, State Hospitals Press, 1939, pp 98–124

Pulver AE, Liang KY: Estimating effects of proband characteristics on familial risk, II: the association between age at onset and familial risk in the Maryland schizophrenia sample. Genet Epidemiol 8:339–350, 1991

Pulver AE, Brown CH, Wolyniec P, et al: Schizophrenia: age at onset, gender, and familial risk. Acta Psychiatr Scand 82:344–351, 1990

Reed SC, Hartley C, Anderson VE, et al: The Psychoses: Family Studies. Philadelphia, PA, WB Saunders, 1973

Ring N, Tantam D, Montague L, et al: Gender differences in the incidence of definite schizophrenia and atypical psychosis—focus on negative symptoms of schizophrenia. Acta Psychiatr Scand 84:489–496, 1991

Risch N: A note on multiple testing procedures in linkage analysis. Am J Hum Genet 48:1058–1064, 1991

Rosanoff A, Handy L, Plesset I, et al: The etiology of so-called schizophrenic psychoses. Am J Psychiatry 91:247, 1934

Rosenthal D: Familial concordance by sex with respect to schizophrenia. Psychol Bull 59:401–421, 1962

Salokangas RKR: Prognostic implications of the sex of schizophrenic patients. Br J Psychiatry 142:145–151, 1983

Samuels L: Reply to Lewine (letter). Schizophr Bull 5:8–10, 1979

Schulz B: Zur Erbpathologie der Schizophrenie [On inherited pathology of schizophrenia]. Zeitschrift für die Gesammte Neurologie und Psychiatrie [Journal of Neurology and Psychiatry] 143:175–293, 1932

Shimizu A, Masayoshi K, Yamaguchi N, et al: Morbidity risk of schizophrenia to parents and siblings of schizophrenic patients. Jpn J Psychiatry Neurol 41:65–70, 1987

Slater E: The monogenic theory of schizophrenia. Acta Genetica Statistica Medica 8:50–56, 1958

Spitzer RL, Endicott J, Robins E: Research Diagnostic Criteria: rationale and reliability. Arch Gen Psychiatry 35:773–782, 1978

Stromgren E: Changes in the incidence of schizophrenia? Br J Psychiatry 150:1–7, 1987

Sturt E, Shur E: Sex concordance for schizophrenia in proband-relative pairs. Br J Psychiatry 147:44–47, 1985

Tsuang MT: A study of pairs of siblings both hospitalized for mental disorder. Br J Psychiatry 113:283–300, 1967

Tsuang MT, Winokur G: The Iowa-500: field work in a 35-year follow-up of depression, mania, and schizophrenia. Canadian Psychiatric Association Journal 20:359–365, 1975

Tsuang MT, Gilbertson MW, Faraone SV: Genetic transmission of negative and positive symptoms in the biological relatives of schizophrenics, in Negative Versus Positive Schizophrenia. Edited by Marneros A, Andreasen NC, Tsuang MT. Berlin, Springer-Verlag, 1991, pp 265–291

Vogel HP: Fertility and sibship size in a psychiatric patient population. Acta Psychiatr Scand 60:483–503, 1979

Wahl OF, Hunter J: Are gender effects being neglected in schizophrenia research? Schizophr Bull 18:313–318, 1992

Wolyniec PS, Pulver AE, McGrath JA, et al: Schizophrenia: gender and familial risk. J Psychiatr Res 26:17–27, 1992

World Health Organization: International Classification of Diseases, 8th Revision. Geneva, World Health Organization, 1968

CHAPTER 10

Gender Differences in Treatment Response in Schizophrenia

Mary V. Seeman, M.D., C.M., F.R.C.P.C.

I s it possible that the relatively favorable outcome in women who have schizophrenia can best be accounted for by superior service provision to women or, alternatively, better response by women to one or more of the current treatments? The first explanation is not further entertained in this chapter because programs for schizophrenia, without exception, report an overwhelming majority of male attendees, enough to raise a legitimate concern that women's needs in this area are being neglected (Perkins and Rowland 1991). A more promising lead to understanding differential outcome between the sexes (at least short-term outcome; there is no convincing evidence that long-term course is superior in women) is to examine treatment response.

To study treatment effectiveness in men and women, many variables must be considered: those known to influence outcome in schizophrenia as well as those suspected of being significantly sexually dichotomized in unaffected men and women. The first category includes factors such as extent and severity of neurodevelopmental mishaps, perinatal complications, enduring presence of neurological soft signs, premorbid health, age at onset, pretreatment duration of symptoms, target symptom responsiveness to neuroleptics, extent of substance use, fidelity of self-monitoring and treatment adherence, familial emotional environment, felt pressure of social expectations, and extent and quality of social supports. In the second category are immune, hormonal, brain laterality and brain perfusion factors, drug metabolism, the ratio of lean body mass to adipose tissue, and sex-specific biosocial development and sociocultural norms. No studies have, as yet, attempted to address all these complex interactive variables in a systematic fashion, although their importance is becoming recognized.

There is a consensus that women with schizophrenia benefit more than men from psychosocial treatments (Keskiner et al. 1973; Mowbray and Chamberlain 1986; Segal and Everett-Dille 1980), which is usually explained from a family interaction or social role perspective. Also, a separate literature suggests that women benefit more than men from neuroleptic drugs (Nedopil et al. 1983; Seeman 1983a, 1989; Yonkers et al. 1992). The explanations for this effect are usually conceptualized in terms of biological differences between the sexes. From another perspective, however, it could equally plausibly be argued that male-female differences in the social and interpersonal realm are biogenetically programmed to subserve evolutionary imperatives, whereas differences in drug response reflect socially sanctioned dependency and compliance in women versus learned autonomy and rebelliousness in men. In other words, the impact of social forces may be biologically based, and response to biological treatments may be learned. Such distinctions are clearly artificial and not helpful to the treating clinician.

The following descriptions of two women being treated for schizophrenia illustrate the current state of knowledge about sex-specific treatment issues but do not in any way resolve etiological questions. Possible determinants of differential response are considered only for their inherent interest and are proposed in full appreciation of their uncertain empirical base.

Alicia

Alicia, now age 26, has been experiencing difficulties since early high school. They were behavioral difficulties at first—school problems, insubordination, and anger. Eventually, they led to a psychiatric assessment, a hospital admission, and a diagnosis of schizophrenia.

Currently, Alicia is trying to complete nursing school. She works diligently and finds her life to be very stressful. She is seeing a psychiatrist regularly and has been taking antipsychotic medication for several years. She has developed severe eye blinking and sporadic, spasmodic tightening of her neck muscles. She smiles very rarely and appears to others to be cold, sullen, and indifferent.

Alicia studies assiduously but is interested in little else. She does not care about her appearance, her food intake, the condition of her room, or the maintenance of friendships from the past. She has difficulty setting personal treatment goals. Her parents have proposed the following goals for her therapy: 1) ensuring her continuation and eventual graduation from nursing school (i.e., vocational rehabilitation); 2) improving her appearance (i.e., mastery of the skills of daily living); 3) ensuring clean, safe housing (i.e., adaptation to family or residential or autonomous living); 4) reversing her tardive dyskinesia (i.e., safe and effective psychopharmacology); 5) working toward marriage and a family (i.e., mastery of psychosocial skills); and 6) anticipating the course of illness (i.e., accurate prognosis).

Gender Differences in Vocational Rehabilitation

Alicia's psychiatrist works very hard, thus far successfully, to keep her in nursing school. Would the effort be justified if the patient were a man (Pakaslahti 1992)? For young men with schizophrenia, the expectation to perform is currently conceptualized as adding to their burdens, contributing to their amotivational state, and influencing the grandiose nature of their delusions and hallucinations. Psychoeducational programs to reduce familial expressed emotion, based primarily on results with male patients (Flaherty and Jobe 1990; Hogarty et al. 1986; Vaughn et al. 1984), routinely advise families to lower expectations for vocational achievement (Birchwood et al. 1992).

Based on the clinical literature, Alicia's chances at success in school are higher because she is a woman. After being hospitalized for schizophrenia, men usually do not succeed scholastically, but this is not true for women. The fact that nursing, for example, requires interpersonal skills would make this course of study even more daunting for a man with schizophrenia.

This theory may be traceable to sex differences in social development. Block (1973, 1983) has described a sequence of developmental stages at which human beings are progressively confronted with problems of ever-increasing complexity. She conceptualizes these problems as solvable either by pursuing individual needs or by attempting to accommodate the goals of the larger social group. Block describes early stages of development in both sexes as being characterized by the pursuit of individual goals. Theoretically, at each sequential stage, individuality-enhancing skills are reinforced in boys, whereas girls are taught social-communal skills. Experimentally, however, it has not been easy to reproduce any solid sex differences in social tendencies (Steinberg 1987). It is possible that it is only the *pace* of social development that differs between the two sexes and that the sex-related deficiency in social skills is especially marked in young men with schizophrenia because they become ill during adolescence before effective socialization has been consolidated (Angermeyer and Kühn 1988; Riecher-Rössler et al. 1992).

Difficulties in socializing result in poor support networks. Other nursing students mingle with one another and use each other for support to buffer the stress of supervisor demands, new learning, life-and-death situations, deadlines, and sleepless nights, but Alicia keeps her distance. She essentially has no friends and communicates with very few people outside the ambit of her therapist and her immediate family. She lacks the social supports with which most individuals buffer stress (Alloway and Bebbington 1987).

Alicia's therapist incorporates cognitive and behavioral techniques into his treatment to help her manage work-related stress. No studies have addressed gender-specific response to such treatment (Liberman and Evans 1985). Because of Alicia's habitual ambivalence, she has difficulty making decisions. Her doctor, therefore, considers nursing a good career choice because of its hierarchical structure that insulates line nurses from having to make purely autonomous decisions. Young men with schizophrenia, although as ambivalent as women, are prone to question rules and to break them (Kay et al.

1988). This automatic opposition to authority makes employment and school options more difficult for male patients.

The shift work required in nursing is an important concern for mental health. Changes in sleep, alimentary, and energy cycles affect mood, hormonal status, and immunity. Whether these transitions are particularly difficult in patients with schizophrenia or more difficult to adapt to in one sex or another is not known. Interestingly, however, the brain's suprachiasmatic nucleus, which controls circadian and other biorhythms, is sexually dimorphic in humans and other mammals (deVries et al. 1984).

Gender Differences in Mastery of Skills of Daily Living

Alicia's parents are most distressed by her neglect of her clothing— her tendency to wear mismatched tops and bottoms and to be careless about matching colors. Alicia often forgets to comb her hair and does not wear makeup. Whenever her mother insists that Alicia wear cosmetics, she applies too much and begins to look eccentric. Although Alicia does not outwardly comply with her mother's wishes, inwardly she rates herself by her mother's standards, and concerns such as weight, hair, skin, nails, and dress code are important to Alicia.

Men with schizophrenia—as a rule—pay much less attention to their hygiene and grooming and, consequently, elicit more avoidance and negative reaction. They become ill so early in life that, in most cases, they are deficient in the domestic skills of laundering, ironing, mending, and shopping. In women, these skills need retooling after an episode of schizophrenia. In men, these skills must be learned for the first time, which is a much more difficult task.

Mention of grooming and external appearance in patients with schizophrenia must include the unfortunate effects of neuroleptic drugs on skin, hair, weight, posture, gait, flexibility, agility, agitation, facial expression, grimacing, sedation, and tremor. For instance, an article by Gopalaswamy and Morgan (1985) with the provocative title "Too Many Chronic Mentally Disabled Patients Are Too Fat" addresses the overweight problem (36% in female patients and 15%

in male patients versus 6%–8% in the general population).

Alicia's deadpan expression is unquestionably caused by her neuroleptics. Her doctor took the trouble of explaining this side effect of medication to Alicia's nursing school instructors who had, until then, thought that her facial blandness was an indication of indifference or even arrogance. Once they learned that, contrary to her appearance, Alicia was a very caring person who was interested in her work and her patients, she overcame a potentially serious obstacle to her continued schooling.

Gender Differences in Accommodation and Family Treatment

As an investment for Alicia's future, her parents bought her a condominium apartment, which they rent out while Alicia lives in the nursing residence. Alicia wants to leave the residence to live in her apartment. At the residence, Alicia has at least superficial contact with others and can eat in the cafeteria. In her own apartment, she would be more isolated and would have to cook for herself. She does not keep her room in the residence very clean, and there is every reason to believe that she would not keep her apartment clean. She does not smoke, but her parents worry, nevertheless, about the possibility of fire. They also worry about how lonely she might be in a self-contained apartment. This decision has become the focus of family treatment involving Alicia and her parents.

The core issue revolves around the relative importance of self-reliance, on one hand, and relatedness on the other. The apartment would be private, and Alicia would have autonomous control. She would, however, be more cut off from other people and would be more lonely. Parental criticism about how she manages the apartment could be expected to increase, but she would have more freedom to keep her private life to herself and in that way, perhaps, incur less criticism. An immediate correct solution is not apparent.

For a male patient, the optimal balance might shift toward a recommendation for sheltered communal living. As mentioned above, domestic skills and social skills are usually too poorly developed in men with schizophrenia to allow comfortable independence. Men are often too dangerously impulsive, and they have difficulty maintaining cleanliness. Because autonomy is so important to men, however, many men with schizophrenia do live alone. The nature of one's accommodations is one of the most important aspects of quality of life; therefore, it is essential to consider in the comprehensive treatment of schizophrenia. A survey in Britain (Conning and Rowland 1991) found that equal numbers of men and women with schizophrenia chose to live alone, independent of hostel or family. These people probably represent the least severely ill and most autonomous but also the very ill who find it impossible to live with others and whom others cannot tolerate. In the survey, of those living with families, the women usually lived with spouses or children; the men lived with parents.

This finding has important implications for family therapy studies, which often select patients residing with their parents as subjects. Thus, most subjects in experimental studies have been men, but the results of family therapy have been extrapolated, perhaps prematurely, to both sexes.

One study of inpatient family treatment for schizophrenia did take gender into account (Glick et al. 1990; Haas et al. 1990). The results were suggestive of superior outcomes for women when a family format intervention was added to standard care during hospital admission. The benefits were present at discharge and still evident at 18-month follow-up for both the severely ill and the more moderately ill women. Men appeared, paradoxically, to be disadvantaged, vis-à-vis control men, by the family therapy intervention.

The sample in this study consisted of 49 men and 43 women consecutively admitted with DSM-III (American Psychiatric Association 1980) schizophrenia disorders. Ages ranged from 18 to 45 years. One randomly assigned group received the family intervention; the other group did not. Both groups also received a partially fixed drug regimen: 150–2,920 mg chlorpromazine equivalents per day. All patients were given therapeutic activity, psychotherapy, group therapy, and a milieu therapy that stressed structure, support, limit setting, social skills, and problem solving. Therapeutic contact time was equalized so that the group receiving the additional family intervention received correspondingly fewer hours of individual psychotherapy.

The family intervention consisted of a brief number (mean, 8.6; mode, 6.0) of family treatments with a central psychoeducational component derived from standard family intervention models, which the authors describe in detail. Explanations for the differential outcome can only be speculative. Family treatment, which stresses cooperation and shared decision making, may require patients to accept a degree of dependency on family, which is generally not acceptable to men in North American culture. At the same time, families may find it more difficult to lower their expectations of sons, regardless of how ill, than of daughters—a readjustment that is necessary for the success of most current family approaches.

A study of 90 female and 97 male (age 19 years) psychology students from mostly intact families in the general population hypothesized that men and women interpret interpersonal behavior differently (Hampson and Beavers 1987). The women endorsed more positive expressions about familial behaviors (e.g., "our family members touch and hug each other")—based on a family inventory. Female scores on positive emotional expressiveness within their families significantly exceeded male scores. Further analysis suggested that, because women perceived more positive emotion, they also saw less conflict, less enmeshment, and less authoritarianism. For instance, when women endorsed statements such as "there was a feeling of togetherness in our family," they did not also endorse "family members found it hard to get away from one another." Men, on the other hand, believed that both statements were true. In the men, scores for positive emotional expression and scores for enmeshment overlapped. The authors concluded that what females experience as warmth, males also perceive but may interpret as intrusion. What women view as interpersonal caring, men may experience as unwanted overinvolvement. This may shed some light on women's superior response to family treatment in schizophrenia.

Gender Differences in Neuroleptic Response

For an acute episode of psychosis, women may require lower doses of neuroleptics than do men to achieve remission (Kolakowska et al.

1985; Nedopil et al. 1983). Differential dose requirements may be accounted for by body size and weight, by activity level and aggressivity, or by active drug concentrations in plasma (Yonkers et al. 1992). Plasma concentrations, in turn, are an end result of many variables; one of these is smoking, which is probably an important variable in patients with schizophrenia (Goff et al. 1992). Neuroleptic concentrations are increased by the concomitant use of antidepressants, which is probably more prevalent in women with schizophrenia than in men (McCreadie et al. 1992). Regional brain blood flow differences may exist between men and women, which may affect the distribution of active drug to neuroleptic-sensitive sites (Seeman 1989). Acute side effects (e.g., dystonia) may be more frequent in men than in women (Casey 1991) because men receive higher doses. Under conditions of fixed dose, women experience more dystonia (Chakos et al. 1992). Subacute side effects, especially akathisia, are more prevalent in women despite the fact that their mean doses are lower (Casey 1991). This may be related to saturation of lipid stores, although several other explanations are possible (Seeman 1989; Yonkers et al. 1992). Because estrogens potentiate the neuroleptic effect, assessments at different periods of the menstrual cycle may affect drug response results (Häfner et al. 1991; Hallonquist et al. 1993).

Women also appear to require lower doses for relapse prevention, at least women under age 40 (Seeman 1983a). One explanation is that the protective effect of estrogens is lost as women approach menopause. Because neuroleptics interfere with the pituitary ovarian feedback loop in a significant proportion of women, it may be that, paradoxically, treatment undermines the protective estrogen effect in women. Loss of the menstrual cycle in neuroleptic-treated women correlates with prescribed dose, which is why it has been suggested that lowering the dose in neuroleptic-refractory women may restore hormonal cyclicity and permit the patient to respond (Häfner et al. 1991; Seeman and Lang 1990). Studies comparing neuroleptic responsiveness in men and women must take not only age but also hormonal status into account. Neuroleptic compliance is acknowledged to be better in women, perhaps because they experience fewer unpleasant side effects (Zito et al. 1985).

Tardive dyskinesia is said to be more prevalent in women than in men, especially in older age groups (Casey 1991), although this has been disputed more recently (Yassa et al. 1992). Estrogen withdrawal after menopause may contribute to this phenomenon. In addition, it has been suggested that patients with affective disorders develop tardive dyskinesia more readily while taking neuroleptics than patients with schizophrenia (Glazer et al. 1990; Yassa et al. 1992). Because more women demonstrate affective symptoms, these two observations may be linked.

Alicia's grimaces and tics are probably a manifestation of neuroleptic withdrawal dyskinesia because her drug dose had been lowered recently. However, adventitious muscle movements antedated and, indeed, precipitated the dosage reduction. The cyclic rise and fall of estrogens may sensitize dopamine receptors and predispose women to tardive dyskinesia (Bedard et al. 1984). If this is the case, estrogen therapy could be attempted in women (Villeneuve et al. 1980). Otherwise, management of tardive dyskinesia for both sexes requires use of neuroleptic doses as low as possible, a long-term strategy that may prove realistic in women because of the relatively benign course of their illness.

Gender Differences in Mastery of Psychosocial Skills Relative to Marriage

More women than men marry after an episode of schizophrenia (Riecher-Rössler et al. 1992; Ritsner et al. 1992). The task of living intimately with another person is relatively more difficult for men with schizophrenia, who often lack the initiative to carry out a successful courtship. Alicia is also quite asocial and has never had a boyfriend. When Alicia's parents asked her therapist about this behavior, he told them that this was unlikely to change but not impossible. Statistically, the men that Alicia is likely to attract would be psychiatrically disabled men encountered at various therapeutic functions (Brown and Heidelberg 1985). Many successful long-term companionships have been known to develop between psychiatric patients, although these partnerships inevitably suffer from financial and emotional burdens. Having children is usually a problem; childbirth itself is a biopsychosocial stressor, and the burden of child rearing is often impossible without adequate therapeutic support

(Apfel and Handel 1992; Waldo et al. 1987; Webster 1990).

Because both men and women with schizophrenia may be victims of sexual abuse (Holbrook 1989), it is important to include sex education in therapy programs (Coverdale and Aruffo 1989; Lukoff et al. 1986). Protection from sexually transmitted disease and from unwanted pregnancy are crucial elements in management (Seeman et al. 1991). This is, perhaps, especially so for women because most investigators agree that women with schizophrenia are more sexually active than men (Friedman and Harrison 1984; Rozensky and Berman 1984). The difference may be explained by the fact that men experience more deficit symptoms and lack the motivation to initiate sexual activity or by the effects of neuroleptics on male libido and sexual performance (Mitchell and Popkin 1980; Segraves 1989; Sullivan and Lukoff 1990).

Gender Differences in Prognosis

Insofar as accurate prediction is part of comprehensive treatment, the lifetime outlook of illness that is communicated to the patient and family must reflect what is known about gender effects on prognosis. Alicia's outlook is brighter than if she were a man. She is likely to be relatively free of symptoms, relatively free of acute psychotic recurrences, and more likely (than if she were a man) to stay in treatment and benefit from it (Salokongas 1983). She is more likely to be employed and to be shielded from the possible negative effects of familial overinvolvement and criticism (Flaherty and Jobe 1990; Goldstein and Kreisman 1988). She is more likely to retain her premorbid skills and to evaluate her life as satisfactory. She is, however, more likely to be beset by anxieties and depression and more likely to die prematurely. Although the suicide rate is higher in schizophrenic men than in schizophrenic women, the ratio of suicide in schizophrenic women to women in the general population is higher than the comparable ratio for men. If she were a man, there might be more entanglements with the law, more frequent crises, and a greater chance of homelessness and estrangement from the family (Heidensohn 1991; Seeman 1986; Watt et al. 1983).

When offering a prognosis, however, the clinician must keep

many other factors in mind. An important factor is age at onset. In Alicia's case, schizophrenia began in her teens so that her course of illness may follow a pattern more typical of males than of females. Disentangling the effect of onset age and gender is a complex task (Riecher-Rössler et al. 1992).

Jane

The case example of Jane illustrates a number of reproductive issues that are especially important in the treatment of women with schizophrenia. Jane gave birth to a premature infant weighing 2 pounds. Jane was homeless at the time she went into labor; she had gone to a hospital emergency department seeking shelter, had been assessed as acutely psychotic (she had a long history of schizophrenia), and had been given an injection of long-acting fluphenazine. Immediately after receiving the injection, she commenced labor. The birth itself was uneventful, but the infant was born with a number of motor and perceptual defects and was kept in the high-risk nursery. Jane was discharged after 3 days.

Because she did not have a home, Jane spent her time in the visitors' lounge at the hospital. She slept there, ate there, and did her laundry there. She talked to herself and said things out loud that were frightening to the other parents. The nursing staff complained that she hovered constantly over her baby and interfered with his care. She also threatened the emergency doctor who had given her the depot injection with a legal suit, claiming that the injection had brought on the premature labor. The social work staff wanted to contact Children's Aid to help plan the baby's posthospital care, but Jane refused. She also refused to see the psychiatrist who had treated her in the past, and she refused to allow social services to help her find a place to live. The reason for her refusal was that she "was waiting for the baby's father." Jane refused to answer any questions about her family and any specific questions about the father of her baby. When asked for names and telephone numbers of friends, she also refused. On 2 separate days, she disappeared from the visitors' lounge and returned the following day, with alcohol on her breath. On those occasions, her behavior seemed even more irrational and disruptive than usual. The staff of the high-risk unit asked for a psychiatric consultation to answer the following questions: 1) Was Jane's mental state caused by her postpartum status (i.e., was it transient or permanent)? 2) Was involuntary hospitalization indicated (i.e., was she dangerous)? 3) Had the neuroleptic injection helped to induce labor? Did her grievance against her doctor have merit? 4) Was it beneficial or harmful for the baby to have Jane in constant attendance? 5) Was alcohol exacerbating Jane's symptoms?

Psychosis of Pregnancy, Labor, and the Puerperium

The rate of postpartum psychosis in schizophrenia is approximately 25% (McNeil 1987). It is highest in those who have been hospitalized at some time in the past and/or who have had an active mental disturbance just before pregnancy. Interestingly, men are not exempt from postpartum psychosis (Harvey and McGrath 1988; Shapiro and Nass 1986; Van Putten and LaWall 1981), but the incidence, as might be expected, is rare.

Any psychotic episode occurring within 2 years of delivery can be conceptualized as puerperal, or birth related. Kendell and colleagues (1987), concluded that, based on an extensive 12-year survey covering 54,087 births, puerperal psychosis usually appears within 3 weeks of childbirth but that psychiatric admissions in women are raised above baseline for 2 years after the birth of a child, most significantly during the first 3 months postpartum. The average rate of psychiatric admission for psychosis during the first postpartum month in their study was 25 times that of the prepregnancy rate for a group of women defined by geographic catchment.

Postpartum psychosis in women may productively serve as a model for understanding the emergence of any psychosis. It occurs at a time of profound endocrine flux (as do puberty-onset psychosis, premenstrual-onset psychosis, and menopause-onset psychosis) (Gitlin and Pasnau 1989; Maggi and Perez 1985). In addition, delivery is frequently accompanied by sleep disturbance, pain, dehydration, fear, dramatic change of self-identity, family tensions, and role shift within the family. There may be accompanying changes in financial, employment, and living arrangements. There are new affections, new loyalties, new bodily experiences, new expectations, and new conflicts. Body weight and the daily rhythm of activity, food intake, and sleep change dramatically. All of these factors may reduce the threshold for psychosis in vulnerable individuals. Jane had experienced psychotic manifestations before and during pregnancy. It is not clear whether labor and delivery worsened her mental state. The injection of long-acting antipsychotic medication should have, in principle, protected her from a postpartum exacerbation of her psychosis. There is no doubt, however, that concern for her baby was aggravating her condition, and, in that sense, she could be expected to improve after the immediate postpartum period and after being reassured about the baby's imminent health.

It is significant that pregnancy itself is probably not a risk period for women with schizophrenia (Apfel and Handel 1992). Most available literature points to an amelioration or stabilization of the schizophrenic process in the mother during pregnancy (Chang and Renshaw 1986), but this generalization is disputed (Krener et al. 1989). If generally true, the protective aspect of pregnancy may be caused by the antidopaminergic and antipsychotic effects of mounting estrogen titers (Seeman 1981), and pregnancy may, therefore, be a period of relatively low risk for neuroleptic-free maintenance. If feasible, this strategy would be an undeniable advantage to the offspring.

Gender Differences in Involuntary Hospitalizations

During an interview, Jane told the psychiatric consultant that she had tried to kill herself many times in the past, once throwing herself in front of a subway train and breaking her leg in the fall. However, she wanted to live now because of the baby. She had no aggressive thoughts connected to the baby, but she did not have a place for the baby to stay after discharge from the hospital, and she did not seem to know very much about how she would feed the baby. "God," she said, "would provide." She told the consultant something particularly worrisome—that God did not approve of all the artificial machinery used in the neonatal unit; that babies were not meant to be hooked up to all this electricity; and that, one day, when no one was looking, she was going to pull the plugs out and disconnect the wires. Jane was assessed as clearly psychotic; her mood was labile, her thoughts were disconnected, and her ideas about God were eccentric. She had grandiose ideas about being special in the eyes of God and paranoid ideas about the doctor who had given her the injection. She was considered both mentally ill and potentially dangerous to the welfare of the infants in the neonatal unit. Because she refused to be admitted to the hospital voluntarily, she fulfilled the criteria for civil commitment and was hospitalized against her will.

The ratio of male-to-female involuntary hospitalization is approximately 3:2 in most studies. Men with psychosis are consistently less willing to agree to admission and consistently perceived as more dangerous (Kastrup 1987; Kay et al. 1988).

Although men are more aggressive in general, infanticide and child kidnapping are behaviors associated with women (Apfel and Handel 1992). Identifying with the baby and therefore "rescuing" him or her from pain is a familiar theme in baby kidnappings and acts of infanticide committed by women. Women may perceive themselves as uniquely capable of fulfilling a baby's needs and therefore become frustrated and furious with themselves (and the baby) when they cannot soothe the baby. Men describe their frustration with a child's crying differently. They become angry at the baby, as if he or she were being willful and crying deliberately. When men hurt a baby, it is often an act of "retaliation" for what they perceive as the baby's aggression. The threat a man with psychosis poses to a child in his care is different from the threat of a woman with psychosis. However, both can be potentially dangerous (Zonana et al. 1990).

Gender-Specific Hormonal Effects of Neuroleptics

There is no specific mention in the literature of neuroleptic injections leading to onset of labor, but clinicians recommend withholding neuroleptics immediately before the expected delivery date (Cohen

et al. 1989; Miller 1991; Oates 1986). Neuroleptics inhibit the dopaminergic suppression of prolactin and cause prolactin levels to rise,
more so in women than in men—and perhaps more so in pregnant
women (Glazer et al. 1981). A steep rise in prolactin levels might be
expected to induce labor. The fact that, in this case, labor followed
so closely on the heels of the depot injection makes the causal connection probable.

Sex-specific neuroleptic side effects should be mentioned in this
context. Not only can side effects differ, but they may be interpreted
differently by men and women (Apfel and Handel 1992; Seeman
1983b). Many women are profoundly affected by neuroleptic-
induced interruption of menses. Depending on their individual
wishes or fears, women may interpret this to mean that they are
pregnant or, alternatively, menopausal with no further chance to
become mothers. They may view the amenorrhea as either defemi-
nizing or liberating, giving them sexual license previously forbidden.
Women may take untoward chances because they believe they are
protected from pregnancy. Many women view menstruation as a
periodic cleansing and may feel unclean without it. Some women
may think, delusionally, that they are becoming men. Whatever the
case, menstruation or the lack of it is a subject of concern to women.
The effects of neuroleptics on the breasts (engorgement, lactation)
also take on special significance. In men, as well as women, breast
effects may take place and cause alarm. Men are especially sensitive
to neuroleptic effects on libido, erection, and ejaculation. Many delu-
sional ideas arise from interference with these emotionally charged
processes. Women also experience changes in ease or range of orgas-
mic responses (Friedman and Harrison 1984; Segraves 1985; Sullivan
and Lukoff 1990).

Neuroleptic drugs cross the placental membrane and are secreted in breast milk (Briggs et al. 1990; Calabrese and Gulledge
1985). An increase in birth defects has been demonstrated in infants
of mothers taking neuroleptics in gestational weeks 6–10 (Edlund
and Craig 1984). In addition, antipsychotic drugs that reach the fetus
or the neonate via either placenta or breast milk can influence behavior long after the drug is eliminated. Drugs can interfere with the
synthesis of neurotransmitter systems and thus cause behavioral
teratogenesis (Coyle et al. 1976). Extrapyramidal symptoms and with-

drawal symptoms in the newborn can interfere with perinatal adaptation and set the scene for future psychological consequences (Cohen et al. 1989).

Is Early Bonding to a
Mother With Psychosis Beneficial?

The conventional wisdom is that newborn and mother need a lot of time together; this early togetherness cements their relationship, and prematurity, with its attendant early separation of mother and infant, is thus potentially detrimental to the optimal health of the child. Mothers of premature infants are encouraged to spend as much time as possible in the nursery and to be present, as much as possible, for feeding and interaction time. Does this hold true for the mother with psychosis? A study by Persson-Blennow and co-workers (1984) indicates that effective bonding does take place between an infant and a mother who has been psychotic. Competency to care for an infant, of course, must be carefully assessed (Stewart and Gangbar 1984). Is it better for an infant to be exposed to the relatively inept and somewhat inconsistent parenting of one constant person or the more efficient but constantly changing parenting of shifts of nurses? Studies of children brought up by mothers with psychosis agree that these children do better, as a group, than children of mothers with depression and that some of these children, paradoxically, turn out "supernormal"—more self-confident, adaptable, and resourceful than their age peers (El-Guebaly and Offord 1980; Kauffman et al. 1979). These are interesting group findings, but the individual background of each such child is so different both genetically and environmentally that it is difficult to formulate any researchable questions about the direct effect of the psychotic mother on her infant.

Jane's behavior and constant presence clearly were having a detrimental effect on the nurses who were caring for her baby. They feared Jane and tended to distance themselves when she was around. This avoidance by the nurses was an additional risk for the baby's health because he required constant monitoring. Therefore, Jane's hospitalization, which separated her from her son, was viewed, on balance, as an advantage for the baby.

Gender Differences in
Substance Abuse in Schizophrenia

Did alcohol exacerbate Jane's psychosis? In both men and women with schizophrenia, alcohol use is widespread. In a United States epidemiological survey (Regier et al. 1990), 47% of individuals meeting criteria for a diagnosis of schizophrenia also qualified for an alcohol dependence or abuse disorder. By comparison, the lifetime rate of alcoholism in the general United States population is 16.4%. Two-thirds of those with a dual diagnosis of alcoholism and schizophrenia also abuse other substances. More than one-quarter of the schizophrenia population in the United States (27.5%) qualify for dependence on a substance other than alcohol. This means that the population who have schizophrenia are three times as likely as the general population to have problems with alcohol abuse.

People with schizophrenia are six times more likely than the general population to have other substance abuse problems. The most common abuse substance, after alcohol, is cannabis. Although the current findings are inconclusive, it has been proposed that cannabis can act as an independent risk factor for schizophrenia. It not only complicates the illness and increases its severity, but cannabis can increase the psychotic features of the illness and diminish the effects of neuroleptics, making patients less responsive to treatment. It is believed that these effects also apply to sniffing glue and other inhalants, cocaine, amphetamines, hallucinogens, and even excessive caffeine intake and excessive tobacco use. Phencyclidine, a more recent drug of abuse, has been less extensively studied but also belongs in this category. Alcohol also tends to contribute to psychotic exacerbations but, paradoxically, those patients who drink are more likely to be socially involved and sexually better adjusted. On the other hand, they are less adherent to treatment regimens and, therefore, in the long run, have a worse outcome of their disease process.

Subjectively, cocaine, alcohol, and cannabis elevate mood. Alcohol and cannabis also allay anxiety. Cocaine increases anxiety. Both cannabis and cocaine increase available energy. Men and women with schizophrenia may use specific substances not only to counteract their interpersonal and motivational problems but also, perhaps, to neutralize the neuroleptic effects of sedation, hypotension, sexual dysfunction, and drug-induced parkinsonism (Schneier and Siris 1987).

More men with schizophrenia than women with schizophrenia drink alcohol and abuse other substances (Arndt et al. 1992; Pulver et al. 1989; Test et al. 1989). Alcohol and drug use may play a significant role in the earlier onset age of schizophrenia in men (Pulver et al. 1989), in their inferior therapeutic response to neuroleptics (Bowers et al. 1990), and in their increased tendencies to violence and impulsivity (Kay et al. 1988). Detoxification and abstinence programs may be especially important to men with schizophrenia.

Summary

In summary, the literature on sex differences in schizophrenia has, for the most part, assumed that course of illness is determined by inherent or developmental differences between men and women. The possibility that the two sexes may respond to a different degree to specific therapeutic interventions has not, as yet, been adequately addressed or explored. This chapter illustrates some questions that need answers. Because comprehensive treatment for schizophrenia encompasses a variety of biopsychosocial intercessions, it may be possible to distinguish among them and to specify which are more effective for each sex. We may find, for instance, that the relatively more benign course of schizophrenia in women is mainly attributable to women's superior response to currently available therapies.

References

Alloway R, Bebbington P: The buffer theory of social support—a review of the literature. Psychol Med 17:91–108, 1987

American Psychiatric Association: Diagnostic and Statistical Manual of Mental Disorders, 3rd Edition. Washington, DC, American Psychiatric Association, 1980

Angermeyer MC, Kühn L: Gender differences in age at onset of schizophrenia: an overview. Eur Arch Psychiatry Neurol Sci 237:351–364, 1988

Apfel RJ, Handel MH: Madness and Loss of Motherhood. Sexuality, Reproduction and Long-Term Mental Illness. Washington, DC, American Psychiatric Press, 1992

Arndt S, Tyrell G, Flaum M, et al: Comorbidity of substance abuse and schizophrenia: the role of pre-morbid adjustment. Psychol Med 22:379–388, 1992

Bedard P, Boucher R, Daigle M, et al: Similar effect of estradiol and haloperidol on experimental tardive dyskinesia in monkeys. Psychoneuroendocrinology 9:375–379, 1984

Birchwood M, Smith J, Cochrane R: Some specific and non-specific effects of educational intervention for families living with schizophrenia. Br J Psychiatry 160:806–814, 1992

Block JH: Conceptions of sex role: some cross-cultural and longitudinal perspectives. Am Psychol 28:512–526, 1973

Block JH: Differential premises arising from differential socialization of the sexes: some conjectures. Child Dev 54:1335–1354, 1983

Bowers MB, Mazure CM, Nelson JC, et al: Psychotogenic drug use and neuroleptic response. Schizophr Bull 16:81–85, 1990

Briggs GC, Freeman RK, Yaffa SJ: Drugs in Pregnancy and Lactation, 3rd Edition. Baltimore, MD, Williams & Wilkins, 1990

Brown K, Heidelberg S: For better or worse: intermarriage in the young adult chronic population. J Psychosoc Nurs Ment Health Serv 23:18–23, 1985

Calabrese JR, Gulledge AD: Psychotropics during pregnancy and lactation: a review. Psychosomatics 26:413–426, 1985

Casey DE: Neuroleptic drug-induced extrapyramidal syndromes and tardive dyskinesia. Schizophr Res 4:109–120, 1991

Chakos MH, Mayerhoff DI, Loebel AD, et al: Incidence and correlates of acute extrapyramidal symptoms in first episode of schizophrenia. Psychopharmacol Bull 28:81–86, 1992

Chang SS, Renshaw DC: Psychosis and pregnancy. Compr Ther 12:36–41, 1986

Cohen LJ, Heller VL, Rosenbaum JF: Treatment guidelines for psychotropic drug use in pregnancy. Psychosomatics 30:25–33, 1989

Conning AM, Rowland LA: Where do people with long-term mental health problems live? A comparison of the sexes. Br J Psychiatry 158 (suppl 10):80–84, 1991

Coverdale JH, Aruffo JA: Family planning needs of female chronic psychiatric outpatients. Am J Psychiatry 146:1489–1491, 1989

Coyle I, Wayne MJ, Singer G: Behavioral teratogenesis: a critical evaluation. Pharmacol Biochem Behav 4:191–200, 1976 deVries GJ, deBruin JPC, Uylings HBM, et al (eds): Progress in Brain Research, Vol 61. Amsterdam, Elsevier, 1984

Edlund MJ, Craig TJ: Antipsychotic drug use and birth defects: an epidemiological reassessment. Compr Psychiatry 25:32–36, 1984

El-Guebaly N, Offord DR: The competent offspring of psychiatrically ill patients. Can J Psychiatry 25:457–467, 1980

Flaherty JA, Jobe TH: Gender, expressed emotion and outcome in schizophrenia. Current Opinion in Psychiatry 3:23–28, 1990

Friedman S, Harrison G: Sexual histories, attitudes, and behavior of schizophrenic and "normal" women. Arch Sex Behav 13:555–567, 1984

Gitlin MJ, Pasnau RO: Psychiatric syndromes linked to reproductive function in women: a review of current knowledge. Am J Psychiatry 146:1413–1422, 1989

Glazer WM, Moore DC, Bowers MB, et al: Serum prolactin and tardive dyskinesia. Am J Psychiatry 138:1493–1496, 1981

Glazer WM, Morgenstern H, Schooler N, et al: Predictors of improvement in tardive dyskinesia following discontinuation of neuroleptic medication. Br J Psychiatry 157:585–592, 1990

Glick ID, Spencer JH, Clarkin JF, et al: A randomized clinical trial of inpatient family intervention, IV: follow-up results for subjects with schizophrenia. Schizophr Res 3:187–200, 1990

Goff DC, Henderson DC, Amico E: Cigarette smoking in schizophrenia: relationship to psychopathology and medication side effects. Am J Psychiatry 149:1139–1194, 1992

Goldstein JM, Kreisman D: Gender, family environment, and schizophrenia. Psychol Med 18:861–872, 1988

Gopalaswamy AK, Morgan R: Too many chronic mentally disabled patients are too fat. Acta Psychiatr Scand 72:254–258, 1985

Haas GL, Glick ID, Clarkin J, et al: Gender and schizophrenia: a clinical trial of an inpatient family intervention. Schizophr Bull 16:277–292, 1990

Häfner H, Behrens S, DeVry J, et al: An animal model for the effects of estradiol on dopamine-mediated behavior: implications for sex differences in schizophrenia. Psychiatry Res 38:125–134, 1991

Hallonquist J, Seeman MV, Lang M, et al: Variation in symptom severity over the menstrual cycle of schizophrenics. Biol Psychiatry 33:207–209, 1993

Hampson RB, Beavers WR: Comparing males' and females' perspectives through family self-report. Psychiatry 50:24–30, 1987

Harvey I, McGrath G: Psychiatric morbidity in spouses of women admitted to a mother and baby unit. Br J Psychiatry 152:506–510, 1988

Heidensohn FM: Women as perpetrators and victims of crime. Br J Psychiatry 158 (suppl 10):50–54, 1991

Hogarty GE, Anderson CM, Reiss DJ, et al: Family psychoeducation, social skills training, and maintenance chemotherapy in the aftercare treatment of schizophrenia, I: one-year effects of a controlled study on relapse and expressed emotion. Arch Gen Psychiatry 43:633–641, 1986

Holbrook T: Policing sexuality in a modern state hospital. Hosp Community Psychiatry 40:75–79, 1989

Kastrup M: Sex differences in the utilization of mental health services. Int J Soc Psychiatry 33:171–184, 1987

Kauffman C, Grunebaum H, Cohler B, et al: Superkids: competent children of psychotic mothers. Am J Psychiatry 136:1398–1402, 1979

Kay SR, Wolkenfeld F, Murrill LA: Profiles of aggression among psychiatric patients, II: covariates and predictors. J Nerv Ment Dis 176:547–557, 1988

Kendell RR, Chalmers JC, Platz C: Epidemiology of puerperal psychosis. Br J Psychiatry 150:662–673, 1987

Keskiner A, Zelman J, Ruppert EH: Advantages of being female in psychiatric rehabilitation. Arch Gen Psychiatry 28:689–692, 1973

Kolakowska T, Williams AO, Ardern M, et al: Schizophrenia with good and poor outcome, I: early clinical features, response to neuroleptics and signs of organic dysfunction. Br J Psychiatry 146:229–246, 1985

Krener P, Simmons MK, Hansen RL, et al: Effect of pregnancy on psychosis: life circumstances and psychiatric symptoms. Int J Psychiatry Med 19:65–84, 1989

Liberman RP, Evans CD: Behavioral rehabilitation for chronic mental patients. J Clin Psychopharmacol 5:85–145, 1985

Lukoff D, Gioia-Hasick D, Sullivan G, et al: Sex education and rehabilitation with schizophrenic male outpatients. Schizophr Bull 12:669–677, 1986

Maggi A, Perez J: Mini review: role of female gonadal hormones in the CNS: clinical and experimental aspects. Life Sci 37:893–906, 1985

McCreadie R, Robertson LJ, Wiles DH: The Nithsdale schizophrenia surveys, IX: akathisia, parkinsonism, tardive dyskinesia, and plasma neuroleptic levels. Br J Psychiatry 161:793–799, 1992

McNeil TF: A prospective study of postpartum psychoses in a high risk group. Acta Psychiatr Scand 75:35–43, 1987

Miller LJ: Clinical strategies for the use of psychotropic drugs during pregnancy. Psychiatr Med 9:275–298, 1991

Mitchell JE, Popkin MK: Antipsychotic drug therapy and sexual dysfunction in men. Am J Psychiatry 139:633–637, 1980

Mowbray CT, Chamberlain P: Sex differences among the long term mentally disabled. Psychology of Women Quarterly 10:383–392, 1986

Nedopil N, Pflieger R, Ruther E: The prediction of acute response, remission, and general outcome of neuroleptic treatment in acute schizophrenic patients. Pharmacopsychiatry 16:201–205, 1983

Oates MR: Psychiatric disorders in pregnancy and the puerperium. Clinics in Obstetrics and Gynecology 13:385–396, 1986

Pakaslahti A: Prediction of Working Disability in Schizophrenia. Publication of the Social Insurance Institution, Finland, Helsinki, ML:119, 1992

Perkins R, Rowland L: Sex differences in service usage in long-term psychiatric care: are women adequately served? Br J Psychiatry 158 (suppl 10):75–79, 1991

Persson-Blennow I, Naslund B, McNeil TF, et al: Offspring of women with nonorganic psychosis: mother-infant interaction at three days of age. Acta Psychiatr Scand 70:149–159, 1984

Pulver AE, Wolyniec PS, Wagner MG, et al: An epidemiological investigation of alcohol-dependent schizophrenics. Acta Psychiatr Scand 79:603–612, 1989

Regier DA, Farmer ME, Rae DS, et al: Comorbidity of mental disorders with alcohol and other drug abuse. JAMA 264:2511–2518, 1990

Riecher-Rössler A, Fatkenheuer B, Löffler W, et al: Is age of onset in schizophrenia influenced by marital status? Soc Psychiatry Psychiatr Epidemiol 27:122–128, 1992

Ritsner M, Sherina O, Ginath Y: Genetic epidemiological study of schizophrenia: reproduction behaviour. Acta Psychiatr Scand 85:423–429, 1992

Rozensky RH, Berman C: Sexual knowledge, attitudes, and experiences of chronic psychiatric patients. Psychosocial Rehabilitation Journal 8:21–27, 1984

Salokongas RKR: Prognostic implications of the sex of schizophrenic patients. Br J Psychiatry 142:145–151, 1983

Schneier FR, Siris SG: A review of psychoactive substance use and abuse in schizophrenia: patterns of drug choice. J Nerv Ment Dis 175:641–652, 1987

Seeman MV: Gender and the onset of schizophrenia: neurohumoral influences. Psychiatric Journal of the University of Ottawa 6:136–138, 1981

Seeman MV: Interaction of sex, age, and neuroleptic dose. Compr Psychiatry 24:125–128, 1983a

Seeman MV: Schizophrenic men and women require different treatment programs. Journal of Psychiatric Treatment and Evaluation 5:143–148, 1983b

Seeman MV: Current outcome in schizophrenia: women vs. men. Acta Psychiatr Scand 73:609–617, 1986

Seeman MV: Prescribing neuroleptics for men and women. Journal of Social Pharmacology 3:219–236, 1989

Seeman MV, Lang M: The role of estrogens in schizophrenia gender differences. Schizophr Bull 16:185–194, 1990

Seeman MV, Lang M, Rector N: Chronic schizophrenia: a risk factor for HIV? Can J Psychiatry 35:765–768, 1991

Segal SP, Everett-Dille L: Coping styles and factors in male/female social integration. Acta Psychiatr Scand 61:8–20, 1980

Segraves RT: Psychiatric drugs and orgasm in the human female. Journal of Psychosomatic Obstetrics and Gynecology 4:125–128, 1985

Segraves RT: Effects of psychotropic drugs on human erection and ejaculation. Arch Gen Psychiatry 46:275–284, 1989

Shapiro S, Nass J: Postpartum psychosis in the male. Psychopathology 19:138–142, 1986

Steinberg L: Recent research on the family at adolescence: the extent and nature of sex differences. Journal of Youth and Adolescence 16:191–197, 1987

Stewart DE, Gangbar R: Psychiatric assessment of competency to care for a newborn. Can J Psychiatry 29:583–589, 1984

Sullivan G, Lukoff D: Sexual side effects of antipsychotic medication: evaluation and interventions. Hosp Community Psychiatry 41:1238–1241, 1990

Test MA, Wallisch SS, Allness DJ, et al: Substance use in young adults with schizophrenic disorders. Schizophr Bull 15:465–476, 1989

Van Putten R, LaWall J: Postpartum psychosis in an adoptive mother and in a father. Psychosomatics 22:1087–1089, 1981

Vaughn C, Sorensen Snyder K, Jones S, et al: Family factors in schizophrenia relapse. Arch Gen Psychiatry 41:1169–1177, 1984

Villeneuve A, Cazejust T, Cote M: Estrogens in tardive dyskinesia in male psychiatric patients. Neuropsychobiology 6:145–151, 1980

Waldo MC, Roath M, Levine W, et al: A model program to teach parenting skills to schizophrenic mothers. Hosp Community Psychiatry 38:1110–1112, 1987

Watt DC, Katz K, Shepherd M: The natural history of schizophrenia: a 5-year prospective follow-up of a representative sample of schizophrenics by means of a standardized clinical and social assessment. Psychol Med 13:663–670, 1983

Webster J: Parenting for children of schizophrenic mothers. Adoption and Fostering 14:37–43, 1990

Yassa R, Nastase C, Dupont D, et al: Tardive dyskinesia in elderly psychiatric patients: a 5-year study. Am J Psychiatry 149:1206–1211, 1992

Yonkers KA, Kando JC, Cole JO, et al: Gender differences in pharmacokinetics and pharmacodynamics of psychotropic medication. Am J Psychiatry 149:587–595, 1992

Zito JM, Routt WW, Mitchell JE, et al: Clinical characteristics of hospitalized psychotic patients who refuse antipsychotic drug therapy. Am J Psychiatry 142:822–826, 1985

Zonana H, Bartel RL, Wells JA, et al: Sex differences in persons found not guilty by reason of insanity. Bull Am Acad Psychiatry Law 18:129–142, 1990

CHAPTER 11

Gender Differences in Eating Disorders

D. Blake Woodside, M.D., M.Sc., F.R.C.P.C.
Sidney H. Kennedy, M.D., F.R.C.P.C.

Often characterized as illnesses exclusive to women, anorexia nervosa and bulimia nervosa, as defined by modern criteria, also affect men. In this chapter, we review gender differences in eating disorders and discuss their possible meaning.

The existence of cases of anorexia nervosa in males had been reported as early as 1694, when Morton recorded the histories of two patients with anorexia nervosa, one male and one female. Periodic case reports on males with anorexia nervosa continued to appear in the literature over the next several centuries (for a review, see Silverman 1991).

More recently, attempts have been made to systematically and scientifically compare male patients with female patients. In this section of the chapter, we concentrate on three comprehensive studies that compare male and female patients who have eating disorders: Crisp and Burns (1991), Edwin and Andersen (1991), and Woodside and colleagues (1991). Crisp and Burns' study compared 36 male patients with 102 female patients; each sample was treated simultaneously. Edwin and Andersen compared 76 male patients with 84 female patients, matched on a variety of demographic variables.

Woodside and colleagues compared 34 male patients with 34 female patients, matched for diagnosis and demographic features. These three studies are the largest reports of comparisons between male and female patients with eating disorders. The majority of other reports in the literature contain 15 or fewer male subjects.

Edwin and Andersen (1991) and Woodside et al. (1991) used DSM-III-R (American Psychiatric Association 1987) criteria to diagnose eating disorders. Crisp and Burns (1991) developed their own criteria that resemble DSM-III-R criteria but are different in that the criteria focus heavily on psychosocial developmental issues. Most of the patients treated by Crisp and Burns appear to have been adolescents; in the other two studies, most patients were over age 18 years.

In all three of these reports, the main finding was that the syndromes were clinically identical for male and female subjects. Crisp and Burns suggested that there was disproportionate athleticism among male subjects compared with female subjects; however, this finding was not unexpected because young men are expected to participate in athletic activity to a greater degree than are young women.

These three studies also compared their groups on a wide variety of psychometric measures, including indices of symptoms, such as the Eating Attitudes Test (EAT; Garner and Garfinkel 1979), specific psychopathology (The Eating Disorders Inventory; Garner et al. 1983), and many other variables. Although each study found a few differences between male and female patients, the differences occurred in a random pattern and were certainly not greater in number than would have been expected to occur by chance based on the large number of comparisons performed. Crisp and Burns examined a range of variables connected to premorbid personality and emotional adjustment and found no evidence of excessive premorbid psychopathology in the male group compared with the female group.

Epidemiology

Virtually all studies of the prevalence of eating disorders have observed the relative scarcity of male patients compared with female patients. According to Pope and associates (1993), the prevalence rate of anorexia nervosa in men in the United States is 0.02%. Many authors suggest that male cases account for about 5% of most treated series. In our own series, men account for approximately 4% of cases during the last 15 years. Attempts have been made to estimate the prevalence of bulimia nervosa in the community. Carlat and Camargo (1991), in a comprehensive review of this topic, quote a rate of 0.2% for bulimia nervosa among men in the community; this figure reflects data from the five most sophisticated studies. Figures for females ranged from 0.3% to 6.0% in these same studies. The authors note that the male-to-female ratio in the community (1/20—1/6) appears to be higher than that found in clinic populations (Carlat and Camargo 1991). Relatively few studies have attempted to estimate the incidence of either disorder in men.

The age at onset of eating disorders has not been studied systematically in men. In our own series ($n = 19$), the average age at onset was 21. This is comparable to the average age at onset of 18.6 years in a sample of 323 female patients we assessed (Woodside et al. 1991). Carlat and Camargo (1991) noted that most studies report a later age at onset for men, a difference of about 2 years. They propose that this difference is accounted for by the differential onset of puberty in girls and boys, with girls, on average, entering puberty several years before boys. Marriage and fertility differences between men and women with eating disorders are unknown.

Sexual Orientation

There is considerable debate as to whether homosexual sexual orientation is overrepresented in men with eating disorders. Examining this question is complicated by a number of factors, including lack of adequate estimates of the community prevalence of homosexual sexual orientation, the frequent equating of lack of any sexual interest (notably in starved anorexic patients) with homosexual sexual orientation, the confusion between femininity and homosexuality, and the possibility that homosexual men are simply more willing than heterosexual men to present for assessment and treatment of an illness that is strongly associated with women. Despite these concerns, some evidence suggests that such an overrepresentation does exist (for a review of this topic, see Herzog et al. 1991). Rates of homosexual sexual orientation cluster around 25% in most series of men with eating disorders (Fichter et al. 1985; Herzog et al. 1984; Schneider and Agras 1987; Woodside et al. 1991), with occasional higher or lower reports. This incidence is likely to be higher than that in the general population, in which a rate of 6%–10% has been suggested (Gadpaille 1989). There does not appear to be any elevation in the rates of homosexuality in female patients with eating disorders; in our series (Woodside et al. 1991), rates of homosexual orientation among our female patients were approximately 5%, not different from the estimated general population prevalence of 2%–4% (Gadpaille 1989).

Disease Course and Outcome

Several studies have examined the course and outcome of eating disorders in men, but, as is often the case in this area, the number of patients studied was very small (Hall et al. 1985; Oyebode et al. 1988). There were no significant differences in either the course or in the long-term outcome. Hall and co-workers believed that the men had a marginally worse outcome than the women, but their sample included only nine patients. In a later report, Crisp and Burns (1991) believed that men who made any type of recovery tended to recover more completely than women; however, their conclusions were tentative and anecdotal. There is currently no compelling reason to believe that these illnesses in men have a worse prognosis than in women.

Treatment Response

No evidence in the literature suggests that treatment for men with eating disorders should be different from that for women. In our setting, a day hospital program, male patients are routinely included in the intensive group therapy program, which includes groups focusing on sexuality, sexual abuse, and body image, among other issues.

Men who have anorexia nervosa or bulimia nervosa tend to require higher caloric levels to gain weight or to stop bingeing behaviors.

However, this difference only reinforces the notion that different individuals require different amounts of food, a concept that avoids rigid, unrealistic definitions of what is "normal." We have not formally analyzed the experience of our male patients, but our clinical sense is that they fared no worse than our female patients in terms of their nutritional and psychological outcome. We have not experienced significant problems integrating male patients into group treatment. When difficulties are handled empathically and sensitively, the opportunity for a woman to perceive a man as nonthreatening and helpful can be a corrective emotional experience, as is described below:

> A female patient had a long history of being sexually abused by her father. She was externally phobic of men and would usually position herself in the group as distantly as possible from a married male co-patient who had children of his own. Over the course of 10 weeks, she began to articulate her fear of being further exploited and her need to recognize that "not all fathers abuse their children."

We were at first concerned about the effect of including male patients in groups focusing on body image and sexuality. Again, this has not proved to be a problem. In most cases, men's concerns about their body shape so closely parallel those of women that there has been minimal effect on groups dealing with body image. Groups focusing on sexuality and sexual abuse are probably affected by the presence of a man. Female patients do report a certain amount of censoring in such a situation; however, they also report appreciating the information they receive directly about male sexuality and the opportunity to discuss some of these issues directly with a male peer. Finally, many of our male patients have also been sexually abused; the revelation of a history of experiencing sexual abuse told by a man has had powerful and beneficial effects on copatients.

It is likely that the most profound effect of including a male patient in such a group is on the male patient himself. Many men report benefit from the treatment experience but have also noted feeling somewhat marginalized and excluded from the group. This appears to be true regardless of the man's sexual orientation. In this respect, male patients appear to resemble female homosexual patients, some of whom have reported similar feelings.

Therefore, no evidence supports the need for separate or segregated treatments for men with eating disorders. For most aspects of these illnesses, the commonalities between male and female patients seem to vastly outweigh the differences.

Our program has both male and female therapists. Our experience suggests that, on the whole, therapist gender is not an issue for most patients with eating disorders. The main exception to this is female patients who have been sexually abused, some of whom are uncomfortable in the presence of male therapists.

In summary, current evidence supports only two gender differences in eating disorders: 1) that these disorders are much more common in women and 2) that more men with eating disorders appear to have a homosexual sexual orientation.

Possible Factors Accounting for Gender Differences in Eating Disorders

Genetic

Considerable evidence from twin (Holland et al. 1984, 1988; Kendler et al. 1992) and family (Strober et al. 1990) studies suggests that a heritable genetic effect may be operating in both anorexia nervosa and bulimia nervosa (for a review, see Woodside 1993). The field is not yet advanced enough to specify potential modes of inheritance or to have established genetic linkage to a specific portion of the genome.

One challenge for researchers in this area is to explain the difference in incidence of eating disorders between men and women. For single-gene models, simple Mendelian patterns of inheritance are inadequate in and of themselves to explain this difference. Sex-linked dominant transmission (a dominant gene carried on the X chromosome) comes the closest. This pattern of inheritance produces a 2:1 predominance of affected women. This inheritance pattern could then be modified (by a factor of 10) by other genetic or environmental effects to produce the usually quoted ratio of 20:1; this amounts to postulating very large differences in the expression of the gene(s) between the two sexes. Alternatively, sex-related effects may cause a single genetic liability to be expressed differently in the two sexes, with women developing eating disorders and depression and men developing another problem such as sociopathy or substance use disorders. The work of Strober and associates (1990) on depression and eating disorders, however, and other work on the genetics of alcoholism (Grove et al. 1990; Merikangas 1990), which all support independent genetic mechanisms for affective and substance use disorders, may make this latter theory untenable. As suggested by Pope and co-workers (1993), a genetic association may exist between eating disorders and body dysmorphic disorder (Phillips et al. 1993). The identification and characterization of a heritable genetic factor in eating disorders may one day explain the difference in incidence between men and women.

Biological

Studies of biological variables in male patients with eating disorders have centered largely around testosterone. Most investigators have found reduced levels of testosterone in male patients with anorexia nervosa (Crisp and Burns 1991; Crisp et al. 1982; Fichter et al. 1985; LeMaire et al. 1983), which is not surprising given the close correlation between testosterone levels and weight. In all but one case (McNab and Hawton 1981), testosterone levels have been reported to return to normal on refeeding.

More recently, some interest has been shown in neuroendocrine response to different neurotransmitter agonists and precursors among male and female volunteer dieters. Prolactin response to L-tryptophan (a precursor to serotonin) was increased in women and unchanged in men after 3 weeks of dieting; this suggests that women may be more sensitive to alterations in serotonin function during dieting compared with men (Goodwin et al. 1987). The possible significance of this finding for increasing our understanding of gender differences in eating disorders is unknown.

The secondary biological effects of dieting appear to affect men and women similarly. In a seminal study of the effects of semistarvation on both physiological and psychological functioning, Keys and co-workers (1950) subjected a sample of healthy young men to a 3-month regimen of semistarvation. By the end of the study period, the group had lost an average 25% of their initial body weight, were exhibiting symptoms of anorexia nervosa (the body image distortion and drive for thinness), and otherwise appeared to react to starvation in the same manner as women with anorexia nervosa.

Social

This topic has been reviewed by Mickalide (1991). There is fairly good evidence that men as a group are exposed to less of society's preoccupation with weight and body shape but are not exempt (Gupta et al. 1993; Pope et al. 1993).

Willingness to access treatment. It has been suggested that men will not present for treatment of an illness that has been largely characterized in the media as a "women's illness." Theories of this nature note that most data concerning different rates of anorexia nervosa and bulimia nervosa are derived from clinic samples. Although these theories are intriguing, two sources of information do not support this view. First, family studies of eating disorders have demonstrated lower rates of eating disorders in male relatives of probands compared with female relatives of probands. In the study by Strober and colleagues (1985), probably the most sophisticated family study of eating disorders to date, rates of eating disorder diagnoses in female relatives were 9.7% versus 0.4% in male relatives—almost the exact 20:1 ratio quoted from clinic series. Second, as has been reviewed above, results from community surveys of bulimic behavior and of formal bulimia nervosa in men support a similar ratio (Carlat and Camargo 1991). It is conceivable that the excess of male homosexual cases observed in clinic settings may be related to a decreased reluctance of this particular population to seek help for the eating disorder, but at present such a theory would be speculative.

Meaning of puberty. Carlat and Camargo (1991) have commented that the later onset of eating disorders in men might be related to the later onset of puberty in boys. However, onset of puberty may have different meanings for boys and girls. For boys, the early onset of puberty may be viewed as a positive step (i.e., one associated with increased power and stature). The onset of adult sexual capacity, including erections, nocturnal emissions, and masturbation to orgasm, may also be viewed by most boys in a generally positive light. The converse situation, that of delayed puberty, is probably viewed negatively by most boys and perhaps also by their families.

The situation is more complex for girls, who may be much more ambivalent about the onset of puberty. For girls, early puberty may signal less, rather than more, safety because it may expose the young girl to unwanted sexual advances from older men, which may include the very frightening possibility of pregnancy and childbirth. Also, female sexuality has frequently been presented in a much less positive light than male sexuality, and thus a young girl experiencing sexual drive may be much more likely to have ambivalent feelings about these impulses. Finally, an early onset of menarche may cause a young girl to feel very out of place with her peers, especially if she is among the first in her group to experience menarche.

Gilligan (1982) has proposed that prepubertal girls and boys have profoundly different foci in their views on relationships; boys are more focused on the external definition of self and girls on defining themselves via their network of relationships. It has been suggested that the diminished weight placed by men on the significance of relationships leaves the adolescent girl with a dilemma: to continue to be highly invested in relationships (and be undervalued by a male-dominated culture that emphasizes external definitions of self) or to attempt to suppress these innate tendencies and thus lose a significant aspect of her identity.

Media attention. There is little argument that the overwhelming media message directed toward women promotes weight loss and a thinner shape as ideal. In more recent years, some authors have attempted to examine the emphases present in media directed toward men (for a review, see Mickalide 1991). Generally, these studies have found that women's magazines focus on dieting, with exercise as an adjunct to the primary goal of weight loss, whereas men's magazines tend to promote physical fitness and exercise without the same emphasis on weight loss. Mickalide (1991) reports on several studies in which the ratio of articles that focus on dieting in women's and men's magazines is about 10:1—approaching the above-mentioned 20:1 ratio for eating disorders.

There is excellent evidence that the focus on a thinner shape for women has increased in the last three decades. Garfinkel and Garner (1982) reviewed height and weight data for *Playboy* centerfolds and Miss America pageant contestants over 20 years, which demonstrated a clear trend toward decreasing weight for height, or a thinner shape. This study was extended recently (Wiseman et al. 1992), and the same trends prevailed. Epidemiological studies continue to show increased dieting behavior among women. Dieting is ubiquitous among adolescent females—75% of girls believe that they are overweight—and very common in girls under age 12, 60% of whom may view themselves as overweight (Maloney et al. 1989). An interesting finding from these two studies is that a significant portion of the young boys and men also believed that they were overweight, but a much smaller proportion of those males were actually engaging in dieting behaviors (63% of females, 16% of males).

Body shape preference. It is commonly assumed that an ectomorphic shape has been traditionally preferred among gay men, despite the absence of studies to directly assess this preference. We have also been informed, usually anecdotally by patients, that since the onset of the acquired immunodeficiency syndrome (AIDS) epidemic, the focus in the homosexual community has shifted away from this ideal to that of a more muscular physique. Carlat and Camargo (1991) reviewed the few studies that examine attitudes toward eating, food, and shape within samples of homosexual men and concluded that there is an excess of concerns about body shape and weight and an increase in dieting behaviors among homosexual men compared with heterosexual men. If the anecdotal reports are true, and preferred body shape is a risk factor, one might expect a gradual diminution of cases of eating disorders in the homosexual male population over time.

Mickalide (1991) reviewed some historical views of men's size and shape. Some evidence suggests that a larger size has historically been associated with greater power and influence for men, perhaps increasingly so as the man ages. The reverse is true for women, in whom a thin shape may remain highly valued throughout their entire life span.

Whereas the ideal body shape for a woman over the years tends toward the ectomorphic (very slender, with no bust or hips), the desired shape for a man tends toward a "V," with broad shoulders tapering to a relatively (but not absolutely) narrow waist.

In our experience, some men with eating disorders do wish to have an extremely lean, slender body, whereas other men are more preoccupied with muscle mass and enter the path of an eating disorder via dieting behavior associated with weight-lifting regimens that emphasize decreased body fat to achieve higher muscular definition. Pope and associates (1993) quote a 2.8% prevalence of anorexia nervosa among male body builders compared with a 0.02% prevalence in the general population of males in the United States.

Occupational. Some evidence suggests that males in certain professions—notably wrestlers and jockeys—are at increased risk for the development of disordered eating behavior. However, Mickalide (1991) believes that individuals in these professions utilize multiple methods of purging to control their weight during the competitive seasons, but they do not display the same attitudes toward weight and shape during the off-season and appear to abandon these practices and return to more normal eating habits.

Multidetermined Nature of Eating Disorders

We believe that any discussion of a possible synthesis of the above factors should proceed from a multidetermined model, as advocated by Garfinkel and Garner (1982). In this model, biological, genetic, psychological, and societal factors are thought to interact to varying degrees in the development of anorexia nervosa or bulimia nervosa. However, the evolution of the specific set of predisposing factors that produces a profound sense of worthlessness and ineffectiveness is common among individuals with eating disorders and eventually leads them to exert control where they can—that is, by dieting, in an attempt to elevate their self-esteem and lessen their sense of worthlessness. Once initiated, the process of coping with psychological, biological, family, and social lack of control through dieting becomes self-perpetuating. As the individual begins to experience the sequelae of an eating disorder, which, in time, only lower self-esteem further and increase feelings of ineffectiveness, he or she is caught in an ongoing self-perpetuating cycle.

For bulimia nervosa, compelling evidence links bingeing behavior to the dieting that inevitably precedes it (Polivy and Herman 1985). Once an individual has invested a significant amount of his or her self-esteem in dietary restraint, the occurrence of binge eating is likely to be viewed as a catastrophe, thus worsening self-esteem, increasing ineffectiveness, and leading to further dietary restraint and possibly purging behaviors in an attempt to reverse the effects of the bingeing.

In attempting to understand why the factors reviewed above might contribute to the excess of eating disorders in women compared with men or to the excess of eating disorders in homosexual men, it is helpful to discuss these factors in the light of the multidetermined model, considering how each factor might lead an individual to that critical first compulsion to diet.

Psychological Factors

Many factors that evoke feelings of helplessness and ineffectiveness in young women are less pronounced in men. Concerns about puberty and the rate of physical maturation are probably less problematic for males because the changes associated with puberty are viewed as more positive in males than in females. Second, much less confusion is likely about the acceptability of the changes in body shape that accompany puberty in young boys. The postpubertal shape for boys is in accordance with societal norms, unlike that for young girls. The same is true for societal attitudes toward the development of an awareness of sexuality; societal norms for males are much more congruent with the biological norms than is the case for females. In the multidetermined model, incongruence with social pressures leads to the need for self-control (i.e., the compulsion to diet).

Biological-Genetic Factors

There is an accepted difference in sex-specific rates of major depression, which is much more common in females than males, although the ratio is not as high as in eating disorders (see Chapters 4 and 5). An episode of depression could trigger increased feelings of worthlessness and helplessness, which lead to dieting. It is conceivable that cyclical changes in weight associated with the menstrual cycle could also cause a young girl to focus attention on weight and shape to a greater extent than a young man would.

One can only speculate about the personality traits encoded by putative contributory genes. One of us has proposed (Woodside 1993) that, for bulimia nervosa, one possibility might be the propensity to binge in response to dietary restraint, as opposed to the more normal response of nonbinge overeating. For anorexia nervosa, there are many heritable possibilities, including alterations in central mechanisms that control hunger and satiety signals or the inheritance of a certain temperament or personality style that facilitates the implementation of extreme dietary restriction.

Societal Factors

Because the multidetermined model described above requires a decision to diet to initiate the illness, any factor that increases that likelihood becomes etiologically important. In this regard, the evidence supporting an increased societal emphasis on a thin shape for women is perhaps the most compelling way to understand the differences in the incidence of the disorders in men and women. This evidence also speaks to the increased incidence of eating disorders in homosexual men, who appear to receive a larger "dose" of our society's preoccupation with a slender shape than do heterosexual men.

Nonetheless, differential propensity to diet is unlikely to be a complete explanation. Despite the increased incidence of dieting behaviors among women compared with men, the differences (roughly fourfold) are not nearly great enough to account for the gender differences in the overall incidence of eating disorders.

Conclusion

It does not appear that any one factor provides an adequate explanation for the most notable difference between men and women with eating disorders—the difference in incidence. Although the differential social pressures to be thin appear to exert a significant effect on incidence, they alone do not appear to be a sufficient explanation. As a point of clarification, the term *social pressures* does not only refer to the media attention focused on thinness but also to a complex constellation of beliefs and attitudes that defines male and female roles in our society, including different attitudes toward male and female sexuality and communication styles.

Because the incidence of dieting behaviors is so much higher than the incidence of eating disorders, certain individuals must be either especially vulnerable to or specifically protected from the development of these disorders. Determining how sex-specific social and maturational pressures might afford such added protection or susceptibility can help to further a greater understanding of these serious illnesses.

References

American Psychiatric Association: Diagnostic and Statistical Manual of Mental Disorders, 3rd Edition, Revised. Washington, DC, American Psychiatric Association, 1987

Carlat DJ, Camargo CA: Review of bulimia nervosa in males. Am J Psychiatry 148:831–843, 1991

Crisp AH, Burns T: Primary anorexia nervosa in the male and female: a comparison of clinical features and prognosis, in Males With Eating Disorders. Edited by Andersen AE. New York, Brunner/Mazel, 1991, pp 77–79

Crisp AH, Hsu LDG, Chen CN, et al: Reproductive hormone profiles in male anorexia nervosa before, during and after restoration of body weight to normal: a study of 12 patients. International Journal of Eating Disorders 1:3–9, 1982

Edwin DH, Andersen AE: Psychometric testing in 76 males with eating disorders, in Males With Eating Disorders. Edited by Andersen AE. New York, Brunner/Mazel, 1991, pp 116–130

Fichter MM, Daser C, Postpischl F: Anorexic syndromes in the male. J Psychiatr Res 19:305–313, 1985

Gadpaille EJ: Homosexuality, in Comprehensive Textbook of Psychiatry, 5th Edition. Edited by Kaplan HI, Saddock BJ. Baltimore, MD, Williams & Wilkins, 1989, pp 1086–1096

Garfinkel PE, Garner DM: Anorexia Nervosa: A Multidimensional Perspective. New York, Brunner/Mazel, 1982

Garner DM, Garfinkel PE: The eating attitudes test: an index of the symptoms of anorexia nervosa. Psychol Med 9:273–279, 1979

Garner DM, Olmsted M, Polivy J: Development and validation of a multidimensional eating disorder inventory for anorexia nervosa and bulimia. International Journal of Eating Disorders 2:15–33, 1983

Gilligan C: In a Different Voice. Cambridge, MA, Harvard University Press, 1982

Goodwin CM, Fairburn CG, Cowen PJ: Dieting changes serotonergic functioning women, not men: implications for the aetiology of anorexia nervosa? Psychol Med 17:839–842, 1987

Grove WM, Eckert ED, Heston L, et al: Heritability of substance abuse and antisocial behaviour: a study of monozygotic twins reared apart. Biol Psychiatry 27:1293–1304, 1990

Gupta MA, Schork NJ, Dhaliwal JS: Stature, drive for thinness and body dissatisfaction: a study of males and females from a non-clinical sample. Can J Psychiatry 38:59–61, 1993

Hall A, Delahunt JW, Ellis PM: Anorexia nervosa in the male: clinical features and follow-up of nine patients. J Psychiatr Res 19:315–321, 1985

Herzog DB, Norman DK, Gordon C, et al: Sexual conflict and eating disorder in 27 males. Am J Psychiatry 141:989–990, 1984

Herzog DB, Bradburn IS, Newman K: Sexuality in males with eating disorders, in Males With Eating Disorders. Edited by Andersen AE. New York, Brunner/Mazel, 1991, pp 40–53

Holland AJ, Hall A, Murray R, et al: Anorexia nervosa: a study of 34 twin pairs and one set of triplets. Br J Psychiatry 145:414–419, 1984

Holland AJ, Sicotte N, Treasure J: Anorexia nervosa: evidence for a genetic basis. Br J Psychiatry 32:561–571, 1988

Kendler KS, MacLean C, Neale M, et al: The genetic epidemiology of bulimia nervosa. Am J Psychiatry 148:1627–1637, 1992

Keys A, Brozek J, Henschel A, et al: The Biology of Human Starvation. Minneapolis, University of Minnesota Press, 1950

LeMaire A, Ardaens K, Lepretre J, et al: Gonadal hormones in male anorexia nervosa. International Journal of Eating Disorders 2:135–144, 1983

Maloney MJ, McGuire J, Daniles SR, et al: Dieting behaviour and eating attitudes in children. Pediatrics 84:482–489, 1989

McNab D, Hawton K: Disturbances of sex hormones in anorexia nervosa in the male. Postgrad Med J 57:254–256, 1981

Merikangas KR: The genetic epidemiology of alcoholism. Psychol Med 20:11–22, 1990

Mickalide AD: Sociocultural factors influencing weight among males, in Males With Eating Disorders. Edited by Andersen AE. New York, Brunner/Mazel, 1991, pp 30–39

Morton R: Phthisologica: Or a Treatise of Consumption. London, S. Smith & B. Walford, 1694

Oyebode F, Boodhoo JA, Schapira K: Anorexia nervosa in males: clinical features and outcome. International Journal of Eating Disorders 1:121–124, 1988

Phillips KA, McElroy SL, Keck PE, et al: Body dysmorphic disorder: thirty cases of imagined ugliness. Am J Psychiatry 150:302–308, 1993

Polivy J, Herman CP: Dieting and bingeing—a causal analysis. Am Psychol 40:193–201, 1985

Pope HG, Katz DL, Hudson JI: Anorexia nervosa and "reverse anorexia" among 108 male body-builders. Compr Psychiatry 34:406–409, 1993

Schneider JA, Agras WS: Bulimia in males: a matched comparison with females. International Journal of Eating Disorders 6:235–242, 1987

Silverman JA: Anorexia nervosa in the male: early historic cases, in Males With Eating Disorders. Edited by Andersen AE. New York, Brunner/Mazel, 1991, pp 3–8

Strober M, Morrell W, Burroughs J, et al: A controlled family study of anorexia nervosa. J Psychiatr Res 18:423–429, 1985

Strober M, Lampert C, Morrell W, et al: A controlled family study of anorexia nervosa: evidence of familial aggregation and lack of shared transmission with affective disorders. International Journal of Eating Disorders 9:239–253, 1990

Wiseman CV, Gray JJ, Mosimann JE, et al: Cultural expectations of thinness in women: an update. International Journal of Eating Disorders 11:85–89, 1992

Woodside DB: Genetics of eating disorders, in Medical Aspects of Eating Disorders. Edited by Kaplan AS, Garfinkel PE. New York, Brunner/Mazel, 1993, pp 193–212

Woodside DB, Garner DM, Rockert W, et al: Eating disorders in males: insights from a clinical and psychometric comparison with females, in Males With Eating Disorders. Edited by Andersen AE. New York, Brunner/Mazel, 1991, pp 100–115

CHAPTER 12

Gender Differences in Sleep Disorders

Eileen P. Sloan, Ph.D.
Colin M. Shapiro, M.B., Ph.D., M.R.C.Psych., F.R.C.P.C.

D isrupted sleep patterns play a significant role in the course, and in some cases the etiology, of a number of psychiatric illnesses (see Table 12–1). Sleep studies are unique in psychiatric practice inasmuch as they allow for simultaneous subjective, objective, and quantitative measures of a behavior disturbance. The results have the potential to act as biological markers and thus to contribute significantly to the field of clinical psychiatry.

Because this book deals with gender issues, one of the best examples of how sleep studies contribute to diagnosis and treatment is in the differentiation of organic from psychological male impotence. In healthy men, penile erections occur during rapid eye movement (REM) sleep, probably reflecting altered autonomic nervous system control. If nocturnal penile tumescence (NPT) recordings show repeated erections during sleep, the likelihood of the impotence having an organic basis becomes minimal (Bancroft 1989). Optimal treatment can then be instituted.

In this chapter, we briefly discuss the physiological function of sleep and outline the variations in human sleep patterns. We then review gender differences in sleep patterns and sleep disorders and

Table 12–1. Psychiatric illnesses associated with disruption of sleep
pattern

Alcoholism	Korsakoff's syndrome
Alzheimer's disease	Manic-depressive illness
Anorexia nervosa	Obsessive-compulsive disorder
Anxiety disorder	Posttraumatic stress disorder
Borderline personality disorder	Panic disorder
Depressive disorders	Schizophrenia

Source. American Sleep Disorders Association 1990.

examine some of the reasons that certain sleep disorders appear to
be more prevalent in women.

Sleep Stages and the Function of Sleep

Sleep is a normal physiological process, accompanied by wide-
ranging changes in brain activity, cardiac function, biochemistry,
body temperature, and hormonal release. Sleep consists of two distinct states—REM and non-REM—which are differentiated on the
basis of changes in electrooculogram (EOG), electroencephalogram
(EEG), and electromyogram (EMG) activity. Throughout the night,
a cycling occurs between the REM and non-REM states, with most
non-REM sleep occurring in the first third of the night and REM
sleep dominating the latter third of the night.

The amount of time spent sleeping and the percentage of sleep
time spent in each sleep stage varies in humans according to age. For
example, newborn babies spend approximately 16 hours per day
sleeping, half of which is REM sleep. In elderly people, sleep time is
greatly reduced, and the composition of sleep is dramatically altered
(Figure 12–1).

Several hypotheses have been advanced to explain the function
of sleep. One popular theory (Fleming and Shapiro 1992) is that sleep,
particularly slow-wave sleep, is a time of restoration for the body. In
adolescents and other populations in whom there would seem to be
an important need for growth (e.g., pregnant women or patients with

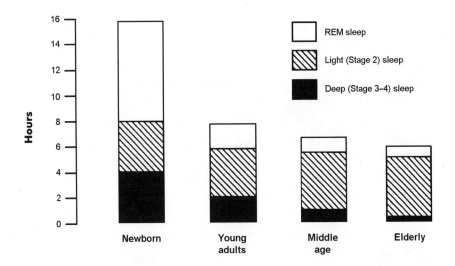

Figure 12–1. Change in sleep time and sleep composition across the life span. REM = rapid eye movement.

anorexia on a refeeding program), there is an increase in the total amount of sleep.

Other theories of sleep function suggest that 1) sleep is necessary for restoration of the central nervous system, 2) sleep is important for energy conservation, 3) memory consolidation takes place during REM sleep, and 4) sleep is necessary for binocular vision.

Gender Differences in Normal Sleep

From a very early age, differences in the sleep patterns of males and females are noticeable. Menna-Barreto and colleagues (1989) examined the sleep-wake cycle of 4- to 14-month-old babies and found that increasing age resulted in a decrease in total sleep time for the entire population studied. After age 10 months, girls tended to sleep more than boys. The reasons for these differences are unclear. One possibility is that they reflect the differential rate of development of the central nervous system.

Changes in sleep (as recorded in the laboratory) across the life span have been studied cross-sectionally by Williams and associates

(1974) (see Table 12–2); within each age group, significant sex differences are apparent. In 3- to 5-year-old children, the TST (time from sleep onset to morning awakening minus time awake during the night) and the average REM cycle length are greater in boys. In 6- to 9-year-old children, non-REM stage 3 latency is greater in girls, whereas in 10- to 12-year-old children, there are a significantly greater number of stages and a higher percentage of stage 3 sleep in boys. In the 13- to 15-year age group, there are no significant gender differences; the sleep patterns are almost identical. At age 16–19 years, the number of REM periods, which have been steadily decreasing since birth, plateaus. The only sex difference noted at this age is that young women have a significantly longer interval between the third and fourth REM period.

In the 20-year span from age 20–39, the sleep patterns of women show no significant changes, whereas men have significant "deterioration" of sleep. Between ages 20 and 29, several trends that separate the sexes appear and continue throughout life. Women have considerably more total sleep time than men. This remains the case throughout adult life. During this period, men have a greater number of awakenings each night. During the 20s, slow-wave sleep begins to decline sharply in men. This is especially the case in men, who continue to show a more rapid decline with increasing age.

In the 30s, there are no significant differences in sleep patterns between the two groups, but the decline in slow-wave sleep that started in men during their 20s continues, whereas in females this decline is just beginning. At this age, women tend to have a longer sleep latency than men and a slightly higher percentage of wakefulness.

Between ages 40 and 59, total sleep time is reduced, and sleep patterns become more disturbed. Sleep may serve a restorative function (Oswald 1980), which is related to diurnal energy expenditure. From middle age onward, energy expenditure usually declines, and the need for sleep may decrease. However, subjective dissatisfaction often arises because one expects the same amount of sleep as before. Disturbance in a variety of physiological functions, such as bladder control, may be responsible for the disturbed sleep patterns in middle-aged and elderly populations.

In women in this age group (40–59), the number of stage changes and the number of awakenings increase significantly. In men, sleep

Table 12–2. Gender differences in sleep architecture across the life span

Age group (years)	Difference in sleep architecture
3–5	TST, REM cycle length, and percentage of stage 2 sleep are higher in males.
6–9	Stage 3 latency is greater in females.
10–12	Number of stages is greater and percentage of stage 3 sleep is higher in males.
13–15	No significant gender differences are apparent.
16–19	Interval between third and fourth REM period is longer in females.
20–29	Short-wave sleep starts to decline steadily in males; a slight decline is noted in females.
30–39	Sleep latency is longer, short-wave and REM sleep are slightly greater, and percentage of wakefulness is higher in females. Short-wave sleep decline continues in males and starts to become evident in females.
40–49	Sleep is more restful and TST is longer in females. Percentage of awake periods during the night is higher and sleep efficiency is dramatically decreased in males.
50–59	Stage 4 sleep is greater in females.
60–69	Awakenings during the night and frequency of stage 1 sleep are greater in males.
70–79	Number of stage shifts are reduced and stage 3 and 4 sleep drop off in males.

Note. TST = time from sleep onset to morning awakening minus time awake during the night; REM = rapid eye movement.

efficiency changes drastically, with an increase in the number of awakenings and the percentage of time spent awake. In the 40–49 age group, women have more restful sleep. Men have a higher percentage of awake periods during the night. In the 50–59 age group, the sleep duration variables are all significantly higher for women, but sleep efficiency is similar in both groups.

In the 60–69 age group, the only gender difference is that men have more awakenings during the night. These changes indicate a continuous trend toward more disturbed sleep in men. In the decade between age 70 and 79, women have a significantly greater number of stage shifts relative to men. According to Williams and colleagues (1974), this finding probably reflects the fact that most women still have all five sleep stages, whereas more than 50% of men have lost stage 3, and almost all have lost stage 4. For men in this group, the length of the third and fourth REM period drops off sharply. It is unclear why men have more awakenings during the night because the incidence of sleep apnea is similar in both sexes at this age. Alcohol, however, is known to disturb sleep (Prinz et al. 1980), and consumption is higher in men (see Chapter 14).

The ability to recover from sleep disruption seems to differ in elderly men and women. For example, Reynolds and co-workers (1986) reported that after 36 hours of sleep deprivation, women had higher sleep efficiency and more slow-wave sleep on the recovery night than in their baseline recordings, whereas male subjects did not show any change in these parameters.

One can conclude that throughout life, significant and quantifiable differences exist between the sleep patterns of men and women. There is no evidence that women have more disturbed sleep or are more prone to sleep disorders than are men. Indeed, it appears that men show greater disturbance in their sleep patterns, with decline in sleep quality beginning at a younger age than in women. On this basis, it is difficult to account for the significantly greater consumption of hypnotic medication by women (see below and also Chapter 15).

Gender Distribution of Sleep Disorders

The International Classification of Sleep Disorders (American Sleep Disorders Association 1990) details the diagnostic and coding procedures for sleep disorders and provides information on the relative frequency with which complaints are diagnosed in each sex. The conditions in which gender differences are known to occur are summarized in Table 12–3.

In addition to those disorders shown in Table 12–3, a number of sleep disorders occur in association with medical or psychiatric conditions. For example, nocturnal cardiac ischemia is more common in men, especially before age 60 years. Rheumatoid arthritis and fibrositis, which are accompanied by severe disturbance in sleep, are more common in women. Rare conditions such as Pok-kuru and Bangugut involve sudden death in young Asian men during sleep, possibly on a cardiac basis. Women appear to be more susceptible to certain psychiatric conditions in which insomnia is often a feature, for example, generalized anxiety disorder, which is two to three times more common in women than in men (see Chapter 6). Because such disorders are almost invariably treated with tranquilizers, this influences the reported prevalence of hypnotic use.

Gender Differences in
Insomnia and Hypnotic Consumption

It is now well established that the rate of hypnotic consumption is significantly higher in women than in men. Cirignotta and others (1985) found that among a large number of respondents from the general population ($n = 5,713$), 9.9% of men and 16.8% of women reported rarely or ever sleeping well. Insomnia was uncommon in people younger than age 20 years, and the prevalence was similar in both sexes up to age 44 years, after which it rose to 23.6% of women and 14.4% of men between ages 45 and 49. The prevalence further diverged to 39.7% of women and 15.3% of men in their early 50s. Karacan et al. (1976) reported that, of the 13.4% of the population who complained of sleeping difficulties "often" or "all the time," older married women of lower social class were the most highly represented group. The findings from more recent studies are similar (Quera-Salva et al. 1991; Weyerer and Dilling 1991).

A preponderance of insomnia in older women may account for the fact that twice as many women as men are prescribed benzodiazepines (Curran and Golombok 1985), a prescribing pattern that is consistent internationally in developed countries (Cooperstock and Parnell 1982).

Holm (1989) examined the weekly prescribing practice of general practitioners and found that of hypnotics (mainly benzodiazepines),

Table 12–3. Sleep disorders for which sex differences are reported in the *International Classification of Sleep Disorders: Diagnostic and Coding Manual*

Sleep disorder	Prevalence within general population	Gender distribution
Psychophysiological insomnia	15% of all insomnias	Higher female prevalence
Obstructive sleep apnea syndrome	1%–2% of general population	Male-to-female ratio of 8:1; equal after menopause
Central sleep apnea syndrome	Prevalence unknown because may be asymptomatic	More prevalent in men; after menopause, difference less apparent
Central alveolar hyperventilation syndrome	General prevalence unknown	More common in men
Restless legs syndrome	Prevalence unknown	More common in women; seen in 11% of pregnant women
Nocturnal leg cramps	16% of healthy people; incidence increasing in the elderly	More common in women; frequently occurs in pregnancy
Rhythmic movement disorder	66% of children at 9 months and 8% at age 4 years	Male-to-female ratio of 4:1
Adjustment sleep disorder	Prevalence unknown	Appears to be more prevalent in women
Insufficient sleep syndrome	2% of cases at sleep clinics; exact prevalence unknown	Slightly more common in men
Sleep onset association disorder	Most prevalent at age 3 and younger, uncommon in adults	Possibly a slightly increased incidence in males
Hypnotic-dependent sleep disorder	General prevalence unknown	More common in women and elderly people

Disorder	Prevalence	Sex difference
Sleep terrors (pavor nocturnus)	3% of children and < 1% of adults	Sex distribution unclear; more common in males
Nightmares	10%–50% of 3- to 5-year-olds and 1% of adults	Sex ratio equal in children; adult female-to-male ratio between 2:1 and 4:1
Sleep paralysis	Occurs at least once in 40%–50% of population and chronically in 3%–6%; occurs in 17%–40% of people with narcolepsy	Familial form more common in women; no sex difference in idiopathic form
Rapid eye movement sleep behavior disorder	Rare in general population, but many cases may masquerade as other parasomnias	Appears more prevalent in men
Sleep enuresis	Occurs in 30% of 4-year-old children and decreases to 3% at age 12; primary enuresis is rare in adults	More prevalent in males
Primary snoring	Prevalence increases with age; occurs in 40%–50% of adults over age 65	More prevalent in males at all ages; habitual snoring occurs in 3%–24% of adult males and in 2.2%–14% of adult females
Infant sleep apnea associated with an apparent life-threatening event	Occurs in at least 1.6/1,000 live births	5%–10% higher incidence in males
Sudden infant death syndrome	Occurs in 1–2/1,000 live births	Male-to-female ratio of 3:2
Kleine-Levin syndrome (recurrent hypersomnia)	Prevalence unknown	Most common in adolescent males; menstrually related hypersomnia has been reported

Source. American Sleep Disorders Association 1990.

68% were prescribed to women and 32% to men. The frequency of prescribing increased markedly with age. According to Holm, the fact that more women have psychiatric disorders that are treated, in part, with hypnotics may explain the discrepancy in prescribing patterns. However, this viewpoint is at variance with that of Cooperstock and Leon (1978), who argue that women are more likely to receive a diagnosis of a psychiatric illness than are men, so women are more often prescribed hypnotics. These investigators suggest that women do not actually have more psychiatric illnesses or insomnia but that doctors are more willing to attach the psychiatric label to women and to use hypnotics for treatment. According to Lennard and Cooperstock (1980), in the elderly population, not only are women at risk for being prescribed tranquilizers but especially women who are poor, disabled, and unattached. The latter attribute probably reflects the fact that many elderly women are widows who have little social support and contact. Their problems may be primarily social but are treated with medicines. Cooperstock (1979) suggests that this compounds the problem because sedative-hypnotics reduce the users' motivation to expand their social network and make them more dependent on the physician. Other explanations for the discrepancy in hypnotic use in men and women have been put forward (see Chapter 15).

The issue of the prescribing habits of family practitioners, and the extent to which they influence the apparent prevalence of insomnia in women, is a complex one. Women may show distress at an earlier stage of insomnia and may seek help more readily. Murray and colleagues (1981) report that women who are prescribed benzodiazepines are less disturbed than men who are given such prescriptions. Whether this reflects a tendency in women to seek help at an earlier and less severe stage of their condition than men or a greater willingness among doctors to resort to medication with female patients at a less severe stage of insomnia remains to be determined.

Evidence suggests that the disturbance in sleep patterns brought on by shift work persists even several years after this type of work has ceased; this suggests that the sleep pattern developed while doing shift work becomes entrained or that some "damage" to the sleep cycle at a young age (which is not initially pronounced in its impact) "reveals" itself years later when the "sleep drive" is less strong (i.e., with the deterioration in sleep pattern that accompanies aging). The prevalence of insomnia in women increases significantly in middle age (Cirignotta et al. 1985). The majority of these women will have had children. Extrapolating from the evidence from shift work, the disturbance to sleep routines brought on by child rearing may have become entrained in certain women. While their children are young, most women are likely to accept disturbed sleep as part of the child-rearing process. However, once the external reason for the disturbance no longer exists, women may feel that their disturbed sleep routines require medical attention.

From a sociological perspective, it is perhaps not surprising that in older women, sleep patterns become disrupted, and they seek medical advice. Relative to their male counterparts, their social status is frequently low, and they generally earn low income and depend on their husbands or partners for financial support. They often find themselves responsible not only for the welfare of their children but also for elderly relatives. In such situations, women may perceive themselves as having little control over their physical and mental health; thus, they accept the doctor's opinion and do not challenge the prescription of hypnotic medication. An additional factor may be that women in their 40s are returning to the work force after having taken time off for childbearing. Such women usually retain domestic responsibilities and are then confronted with "double work." The added stress may lead to sleep disruption and hypnotic use.

From Table 12–3, it appears that apart from disorders associated with pregnancy, sleep disorders that are more prevalent in women seem to have a more psychological basis, whereas the causes of sleep disorders that are more prevalent in men could be considered more physiological or anatomical. In the case of insomnia, Hauri and Esther (1990) propose three etiological categories: 1) insomnia related to mental disorders, such as depression and anxiety; 2) primary insomnia (e.g., learned psychophysiological insomnia and insomnia complaints without objective findings); and 3) insomnia related to known organic factors, such as sleep apnea. Qualitative differences may exist between the insomnia experienced by men and women; in women, insomnia is treated with hypnotics, whereas in men, insomnia is treated with therapeutic approaches such as continuous positive airway pressure.

Hormonal Effects on Sleep

Events that are unique to women, such as menstruation and pregnancy, can disrupt sleep patterns. Lee and co-workers (1990) found no differences in the percentage of the various sleep states between the luteal (postovulatory) phase and the follicular (preovulatory) phase of the menstrual cycle. However, women who had depressive symptoms during the premenstruum had significantly reduced slow-wave sleep during both phases. This may constitute a degree of sleep deprivation, which in depressed women makes them more sensitive to monthly hormonal fluctuations. Alternatively, Lee and co-workers (1990) suggest that the symptomatic women who experience less slow-wave sleep may have an underlying physiological deficit that is accentuated by monthly gonadal hormone fluctuations. Relatively little research has been done on changes in sleep across the menstrual cycle, and the extent to which changes vary according to age in women is still unclear.

In women, sleep-related breathing disorders, such as sleep apnea syndrome, become more prevalent after menopause. This may be related to decreases in the level of progesterone, a respiratory stimulant. Block and associates (1980) found that 60% of postmenopausal women had sleep events, such as apnea or oxygen desaturation, whereas only 11% of younger women showed such events. This evidence suggests that the respiratory-stimulating effects of circulating progesterone or the ratio of progesterone to androgenic hormones may protect younger women from sleep-related breathing disorders. Once menopause occurs and progesterone levels decrease, the protective mechanism no longer operates, and sleep-related breathing disorders develop. Consequently, the prevalence in this age group is similar for men and women, whereas in younger age groups, the prevalence is significantly higher in men. However, the nature of the disorder may vary according to gender. Leech and colleagues (1988) found that women tend to experience hypopneas rather than complete apneas and, when apneas *are* present, they tend to be shorter than those in men, perhaps reflecting a difference in upper-airway anatomy or physiology. Valencia-Flores and others (1992) report that women with sleep apnea have longer sleep latencies, greater amounts of slow-wave sleep, and fewer awakenings during the night than men with the condition. These differences are in accordance with known gender differences in sleep architecture.

A high proportion of women report the development of hot flashes at the onset of menopause. At the same time, they may begin to complain of sleep problems (i.e., trouble falling asleep, frequent waking at night, and increased daytime tiredness). The appearance of hot flashes may result in disrupted sleep patterns.

For many women, disrupted sleep patterns are a feature of pregnancy and early motherhood. Nocturnal events such as fetal movement, uterine contractions, urinary frequency, position-related indigestion, breathing disturbances, and leg cramps contribute to disrupted sleep patterns. In a sample of 100 pregnant women, Fast and associates (1989) found that 67% experienced backache at night before going to sleep, 36% reported that backache actually wakened them, and 60% experienced leg cramps during the night that also compromised their sleep. In a group of women recorded sequentially in each trimester of pregnancy and in the first month postpartum, Driver and Shapiro (1992) showed that slow-wave sleep progressively increases throughout pregnancy and the postpartum period compared with age-matched control subjects. However, Karacan and colleagues (1968), in a cross-sectional study, reported that there is a reduction in slow-wave sleep in late pregnancy, with sleep recovery starting on the first night postpartum. In the postpartum period, the recovery of deep sleep may be especially important for restoration. Evidence suggests, however, that factors related to the hospital environment, such as bright light, noise, and nursing activities, interfere with the new mother's ability to attain deep sleep (Lentz and Killien 1991). The unpredictable sleep-wake patterns of the newborn baby also frequently disrupt maternal sleep (Campbell 1986).

Other Factors in Sleep and Sleep Disorders

Several influences on sleep appear to be sex specific. Our studies on the impact of exercise and fitness on sleep lead to different conclusions depending on whether the subjects are male or female. Meintjes and co-workers (1989) found that, in men, improved physical fitness led to improved sleep quality, but a similar effect was not found in women (Shapiro et al. 1984). The results of studies by other groups of researchers support these observations.

There is a clear effect of body composition on sleep (Shapiro et al. 1987). Body fat is higher in women, but no comparative studies across gender have examined whether it is relevant to sleep patterns. A relationship between body composition and sleep has been observed in female subjects with anorexia and young women of normal weight but not in obese women (Shapiro et al. 1990).

Important changes occur in sleep during puberty. Luteinizing hormone is first released during the sleeping period. It is interesting that in people with anorexia who regain weight, this sequence of pubertal evolution is replayed (Kapen et al. 1974). However, many of the studies on sleep physiology have used male subjects exclusively (e.g., those on growth hormone release during sleep and particularly after sleep deprivation), which limits any appreciation of gender-specific physiological effects.

There are differences in relation to dream and dream recall across gender. Kramer and co-investigators (1981) reported significant differences in the dream content of male and female subjects ages 20–25 years. For example, women's dreams reflected more cognitive activity and stronger intensity or emotionality, whereas men's dreams were more filled with objects of large sizes, old age references, fullness, and crookedness. The sexes did not differ in their references to aggression, misfortune to self or others, or social interactions. The investigators speculate that these findings indicate that some of the traditional gender differences in dream recall, such as the expression of aggression, have disappeared, perhaps as a result of increased sexual equality. Some new differences have emerged, such as male concerns with intimacy, whereas others, such as the increased emotionality of women, have not changed.

In some circumstances, it is almost impossible to find appropriate male control subjects for studies of female populations—for example, the impact of rape or sexual abuse on sleep. Other issues, such as the effect of gender on treatment response and outcome, have not been addressed. Evidence suggests that oral contraceptives may affect the metabolism of some benzodiazepines (Ellinwood et al. 1983). Consideration also must be given to the possible effects of menstrual phase on the effectiveness of psychopharmacological agents.

Conclusion

Sleep is a normal biological process that is different in men and women. The disruption of sleep may lead to psychiatric illness (as well as being a manifestation of psychiatric illness). The physiological and pathophysiological influences on sleep are different for men and women. In addition to pathophysiological causes of sleep disruption, a number of social and cultural factors may lead to sleep changes in women, which, in turn, may place women, especially those who are middle aged, at greater risk for psychiatric illness.

There is a dearth of information about many relevant aspects of sleep differences between men and women. An awareness of gender-related effects on sleep disruption (e.g., "estrogen deficiency" producing insomnia in postmenopausal women and the impact of sleep disruption in triggering psychiatric ill health) is necessary before optimal care can be provided. In addition to critical studies of particular facets of sleep physiology and pathology, wider, more detailed, systematic review of the information that does exist is essential.

References

American Sleep Disorders Association: International Classification of Sleep Disorders: Diagnostic and Coding Manual. Rochester, MN, Allan Press, 1990

Bancroft J: Human Sexuality and Its Problems. Edinburgh, Churchill Livingstone, 1989

Block AJ, Wynee JW, Boysen PG: Sleep disordered breathing and nocturnal oxygen desaturation in postmenopausal women. Am J Med 69:76–79, 1980

Campbell I: Postpartum sleep patterns of mother-baby pairs. Midwifery 2:193–201, 1986

Cirignotta F, Mondini S, Zucconi M, et al: Insomnia: an epidemiological survey. Neurophysiol Clin 8 (suppl 1):549–554, 1985

Cooperstock R: A review of females' psychotropic drug use. Can J Psychiatry 24:29–34, 1979

Cooperstock R, Leon JS: Prescriptions to the Elderly in Family Practice. Toronto, Addiction Research Foundation, 1978

Cooperstock R, Parnell P: Research on psychotropic drug use: a review of findings and methods. Soc Sci Med 16:1179–1196, 1982

Curran V, Golombok S: Bottling It Up. London, Faber & Faber, 1985

Driver HS, Shapiro CM: A longitudinal study of sleep stages in young women during pregnancy and post-partum. Sleep 15:449–453, 1992

Ellinwood EH, Easier ME, Linnoila M, et al: Effects of oral contraceptives on diazepam-induced psychomotor impairment. Clinical Pharmacological Therapy 35:360–366, 1983

Fast A, Weiss L, Parikh S, et al: Night backache in pregnancy—hypothetical pathophysiological mechanisms. Am J Phys Med Rehabil 69:227–229, 1989

Fleming J, Shapiro CM: Sleep Function and Insomnia Assessment. Montreal, Kommunicom Publications, 1992

Hauri PJ, Esther MS: Insomnia. Mayo Clin Proc 65:869–882, 1990

Holm M: Prescription of psychopharmaceuticals in general practice. Ugeskr Laeger 151:2130–2133, 1989

Kapen S, Boyar RM, Finkelstein JW, et al: Effect of sleep-wake cycle reversal on luteinizing hormone secretory pattern in puberty. J Clin Endocrinol Metab 39:293–299, 1974

Karacan I, Heine W, Harman WA, et al: Characteristics of sleep patterns during late pregnancy and the postpartum periods. Am J Obstet Gynecol 101:579–586, 1968

Karacan I, Thornby JI, Anch M, et al: Prevalence of sleep disturbance in a primarily urban Florida county. Soc Sci Med 10:239–244, 1976

Kramer M, Kinney L, Scharf M: Sex differences in dreams. The Psychiatric Journal of the University of Ottawa 8:1–4, 1981

Lee KA, Shaver JF, Giblin EC, et al: Sleep patterns related to menstrual cycle phase and premenstrual affective symptoms. Sleep 13:403–409, 1990

Leech LA, Onal E, Dulberg C, et al: A comparison of men and women with occlusive sleep apnea syndrome. Chest 94:983–988, 1988

Lennard HL, Cooperstock R: The social context and functions of tranquillizer prescribing, in Prescribing Practice and Drug Usage. Edited by Mapes R. London, Croom Helm, 1980, pp 72–82

Lentz MJ, Killien MG: Are you sleeping? Sleep patterns during postpartum hospitalization. Journal of Perinatal and Neonatal Nursing 4:30–38, 1991

Meintjes AF, Driver HS, Shapiro CM: Improved physical fitness failed to alter the EEG patterns of sleep in young women. Eur J Appl Physiol 59:123–127, 1989

Menna-Barreto L, Montagner H, Soussignan R, et al: The sleep/wake cycle in 4- to 14-month children: general aspects and sex differences. Braz J Med Biol Res 22:103–106, 1989

Murray J, Dunn G, Williams P, et al: Factors affecting the consumption of psychotropic drugs. Psychol Med 11:551–560, 1981

Oswald I: Sleep as a restorative process: human clues. Prog Brain Res 50:279–287, 1980

Prinz PN, Roberts TA, Vitaliano PP, et al: Effects of alcohol on sleep and nighttime plasma growth hormone and cortisol concentrations. J Clin Endocrinol Metab 51:759–764, 1980

Quera-Salva MA, Orluc A, Goldenberg F, et al: Insomnia and use of hypnotics: study of a French population. Sleep 14:386–391, 1991

Reynolds CF, Kupfer DJ, Hoch CC, et al: Sleep deprivation in healthy elderly men and women: effects on mood and on sleep during recovery. Sleep 9:492–501, 1986

Shapiro CM, Goll CC, Cohen G, et al: Heat production during sleep. J Appl Physiol 56:671–677, 1984

Shapiro CM, Catterall J, Warren P, et al: Lean body mass correlates with non-REM sleep. BMJ 294:22, 1987

Shapiro CM, Driver H, Cheshire K, et al: Sleep and body composition. Basic Life Sci 55:231–235, 1990

Valencia-Flores M, Bliwise DL, Guilleminault C, et al: Gender differences in sleep architecture in sleep apnoea syndrome. Journal of Sleep Research 1:51–53, 1992

Weyerer S, Dilling H: Prevalence and treatment of insomnia in the community: results from the Upper Bavarian Field study. Sleep 14:392–398, 1991

Williams RL, Karacan I, Hursch CJ: Electroencephalography of Human Sleep: Clinical Applications. New York, Wiley, 1974

CHAPTER 13

Gender Differences in Somatoform Disorders

Brenda B. Toner, Ph.D.

D SM-II (American Psychiatric Association 1968) included a detailed section labeled "psychophysiological disorders that were defined as physical disorders of psychogenic etiology." DSM-III and DSM-III-R (American Psychiatric Association 1980, 1987) deleted this classification on the grounds that it reflected an artificial dichotomy between "psychophysiological" and "physical" disorders. In DSM-III, individuals who would have received a DSM-II diagnosis of psychophysiological disorder were classified as having either 1) psychological factors affecting physical conditions or 2) somatoform disorders. According to DSM-III-R, psychological factors affecting physical conditions could not be used in cases of somatoform disorders, which were regarded as disturbances in which the specific pathophysiological process involved in the disorder was not demonstrable by existing standard laboratory procedures. The same distinction is maintained in DSM-IV (American Psychiatric Association 1994).

Somatoform disorder best encompasses three illnesses that have received increasing attention during the last decade: 1) irritable bowel syndrome (IBS), 2) chronic fatigue syndrome (CFS), and 3) fibromyalgia syndrome (FMS) (Table 13–1). However, some investigators conceptualize these syndromes as medical conditions affected by psychological factors. Other investigators suggest that no DSM-IV classification accurately captures these "functional somatic disorders" (Kirmayer and Robbins 1991). Moreover, Taylor (1993) argues that the dichotomization of illness into organic and functional categories is inconsistent with contemporary views of psychosomatic medicine.

These three syndromes are all more prevalent in women than in men, but the epidemiological rates are based on treatment samples rather than community samples. Therefore, these rates may be affected by gender differences in help-seeking behaviors and diagnostician bias.

In this chapter, I use IBS as an example of somatoform disorder because most of the issues I discuss also apply to the related disorders of FMS and CFS. In fact, as I discuss later in this chapter, some in-

Table 13–1. DSM-IV diagnostic criteria for undifferentiated somatoform disorder

---

A. One or more physical complaints (e.g., fatigue, loss of appetite, gastrointestinal or urinary complaints).
B. Either (1) or (2):
    (1) after appropriate investigation, the symptoms cannot be fully explained by a known general medical condition or the direct effects of a substance (e.g., a drug of abuse, a medication)
    (2) when there is a related general medical condition, the physical complaints or resulting social or occupational impairment is in excess of what would be expected from the history, physical examination, or laboratory findings
C. The symptoms cause clinically significant distress or impairment in social, occupational, or other important areas of functioning.
D. The duration of the disturbance is at least 6 months.
E. The disturbance is not better accounted for by another mental disorder (e.g., another somatoform disorder, sexual dysfunction, mood disorder, anxiety disorder, sleep disorder, or psychotic disorder).
F. The symptom is not intentionally produced or feigned (as in factitious disorder or malingering).

Source. Reprinted from American Psychiatric Association: *Diagnostic and Statistical Manual of Mental Disorders, 4th Edition.* Washington, DC, American Psychiatric Association, 1994, p. 451. Used with permission.

vestigators have recently suggested that all three of these disorders are similar and that their specific diagnostic categorizations are arbitrary and serve no useful clinical or research purpose (Moldofsky and Lue 1993).

Despite the repeated finding that IBS is diagnosed significantly more frequently in women than in men, little attention has been devoted to gender issues in either the conceptualization or clinical management of the disorder. This chapter has two major objectives: 1) to provide an overview of what clinicians know and do not know about IBS and 2) to discuss the role of gender in the prevalence, expression, diagnosis, and treatment of this disorder.

Definition and Symptoms

A *functional disorder* is defined as a variable combination of chronic or recurrent symptoms not explained by structural or biochemical abnormalities. IBS is defined as a functional gastrointestinal (GI) disorder referable to the intestines and associated with continuous or recurrent symptoms for at least 3 months (Drossman et al. 1990a). Manning and colleagues (1978) found that the following five physical symptoms occurred significantly more often in IBS than in organic GI disorders: abdominal pain that is relieved with bowel movement, loose and more frequent stool with pain onset, mucus per rectum, feeling of incomplete evacuation, and abdominal distention. However, some studies have found that the Manning criteria are less predictive of IBS in men than in women (Smith et al. 1991; Talley 1991; Talley et al. 1990).

Epidemiology

There is general agreement that IBS is the most common functional GI disorder (Thompson et al. 1989) and the most common disorder of the digestive tract (Sammons and Karoly 1987). It is estimated to affect 8%–19% of the general adult population in a given year (Drossman et al. 1982; Thompson and Heaton 1980; Welch et al. 1985).

Although most individuals do not come to medical attention, patients who do seek consultation and treatment for the disorder make extensive use of the health care system. This common syndrome accounts for 20%–70% of all referrals made to gastroenterologists in Western societies (Ferguson et al. 1977; Harvey et al. 1983; Latimer 1983; C. M. Mitchell and Drossman 1987b). The syndrome is usually reported as chronic without long symptom-free periods (Waller and Misiewicz 1969). This disorder leads to more than 2 million prescriptions per year in the United States (Sandler 1990), and it is associated with unnecessary and often harmful tests, procedures, and surgeries (Thompson et al. 1989). Of particular concern, Whitehead and associates (1990) found that 21% of IBS patients in their sample had undergone hysterectomies without benefit. This rate is significantly higher than the national United States average of 5.5%. In addition to the cost to the health care system, the general economic impact of IBS is considerable. IBS has been ranked as the second most common cause of industrial absenteeism due to illness (Young et al. 1976).

Conceptual Model

To date, no physiological or psychosocial markers of IBS have been identified. Rather, several predisposing, precipitating, and perpetuating factors have been considered as contributory. IBS is best conceptualized using a biopsychosocial framework. Symptoms may be generated from physiological disturbances (enhanced intestinal motility and visceral sensation), which are closely connected to central nervous system (CNS) activity (via the CNS-ENS [enteric nervous system] axis). The clinical expression of these symptoms (e.g., a person's illness behavior, the decision to take medication or seek health care) is strongly influenced by psychosocial factors. For this reason, the high frequency of psychosocial disturbance (e.g., high life stress, psychiatric diagnoses, sexual abuse history) in the absence of modulating factors (e.g., social support, coping strategies) reported among IBS patients may, in part, relate to their self-selection into referral practices. To support this conclusion, several studies have found that persons with IBS who do not seek health care (IBS nonpatients) are indistinguishable from healthy control subjects on several psychological parameters (Drossman et al. 1988; Whitehead et al. 1988).

Physiological Factors

IBS patients experience a heightened colonic motility response to ingestion of food, balloon distention of the colon, stress, and emotional arousal (Welgan et al. 1988). Latimer and co-workers (1981), however, found that an IBS group did not differ significantly from a non-IBS "neurotic" control group on measures of either myoelectric or colonic activity. This finding implies that colon reactivity may not be specific to IBS patients but may be a general finding in patients with psychological distress.

Recent interest has shifted from motility to investigations of abnormal pain perception in physiological studies of IBS (Whitehead 1992). Whitehead (1992) reported that several laboratories have found abnormal pain thresholds in IBS patients, including low thresholds for experiencing sensations of gas, rectal fullness, and urgency to defecate. Physiological factors have not been found, however, to be associated with frequency or intensity of IBS symptoms or with the decision to seek medical care for symptoms. Thus, it is not surprising that treatments that focus primarily on modifying intestinal physiology (e.g., antimotility drugs) have been no more effective than placebo (Klein 1988).

Psychological Factors

Research has repeatedly demonstrated a significant psychological component in patients who seek repeated medical consultation for IBS. In particular, numerous studies have demonstrated a high prevalence of psychiatric illness (50%–100%) in IBS patients who are seen in a treatment setting (Latimer 1983; Toner et al. 1990a, 1990b; Walker et al. 1990; Young et al. 1976). In addition to the high frequency of psychiatric illness, various psychological symptoms, characteristics, and behaviors have been reported in IBS patients.

Anxiety and depression scores are elevated (Esler and Goulston 1973; Latimer et al. 1981). Esler and Goulston (1973) and Latimer et al. (1981) have reported more neuroticism and introversion in IBS patients than in nonclinical community samples. Patients with IBS have also been described as compulsive, overconscientious, dependent, sensitive, guilty, worried, unassertive, and exhibiting an increased need for approval and social desirability (Blanchard et al. 1987; Latimer 1983; Toner et al. 1990a, 1990b). These characteristics may more accurately describe women than men in Western society, for reasons that I discuss later in this chapter.

Physiological Interventions

Klein (1988) performed a critical review of 43 randomized, double-blind, placebo-controlled treatment trials for IBS involving the following agents: antispasmodics, barbiturates, antidepressants, bulking agents, carminatives, dopamine antagonists, opioids, tranquilizers, and miscellaneous treatments including timolol, phenytoin, and diltiazem. Klein (1988) concluded that many agents are available to treat IBS symptoms, but, in adequately controlled trials, none has been shown to be superior to placebo. Methodological issues that further limit interpretation of the efficacy of work in this area include 1) an inadequate operational definition of IBS, 2) use of a global self-report of treatment satisfaction as the only measure of treatment outcome, 3) short trial duration (most studies are less than 8 weeks), 4) high placebo response, and 5) inappropriate statistical techniques of analysis.

Psychological Interventions

The importance of psychological factors in patients who seek repeated specialized consultation for IBS has been well documented in the literature (C. M. Mitchell and Drossman 1987a), as has the disproportionate number of women who are referred to specialists for this condition. However, it is surprising that few controlled studies have investigated psychological treatments for IBS patients, and no work has been published on gender issues in treatment. Psychosocial approaches to treatment have included supportive psychotherapy (Apley and Hale 1973), insight-oriented psychotherapy (Svedlund et al. 1983), hypnotherapy (Whorwell et al. 1984), and various behavior (K. R. Mitchell 1978; Schwarz et al. 1986; Whitehead and Schuster 1985; Youell and McCullum 1975) and cognitive-behavior therapies (Harrell and Beiman 1978; Litt and Baker 1987). In summary, outcome in uncontrolled studies is promising, with improvements seen in IBS symptoms on a variety of psychological parameters (Blanchard et al. 1987). However, interpretation of the efficacy of treatments based on case studies and uncontrolled trials is problematic, especially in light of the reportedly high placebo response among IBS patients in drug trials (Whitehead and Schuster 1985). I am aware of only seven controlled studies of psychological treatment for IBS patients (Bennett and Wilkinson 1985; Blanchard et al. 1992; Guthrie et al. 1991; Lynch and Zamble 1989; Neff and Blanchard 1987; Svedlund et al. 1983; Whorwell et al. 1984). These studies are promising in that they support the efficacy of psychological intervention for IBS, but they all have substantial methodological flaws that limit interpretation of their findings.

Relation to Other DSM-IV Disorders

As mentioned earlier in this chapter, several studies have documented that a substantial percentage of patients receiving a diagnosis of IBS also meet DSM-IV criteria for a psychiatric disorder, most commonly an affective or anxiety disorder. As indicated in other chapters in this book, women also receive diagnoses of anxiety and depressive disorders at a higher rate than men. There is much debate about the relationship between psychophysiological disorders, anxiety, and depression (e.g., cause, consequence, or co-occurrence). Some investigators have suggested that IBS represents a physiological expression of an affective disorder (Hislop 1971) or that it is part of an affective spectrum of disorders (Hudson and Pope 1990). However, investigators have not examined how patients with IBS may be unique from patients with affective disorder. My group was particularly interested in comparing the self-schema of patients with IBS presenting to gastroenterologists with patients with major depression presenting to mental health professionals (Toner et al. 1990b). Self-schema refers to a cognitive framework of the individual's beliefs, attitudes, and self-perceptions that is stored in memory and influences incoming information (Beck 1976). It has been repeatedly reported that individuals with a diagnosis of major depression process information in the context of a self-schema that contains mainly negative ideas about the self (Beck et al. 1979; Kuiper and MacDonald 1983; MacDonald and Kuiper 1984). We predicted that the two groups might share depressive symptoms, but the IBS group would not demonstrate the self-schemata found in depressed patients. We found that IBS patients endorse some depressive symptoms, but they do not have the negative view of themselves that is characteristic of patients being treated for major depression.

In related work, my group (Toner et al. 1990a) confirmed other investigators' findings (Latimer et al. 1981; Palmer et al. 1974) that IBS patients have elevated L scores on the Eysenck Personality Inventory (EPI; Eysenck and Eysenck 1968); this suggests that these patients may have a response tendency for social desirability (Latimer et al. 1981; Lynch and Zamble 1989). The construct of social desirability has been viewed as a personality variable as well as a response tendency (e.g., need for social approval or defensiveness, respectively) (Blankstein and Toner 1987). The literature on social desirability suggests that subjects concerned with positive self-presentation describe themselves as unrealistically positive and well-adjusted (Crowne and Marlowe 1964). In particular, we found that a subgroup of IBS patients who also met DSM-IV criteria for major depression had higher EPI-L scores than a group of psychiatric outpatients with major depression. This pattern was recently confirmed by our group (Toner et al. 1992) with a scale that was specifically designed to measure the construct of social desirability. We found that IBS patients scored higher than both depressed and nonclinical control groups on the Marlowe-Crowne Social Desirability Scale (Crowne and Marlowe 1964). Based on these results, we proposed that the construct of social desirability may be key to understanding why some IBS patients do not attend to psychological aspects of their symptoms (Toner et al. 1992). Emphasis on physiological attributions for IBS symptoms may protect patients from the stigma associated with psychological attributions.

This work must be replicated and expanded. In addition, future research must examine self-schema of IBS patients relative to patients who present with anxiety disorders. Beck (1976) proposed that individuals with anxiety disorders process information with a self-schema containing ideas of threat or danger. Although possible neuroanatomical and pathophysiological links between IBS and anxiety disorders have been recently discussed in the literature, common or unique psychological mechanisms have not been identified (Latimer 1983).

Chronic Fatigue Syndrome and Fibromyalgia

Kirmayer and Robbins (1991) suggest that IBS, CFS, and FMS (three functional somatic syndromes seen by three different medical specialties), have much symptomatic overlap—these three syndromes share many symptoms, psychopathological profiles, and illness behaviors. Other investigators have also documented a substantial overlap in symptoms and behaviors among patients with these disorders (Maxton et al. 1991; Veale et al. 1991; Wessley and Powell 1989; Whorwell et al. 1986; Yunus et al. 1989). Moldofsky and Lue (1993) suggested that sleep disturbances, musculoskeletal pain, fatigue, bowel dysfunction, and mood symptoms are often described by patients who have received the diagnostic labels of FMS, CFS, or IBS. They suggest that the assignment of these diagnostic labels is arbitrary and propose that this constellation of symptoms is influenced or modulated by the sleep-waking brain. The demographics of these three disorders with respect to gender and age are remarkably similar. The majority of published studies indicate that 70%–90% of the patients are women, and the mean age is 38–40 years (for a review, see Moldofsky and Lue 1993). However, as mentioned earlier in this chapter, epidemiological rates are based on treatment samples rather than community samples.

Gender Issues

Gender differences in treatment prevalence might be explained by five different perspectives.

1. *Help-seeking behavior:* The first is the acknowledged difference between men and women with respect to seeking help. Women are more likely to report physical and mental problems and seek and receive medical care than are men (Pennebaker 1982; Strickland 1988). Several factors have been postulated as possible explanations for this gender discrepancy. Utilization figures include nonillness health care use, such as childbirth, or preventive procedures, such as breast biopsies. In addition, women may have easier access to medical facilities than men if they do not work full-time. Some have suggested that women are more attentive to their internal state than are men (Pennebaker 1982). Women are more likely than men to be socialized to pay attention to and deal directly with symptoms of illness because women have traditionally taken primary responsibility for health care in families (Lips 1993). Furthermore, admitting psychological and physical weakness and seeking help is an acceptable part of the traditional feminine role, which makes it easier for women to seek professional consultation (Verbrugge 1979). The repeated finding that women utilize preventive health services more than men do may help account for their higher prevalence in clinically collected samples and their lower mortality (Lips 1993).

2. *Cultural differences:* The second important perspective is cultural. Only in Western countries are women significantly more likely to seek medical consultation and to receive a diagnosis of IBS than men (Thompson et al. 1989). Of individuals who receive a diagnosis of IBS, 70%–90% in the West versus only 20%–30% in the East are women.

3. *Sexual and physical abuse:* Third, pain syndromes have been related to sexual and physical abuse (Walker et al. 1988). Drossman and colleagues (1990b) found that a history of sexual and physical abuse is common, yet often undetected, in women seen in gastroenterology clinics and is particularly common in patients with functional GI dis-

orders. Specifically, in a consecutive sample of 206 women seen in a referral-based gastroenterology practice, Drossman and colleagues (1990b) found a 44% prevalence of sexual and physical abuse. Almost one-third of the abused patients had never discussed their experiences with anyone, and only 17% had informed their doctors. Women with functional GI disorders were significantly more likely than those with organic diseases to report forced intercourse, frequent physical abuse, incest, chronic or recurrent abdominal pain, and more lifetime surgeries. Abused women were more likely than nonabused women to report pelvic pain, multiple somatic symptoms, more lifetime surgeries, and more health care utilization. The frequency of abuse found in this study is similar to that reported in studies of women with laparoscopy-negative chronic pelvic pain (Walker et al. 1988).

The high prevalence of patients with a history of abuse may, in part, reflect a self-selection bias of women who seek medical consultation and are referred to tertiary-care facilities. Studies are needed to investigate the prevalence of abuse among women with functional pain symptoms in the community.

These findings have clinical implications for both the assessment and treatment of women with functional disorders. It is important to establish whether there is history of abuse and to integrate this information into the conceptualization and clinical management.

4. *Conflict with gender role:* A fourth aspect to consider is the degree of conflict with one's gender role. Femininity has traditionally been equated with dependence, intuition, submissiveness, and emotionality (Long 1991). As a result of social pressures, boys may perceive themselves as stronger, more powerful, and more dominant than girls (Maccoby and Jacklin 1974). The consistently different treatment by others that is elicited by the two sexes may result in feelings of greater control for boys but greater helplessness for girls (Dweck et al. 1987). Thus, women's belief in their relative inability to control life events may be established at an early age and reinforced throughout life.

Although the acquisition of sex-typed behaviors and characteristics has been considered a prerequisite to mental health, mental health professionals themselves, as well as society in general, have consistently valued masculine traits more positively than feminine traits

(Broverman et al. 1970). This undervaluing of women's roles by both society and mental health professionals may contribute to the difficulties that women seem to experience with issues of self-devaluation. In a concise literature review, Long (1991) found empirical evidence that women discredit their own abilities, have lower expectancies of their abilities, attribute their success to factors other than their own competency, and experience fear of success. The literature has also related women's fear of success to the belief that success is incompatible with femininity and women's feminine gender role (Sohn 1982). In fact, assimilating a feminine identity has been associated with anxiety, low self-esteem, and poor emotional adjustment (Kleinplatz et al. 1992).

Ground-breaking research in the 1970s cast doubt on the earlier assumptions that masculinity and femininity are mutually exclusive personality dimensions on a dichotomous bipolar continuum. This research resulted in the emergence of the concept of *psychological androgyny* (Bem 1974). Although androgyny has been associated with favorable mental health in women, the *masculine* dimension of androgyny is the positive predictor (Bassoff and Glass 1979; Deaux 1984; Pyke 1985). The society-valued competency-oriented masculine traits have been correlated with high self-esteem in both men and women. Feminine traits are either irrelevant or correlate negatively with the self-esteem measure (Bassoff and Glass 1979). At the same time, it has been reported that femininity and occupational achievement are two desirable but mutually exclusive aspirations for women in Western society; women who fail in an occupation are rated more positively and are perceived to be more feminine by both sexes than those who succeed (Feather and Simon 1975).

Thus, the conflict for women is clear. In a world that is changing and increasingly demanding more from women—to act not only relationally as wives and mothers but also professionally as wage earners—this conflict appears to be intensifying. Because masculine attributes are more highly valued, women will rightfully want to incorporate them, but, in doing so, they risk experiencing greater gender role conflict. Because feminine attributes are less valued, men are less likely to aspire to them. Thus, gender role conflict may be seen as a potentially more relevant issue for women than for men in Western society.

Admitting weakness, especially psychological vulnerability, is not socially desirable in Western culture. As discussed earlier in this chapter, patients with IBS score higher on measures of social desirability than psychiatric and nonclinical groups. This undoubtedly results in a gender role socialization conflict for these women. IBS has recently received the dubious label of "career women's disease" in the popular press (Sandmaier 1991). Female patients with functional GI disorders have been found to be more ambitious in terms of work and career goals than a nonclinical community sample of women (Craig and Brown 1984). Abbey and Garfinkel (1991) suggested that women who present with CFS also feel conflict about the difficulty of balancing career, family, and personal wishes. I believe that vulnerability to certain expressions of psychological distress through physical symptoms may be related to difficulties in dealing with contradictions between interpersonal and achievement-oriented concerns. An overemphasis on either of these areas of life to the exclusion of the other may lead to emotional distress (Beck 1976), but attempting to reconcile their inherent contradictions may lead to conflict that is expressed as somatic symptoms. Further research must assess the acceptability of and adherence to feminine gender role socialization in women who seek consultation from mental health professionals for anxiety and depression compared with women who consult medical specialists for functional somatic disorders (IBS, CFS, FMS). I postulate that women seeking emotional help would score higher on a femininity scale and respond with less gender role conflict than women presenting with functional somatic syndromes. We are developing a gender role conflict scale that reveals the conflicting messages that women experience, possible risk factors in the expression of certain patterns of psychosocial distress, and bodily symptoms.

Davis and Padesky (1989) identified common dysfunctional thoughts concerning body functioning in female patients. These thoughts often center around fears of losing control, doing something publicly unacceptable, appearing less than perfect, having something terribly wrong with their body, and not being able to influence body functions via thoughts or behavior. A common clinical presentation is a hypervigilance or hyperawareness of any notable body sensation with corresponding hyperconcern over the potential meaning of that sensation. Both men and women may develop these thoughts and attitudes. However, girls undergo a socialization process that is more likely to emphasize appearance and self-control and restraint in physical activity (Davis and Padesky 1989). Physical appearance and function have a great impact on a woman's sense of social worth. Davis and Padesky advise that an understanding of a woman's dysfunctional thoughts about her body may be enhanced by recognizing the social and cultural reinforcement she experiences. For example, in regard to GI function, belching and passing gas are not usually socially desirable in public for either sex, but females are socialized into believing that they are especially not ladylike (e.g., "belching and farting" contests are frequent among male adolescents but very rare in females).

Davis and Padesky further suggest that several underlying beliefs consistently reemerge among women. First, physical appearances are more important than physical functions. Physical functions are viewed as a source of embarrassment or devaluation or as a loss of control. Also, the prevalent belief is that it is wrong, bad, or unimportant for a woman to place a priority on nurturing of her physical self, except in the interest of making herself more attractive to others (Davis and Padesky 1989). Barsky and associates (1988) suggest that patients with unexplained medical symptoms are often quite surprised to realize how poorly they care for themselves. These investigators suggest that patients with somatic complaints often go out of their way to help others but do not take time to self-nurture.

We have identified a number of these dysfunctional cognitions in cognitive-behavioral groups of women with IBS (Toner et al., in press), which can be categorized into IBS-related cognitions and non-IBS cognitions. The most common IBS-related thoughts center around public embarrassment and humiliation and perfectionistic or rigid views of bodily functions. The most common non-IBS cognitions focus on a heightened need for approval or acceptance, extreme competence, and control or certainty.

5. *Hormonal factors:* A fifth perspective on gender differences is hormonal. For instance, hormonal factors have been suggested to influence the expression of IBS (Talley 1991). Specifically, female gonadal hormones have been found to slow gastric emptying and increase the mouth-to-cecum transit time. This effect, in part, may explain why bloating is much more common in female patients with IBS (Talley et al. 1989; Wald et al. 1981). These hormonal factors have also been shown to be associated with a reduction of the lower esophageal sphincter pressure and slower emptying of the gallbladder (Braverman et al. 1980; Van Thiel et al. 1976). Moreover, female hormones may slow colonic transit (Hinds et al. 1989).

Future research will need to systematically investigate whether IBS symptoms coincide with specific reproductive events such as menstrual cycle phase, pregnancy, and menopause. We are documenting this information in current studies. The clinical literature and our experience suggest that IBS symptoms are more frequent and intense premenstrually. Moreover, some of my GI colleagues have noted that IBS symptoms seem to disappear during pregnancy and reappear after childbirth. These clinical observations must be investigated in treated and community samples.

The role gender plays in the expression and maintenance of psychophysiological symptoms must be incorporated into clinical management. To date, no study has examined gender differences in the treatment or prognosis of IBS. One methodological barrier to systematically examining gender differences in treatment studies is that the sample size would be so low for men in most centers that meaningful comparisons would be difficult. In order to have adequate sample sizes for men, large, multicentered treatment protocols will be necessary.

Treatment Implications

Various theoretical perspectives can integrate gender issues into treatment protocols, and we have found that this approach is especially compatible with cognitive-behavior therapy. Very briefly, the treatment protocol we have used in our work with IBS patients is derived from that of Beck and co-workers (Beck and Emery 1974; Beck et al. 1979, 1985) for depressive and anxiety disorders. We (Toner et al., in press) have adapted this protocol to the treatment of IBS patients. This protocol integrates recent theoretical and empirical work on the influence of attention, personal appraisal style, and illness attribution in chronic pain and psychosomatic disorders (Salkovskis and Warwick 1986; Sharpe et al. 1992; Turk et al. 1978).

Our future work with female IBS patients will highlight the importance of gender in the development and organization of cognitive schemata (Markus et al. 1982). Therapists will explore the ways in which women's thoughts and behaviors are influenced by their social realities. In addition to common dysfunctional thoughts about body functioning mentioned earlier in this chapter, common underlying schemata for women in relation to assertion problems will be explored. Specific techniques for assertiveness training for women are adapted from the work of Lange and Jakubowski (1976). The protocol includes 10–12 weekly sessions. The major purpose of the first session is to begin teaching patients about the theoretical and therapeutic rationale for cognitive-behavior therapy. A second purpose is to establish initial rapport with the patient and to identify goals. At each session, a general theme is established in collaboration with the patient. Themes include thoughts, feelings and symptoms, coping with stress, anxiety, assertion, anger, social approval, perfectionism, and control.

Summary

This chapter has focused on IBS as an example of a somatoform disorder that has been diagnosed significantly more often in women than in men. Many of the issues described here are applicable to related disorders that disproportionately affect women, such as CFS and FMS. Future research must further identify and integrate gender-related variables into the conceptualization and treatment of these disorders. Of primary importance, gender-related variables such as symptom perception and expression, gender role conflict, history of physical and sexual abuse, and hormonal influences must be examined in community and treated samples.

References

Abbey SE, Garfinkel PE: Neurasthenia and chronic fatigue syndrome: the role of culture in the making of a diagnosis. Am J Psychiatry 148:1638–1646, 1991

American Psychiatric Association: Diagnostic and Statistical Manual of Mental Disorders, 2nd Edition. Washington, DC, American Psychiatric Association, 1968

American Psychiatric Association: Diagnostic and Statistical Manual of Mental Disorders, 3rd Edition. Washington, DC, American Psychiatric Association, 1980

American Psychiatric Association: Diagnostic and Statistical Manual of Mental Disorders, 3rd Edition, Revised. Washington, DC, American Psychiatric Association, 1987

American Psychiatric Association: Diagnostic and Statistical Manual of Mental Disorders, 4th Edition. Washington, DC, American Psychiatric Association, 1994

Apley J, Hale B: Children with recurrent abdominal pain: how do they grow up? BMJ 3:7–9, 1973

Barsky AJ, Geringer E, Wool CA: A cognitive-educational treatment for hypochondriasis. Gen Hosp Psychiatry 10:322–327, 1988

Bassoff ES, Glass GV: The relationship between sex roles and mental health: a metaanalysis of twenty-six studies. The Counseling Psychologist 10:105–116, 1979

Beck AT: Cognitive Therapy and the Emotional Disorders. New York, International University Press, 1976

Beck AT, Emery G: Cognitive Therapy of Anxiety and Phobic Disorders. Philadelphia, PA, Centre for Cognitive Therapy, 1974

Beck AT, Rush AJ, Shaw BF, et al: Cognitive Therapy of Depression: A Treatment Manual. New York, Guilford, 1979

Beck AT, Emery G, Greenberg R: Anxiety Disorders and Phobias. New York, Basic Books, 1985

Bem SL: The measurement of psychological androgyny. J Consult Clin Psychol 42:155–162, 1974

Bennett P, Wilkinson S: A comparison of psychological and medical treatment of the irritable bowel syndrome. Br J Clin Psychol 24:215–216, 1985

Blanchard EB, Schwarz SP, Radnitz CR: Psychological assessment and treatment of irritable bowel syndrome. Behav Modif 2:348–372, 1987

Blanchard EB, Schwarz SP, Suls JM, et al: Two controlled evaluations of a multi-component psychological treatment of irritable bowel syndrome. Behav Res Ther 2:175–189, 1992

Blankstein KR, Toner BB: Influence of social desirability responding on the Sarasontest Anxiety Scale: implications for selection of subjects. Psychol Rep 61:63–69, 1987

Braverman DZ, Johnson ML, Kern F: Effects of pregnancy and contraceptive steroid on gallbladder function. N Engl J Med 302:362–364, 1980

Broverman IK, Broverman DM, Clarkson FE, et al: Sex-role stereotypes and clinical judgements of mental health. J Consult Clin Psychol 34:1–7, 1970

Craig TKG, Brown GW: Goal frustration and life events in the aetiology of painful gastrointestinal disorder. J Psychosom Res 28:411–421, 1984

Crowne D, Marlowe D: The Approval Motive: Studies in Evaluative Dependence. New York, Wiley, 1964

Davis D, Padesky C: Enhancing cognitive therapy with women, in Comprehensive Handbook of Cognitive Therapy. Edited by Freeman A. New York, Plenum, 1989, pp 535–557

Deaux K: From individual differences to social categories: analysis of a decade's research on gender. Am Psychol 39:105–116, 1984

Drossman DA, Sandler RS, McKee DC, et al: Bowel patterns among subjects not seeking health care: use of a questionnaire to identify a population with bowel dysfunction. Gastroenterology 83:529–534, 1982

Drossman DA, McKee DC, Sandler RS, et al: Psychosocial factors in the irritable bowel syndrome: a multivariate study of patients and non-patients with irritable bowel syndrome. Gastroenterology 95:701–708, 1988

Drossman DA, Funch-Jensen P, Janssens J, et al: Identification of subgroups of functional bowel disorders. Gastroenterology International 3:159–172, 1990a

Drossman DA, Leserman J, Nachman G, et al: Sexual and physical abuse in women with functional or organic gastrointestinal disorders. Ann Intern Med 113:828–833, 1990b

Dweck CS, Davidson W, Nelson S, et al: Sex differences in learned helplessness, II: the contingencies of evaluative feedback in the classroom. Developmental Psychology 14:268–276, 1987

Esler MD, Goulston KL: Levels of anxiety in colonic disorders. N Engl J Med 288:16–20, 1973

Eysenck JH, Eysenck SBG: Eysenck Personality Inventory. San Diego, CA, Educational and Industrial Testing Service, 1968

Feather NT, Simon JG: Reactions to male and female success and failure in sex-linked occupations: impressions of personality, causal attributions, and perceived likelihood of different consequences. J Pers Soc Psychol 31:20–31, 1975

Ferguson A, Sircus W, Eastwood MA: Frequency of "functional" gastrointestinal disorders. Lancet ii:613–614, 1977

Guthrie E, Creed F, Dawson E, et al: A controlled trial of psychological treatment for the irritable bowel syndrome. Gastroenterology 100:450–457, 1991

Harrell TH, Beiman I: Cognitive-behavioral treatment of the irritable colon syndrome. Cognitive Therapy and Research 2:371–375, 1978

Harvey RF, Salih SY, Read AF: Organic and functional disorders in 2000 gastroenterology outpatients. Lancet i:632–634, 1983

Hinds JP, Stoney B, Wald A: Does gender or the menstrual cycle affect colonic transit? Am J Gastroenterol 82:123–126, 1989

Hislop JG: Psychological significance of the irritable colon syndrome. Gut 8:221–229, 1971

Hudson JI, Pope HG: Affective spectrum disorder: does antidepressant response identify a family of disorders with a common psychopathology? Am J Psychiatry 147:552–564, 1990

Kirmayer LJ, Robbins JM: Functional somatic syndromes, in Current Concepts of Somatization: Research and Clinical Perspectives. Edited by Kirmayer LJ, Robbins JM. Washington, DC, American Psychiatric Press, 1991, pp 79–105

Klein KB: Controlled treatment trials in the irritable bowel syndrome: a critique. Gastroenterology 95:232–241, 1988

Kleinplatz P, McCarrey M, Kateb C: The impact of gender role identity on women's self-esteem, lifestyle satisfaction and conflict. Canadian Journal of Behavioural Science 24:333–347, 1992

Kuiper NA, MacDonald MR: Schematic processing in depression: the self based consensus bias. Cognitive Therapy Research 7:469–484, 1983

Lange A, Jakubowski P: Responsible Assertive Behavior: Cognitive/Behavioral Procedures for Trainers. Champaign, IL, Research Press, 1976

Latimer P: Functional Gastrointestinal Disorders: A Behavioral Medicine Approach. New York, Springer, 1983

Latimer PR, Sarna SK, Campbell D, et al: Colonic motor and myoelectric activity: a comparative study of normal subjects, psychoneurotic patients and patients with irritable bowel syndrome (IBS). Gastroenterology 80:893–901, 1981

Lips HM: Sex and Gender: An Introduction. Mountain View, CA, Mayfield Publishing, 1993

Litt MD, Baker LH: Cognitive-behavioral interventions for irritable bowel syndrome. J Clin Gastroenterol 2:208–211, 1987

Long WO: Gender role conditioning and women's self-concept. Journal of Humanistic Education and Development 30:19–29, 1991

Lynch PM, Zamble E: A controlled behavioral treatment study of irritable bowel syndrome. Behavior Therapy 20:509–523, 1989

Maccoby EE, Jacklin CN: The Psychology of Sex Differences. Stanford, CA, Stanford University Press, 1974

MacDonald MR, Kuiper NA: Self-schema decision consistency in clinical depressives. Journal of Social and Clinical Psychology 2:264–272, 1984

Manning AP, Thompson KW, Heaton KW, et al: Toward positive diagnosis of the irritable bowel. BMJ 2:653–654, 1978

Markus H, Crane M, Bernstein S, et al: Self-schemas and gender. J Pers Soc Psychol 42:38–50, 1982

Maxton DG, Morris J, Whorwell PJ: More accurate diagnosis of irritable bowel syndrome by the use of "non-colonic" symptomatology. Gut 32:784–786, 1991

Mitchell CM, Drossman DA: The irritable bowel syndrome: understanding and treating a biopsychosocial illness disorder. Annals of Behavioural Medicine 9:13–18, 1987a

Mitchell CM, Drossman DA: Survey of the AGA membership relating to patients with functional gastrointestinal disorders. Gastroenterology 92:1228–1245, 1987b

Mitchell KR: Self-management of spastic colitis. J Behav Ther Exp Psychiatry 9:269–272, 1978

Moldofsky H, Lue F: Disordered sleep, pain, fatigue, and gastrointestinal symptoms in fibromyalgia, chronic fatigue and irritable bowel syndromes, in Basic and Clinical Aspects of Chronic Abdominal Pain. Edited by Mayer EA, Raybould HE. Amsterdam, Elsevier, 1993, pp 249–255

Neff DF, Blanchard EB: A multi-component treatment for irritable bowel syndrome. Behavior Therapy 18:70–83, 1987

Palmer RL, Stonehill E, Crisp AH, et al: Psychological characteristics of patients with the irritable bowel syndrome. Postgrad Med J 50:416–419, 1974

Pennebaker JW: The Psychology of Physical Symptoms. New York, Springer-Verlag, 1982

Pyke S: Androgyny: an integration. International Women's Studies 8:529–539, 1985

Salkovskis P, Warwick HMC: Morbid preoccupations, health anxiety and reassurance: a cognitive-behavioral approach to hypochondriasis. Behav Res Ther 24:597–602, 1986

Sammons MT, Karoly P: Psychosocial variables in irritable bowel syndrome: a review proposal. Clinical Psychology Review 7:187–206, 1987

Sandler RS: Epidemiology of irritable bowel syndrome in the United States. Gastroenterology 99:409–415, 1990

Sandmaier M: "What's stress got to do with it?" Working Woman, February 1991, p 90

Schwarz SP, Blanchard EB, Neff DB: Behavioral treatment of irritable bowel syndrome: a 1-year follow-up study. Biofeedback Self Regul 11:189–198, 1986

Sharpe M, Peveler R, Mayou R: The psychological treatment of patients with functional somatic symptoms: a practical guide. J Psychosom Res 36:515–529, 1992

Smith RC, Greenbaum DS, Vancouver JB: Gender differences in Manning criteria in irritable bowel syndrome (abstract). Gastroenterology 98:396, 1991

Sohn D: Sex differences in achievement self-attributions: an effect-size analysis. Sex Roles 8:345–357, 1982

Strickland BR: Sex related differences in health and illness. Psychology of Women Quarterly 12:381–399, 1988

Svedlund J, Sjodin I, Ottosson J, et al: Controlled study of psychotherapy in irritable bowel syndrome. Lancet ii:589–592, 1983

Talley NJ: Diagnosing an irritable bowel: does sex matter? Gastroenterology 110:834–837, 1991

Talley NJ, Shuter B, McCrudden G, et al: Lack of association between gastric emptying of solids and symptoms in non-ulcer dyspepsia. J Clin Gastroenterol 11:625–630, 1989

Talley NJ, Phillips SF, Melton LJ, et al: Diagnostic value of the Manning criteria in irritable bowel syndrome. Gut 31:77–81, 1990

Taylor GJ: Review of Shorter E's book titled: From Paralysis to Fatigue: A History of Psychosomatic Illness in the Modern Era. Psychosom Med 55:88–89, 1993

Thompson WG, Heaton KW: Functional bowel disorders in apparently healthy people. Gastroenterology 79:283–288, 1980

Thompson WG, Dotevall G, Drossman DA, et al: Irritable bowel syndrome: guidelines for the diagnosis. Gastroenterology International 2:92–95, 1989

Toner BB, Garfinkel PE, Jeejeebhoy KN: Psychological factors in irritable bowel syndrome. Can J Psychiatry 35:158–161, 1990a

Toner BB, Garfinkel PE, Jeejeebhoy KN, et al: Self-schema in irritable bowel syndrome. Psychosom Med 52:149–155, 1990b

Toner BB, Koyama E, Garfinkel PE, et al: Social desirability and irritable bowel syndrome. Int J Psychiatry Med 22:99–103, 1992

Toner BB, Segal ZV, Garfinkel PE, et al: Functional Gastrointestinal Disorders: Cognitive-Behavioral Perspective. New York, Guilford (in press)

Turk DC, Meichenbaum D, Genest M: Pain and Behavioural Medicine. A Cognitive–Behavioural Perspective. New York, Guilford, 1978

Van Thiel DH, Gavaler JS, Stremple J: Lower esophageal sphincter pressure in women using sequential oral contraceptives. Gastroenterology 71:232–235, 1976

Veale D, Kavanagh G, Fielding JF, et al: Primary fibromyalgia and the irritable bowel syndrome: different expressions of a common pathogen process. Br J Rheumatol 30:220–222, 1991

Verbrugge LM: Female illness rates and illness behavior: testing hypotheses about sex differences in health. Women Health 4:61–79, 1979

Wald A, Van Theil DH, Hoechstetter L, et al: Gastrointestinal transit: the effect of the menstrual cycle. Gastroenterology 80:1497–1500, 1981

Walker E, Katon WJ, Harrop-Griffiths J, et al: Relationship of chronic pelvic pain to psychiatric diagnosis and childhood sexual abuse. Am J Psychiatry 145:75–80, 1988

Walker EA, Roy-Byrne PP, Katon WJ: Irritable bowel syndrome and psychiatric illness. Am J Psychiatry 147:565–572, 1990

Waller SI, Misiewicz JJ: Prognosis in irritable bowel syndrome. Lancet ii:735–756, 1969

Welch GW, Hillman LC, Pomare EW: Psychoneurotic symptomatology in the irritable bowel syndrome: a study of reporters and non-reporters. BMJ 291:1382–1384, 1985

Welgan P, Meshkinpour H, Beeler M: Effect of anger on colon motor and myoelectric activity in irritable bowel syndrome. Gastroenterology 94:1150–1156, 1988

Wessley S, Powell R: Fatigue syndromes: a comparison of chronic "postviral" fatigue with neuromuscular and affective disorders. J Neurol Neurosurg Psychiatry 52:940–948, 1989

Whitehead WE: Behavioral medicine approaches to gastrointestinal disorders. J Consult Clin Psychol 60:605–612, 1992

Whitehead WE, Schuster MM: Gastrointestinal Disorders: Behavioral and Physiological Basis for Treatment. New York, Academic Press, 1985

Whitehead WE, Bosmajian L, Zonderman AB, et al: Symptoms of psychologic distress associated with irritable bowel syndrome: comparison of community and medical clinic samples. Gastroenterology 95:709–714, 1988

Whitehead WE, Cheskin LJ, Heller BR, et al: Evidence for exacerbation of irritable bowel syndrome during menses. Gastroenterology 98:1485–1489, 1990

Whorwell PJ, Prior A, Farager EB: Controlled trial of hypnotherapy in the treatment of severely refractory irritable bowel syndrome. Lancet ii:1232–1233, 1984

Whorwell PJ, McCallum M, Creed FH, et al: Non-colonic features of irritable bowel syndrome. Gut 27:37–40, 1986

Youell KJ, McCullum JP: Behavioral treatment of mucous colitis. J Consult Clin Psychol 43:740–745, 1975

Young SJ, Alpers DH, Norland CC, et al: Psychiatric illness and the irritable bowel syndrome. Gastroenterology 70:162–166, 1976

Yunus MB, Masi AT, Aldag JC: A controlled study of primary fibromyalgia syndrome: clinical features and association with other functional syndromes. J Rheumatol 19:62–71, 1989

CHAPTER 14

Alcohol and Other Psychoactive Substance Dependence in Women and Men

Barbara W. Lex, Ph.D., M.P.H.

In this chapter, I selectively discuss current findings about gender differences in alcohol, marijuana, opiate, and cocaine abuse and dependence. Studies reviewed provide a broad spectrum of information about psychological, biological, and sociocultural aspects of substance abuse but are by no means exhaustive. Much of this review focuses on alcohol, largely because it is well documented that women and men differentially absorb and metabolize alcohol and exhibit different alcohol consumption patterns. Typically, onset and course of alcohol and other psychoactive substance dependence in women appear accelerated or "telescoped."

This research was supported in part by grants DA 0064, DA 04870, and DA 07252 from the National Institute on Drug Abuse and grants AA 06252 and AA 06794 from the National Institute on Alcohol Abuse and Alcoholism, of the Alcohol, Drug Abuse and Mental Health Administration. The author is grateful to Janice R. Norris who prepared the manuscript, to Eleanor DeRubeis for her editorial expertise, and to Michel Wapler, M.D., Noelle Lawler, and Sandy Springer for their helpful comments.

Limitations of Research Methodologies

Assumptions about factors that influence drinking behavior as well as definitions of *problem drinking, alcoholism, alcohol abuse,* and *alcohol dependence* have varied through time and across disciplines. Estimates of the prevalence of psychoactive substance use disorders generally have been obtained from self-reports in cross-sectional household surveys, although other information comes from treated populations or mortality data.

Methodological limitations should be recognized insofar as use of disparate assumptions, definitions, and instruments may bias findings (Lex 1987; Lex et al. 1988; Westermeyer 1990). Survey instruments that require retrospective self-reports are likely to underestimate frequency of consumption and quantity of alcohol or other drug use as well as incidence and severity of associated behaviors. Community surveys of use and abuse patterns may have oversampled persons living in fixed places of residence and undercounted individuals who are estranged from their families, institutionalized, or homeless. Specifications of cutoff points for hazardous consumption quantities or frequencies (e.g., "heavy drinking") typically vary between women and men, but these categories rarely have been adjusted for gender. Men and women also may identify different consequences and problems associated with substance abuse (Robbins 1989). Thus, recognition of gender differences must be better integrated into interview schedules.

Toward Operational Criteria

It is useful to review the various diagnostic criteria that have been adopted, revised, and discarded for drug dependence and alcoholism categories because women and men occupy different social roles and may experience different physiological effects from psychoactive substance use. Development of nosology and taxonomy as related to alcohol is focal in this discussion for several reasons: 1) alcohol is the most widely abused substance in American society, 2) consequences of excessive alcohol intake have generated the largest number of studies, and 3) understanding tolerance to and dependence on alcohol provides a heuristic method for understanding other drug use (Edwards 1977; Edwards and Gross 1976).

DSM-III and Beyond: Social Consequences and Patterns of Pathological Use

For both alcohol abuse and alcohol dependence criteria, DSM-III (American Psychiatric Association 1980) listed examples of impaired social and occupational functioning due to alcohol use: violence while intoxicated, absence from work, loss of job, legal difficulties, and arguments or difficulties with family or friends because of excessive alcohol use. In DSM-III-R (American Psychiatric Association 1987), however, alcohol dependence was subsumed under psychoactive substance dependence. Psychoactive substance dependence is understood to include biological, social, and behavioral components associated with impaired control of substance use and constriction of individual behavior such that salience of substance-taking behavior becomes dominant in daily life.

In DSM-IV (American Psychiatric Association 1994), both alcohol abuse and alcohol dependence, along with 10 other classes of drugs, are subsumed under substance use disorders. Substance dependence includes cognitive, behavioral, and physiological symptoms associated with maladaptive repeated self-administration of a drug that causes impairment or distress over a minimum 12-month interval. Three or more of seven criteria are required for a DSM-IV diagnosis of substance dependence. However, two of the seven criteria—indications of tolerance (the need for increased doses to attain a desired effect or a lessened effect at the same dose) and withdrawal signs (tissue changes and ensuing disruptions of behavior that occur when prolonged heavy use is ceased)—are *not* necessary for the diagnosis of substance dependence. Presence or absence of tolerance or withdrawal changes associated with substance dependence are indicated diagnostically by "specifiers" of "with physiological dependence" or "without physiological dependence" (pp. 178–179).

Social Consequences

In addition to physiological changes involved in the tolerance and withdrawal criteria, psychological changes are reflected in two criteria: loss of control of amount of the substance or duration of time or use; and inability to cut down or to otherwise control use. The three social and occupational criteria for DSM-IV substance dependence include the following consequences:

1. A disproportionate amount of time expended to obtain, consume, and recover from effects of the substance
2. Curtailment or relinquishment of important social, occupational, or recreational activities because of the use of the substance
3. Continued substance use despite knowledge of deleterious physical or psychological effects caused or exacerbated by use of the substance

A national survey of drinking patterns and drinking problems among women ($N = 917$) conducted in 1981 investigated drinking consequences, such as driving while intoxicated, belligerence, and conflict with spouse, as well as events more pertinent to women, such as problems with children, interference with role performance in the home, and home accidents (Wilsnack et al. 1986). It is surprising that among women who used alcohol, the most frequently reported problem was driving while intoxicated (17%), followed by fighting with spouse (11%), and request by spouse to cut down drinking (5%). Only 3% acknowledged that drinking had disrupted housework, and 2% reported that drinking had created problems with their children. Frequencies of problems among men exceeded those for women but generally followed the same rank ordering (Wilsnack et al. 1986).

Consumption and Tolerance

The same national survey of women's drinking patterns and drinking problems (Wilsnack et al. 1986) also inquired about alcohol dependence symptoms, such as memory lapses ("blackouts"), gulping drinks, morning drinking, inability to abstain or cut down use, and inability to stop drinking until intoxicated. Among women who used alcohol, memory lapse (10%) was the most frequently reported symptom, followed by gulping drinks (8%), and morning drinking (2%); only 2% of the women acknowledged inability to abstain or cut down use, and 3% reported inability to stop drinking until intoxicated (Wilsnack et al. 1986). Again, frequencies of drinking problems for men exceeded those for women but generally followed the same rank ordering.

For both alcohol abuse and alcohol dependence criteria, DSM-III listed examples of "patterns of pathological use." These included "need for daily use for adequate functioning; inability to cut down or stop drinking; repeated efforts to control or reduce excess drinking by going on the wagon . . . or restricting drinking to certain times of the day . . . ; binges . . . ; occasional consumption of a fifth of spirits (or its equivalent in wine or beer); . . . (blackouts); continuation of drinking despite a serious physical disorder that the individual knows is exacerbated by alcohol use; and drinking of non-beverage alcohol" (American Psychiatric Association 1980, pp 169–170).

In DSM-IV, substance abuse, including alcohol abuse, is marked by maladaptive substance use under recurrent and significantly adverse circumstances (pp. 182–183). Diagnosis of substance abuse specifically excludes any criteria for substance dependence. Substance abuse criteria include distress or impairment associated with 1) failure to fulfill important social roles (e.g., substance-related performance impairment, absences, or expulsions from work or school; neglect of care for children or household), 2) recurrent substance use in physically hazardous contexts (e.g., drives or operates machinery while impaired), 3) repeated substance-related legal problems (e.g., arrest for disorderly conduct), and 4) continued substance use despite persistent or recurrent social or interpersonal problems caused by or exacerbated by substance use (e.g., arguments with spouse about substance use, physical fights).

It was argued that requiring criteria involving social and occupational consequences of substance abuse and dependence, as in DSM-III, might miss diagnoses in persons able to "hide" problems and thus buffer themselves in their social and occupational realms (examples given are housewives or impaired physicians) (Rounsaville and Kranzler 1989; Rounsaville et al. 1986). Empirical difficulty in disentangling cause-and-effect relationships between substance use and associated social impairment also was a pertinent factor in shifting to the new criteria.

Potential Gender Bias

The DSM-IV criteria do not appear overtly gender biased. However, for treatment planning, it may be necessary to adopt probes for women, as evidenced by two studies of women's drinking in Ireland and in England (Corrigan and Butler 1991; Thom 1986). Thom (1986) examined barriers to help seeking in 25 male and 25 female first admissions to an alcohol clinic in England. Women tended to deny alcohol problems. Four times more women than men claimed that drinking was not their main problem. Women worried about public opinion regarding their attendance at the clinic. Women and men differed in the extent to which their self-image was integrated with a perception of alcohol problems. Women emphasized that drinking had not compromised their major social roles—as wives and mothers. Women focused on their role as food provider and claimed that they always managed to feed babies or prepare a family meal (Thom 1986).

Corrigan and Butler (1991) studied consequences of substance use in a series of 114 Irish women of varied education and income in alcoholism treatment in the Dublin area. Use of other psychoactive substances was common among the women with alcoholism in this sample: 58% used tranquilizers, 55% used "sleeping pills," and 13% used marijuana. Most (75%) drank alone at home; 86% believed that women receive more opprobrium than men for drinking; and 53% continued to "hide" their drinking before admission for treatment. Dependence symptoms affected more than half of the women, with 86.8% reporting loss of control of alcohol intake, 82.5% reporting memory lapses, and 77.2% attempting temporary abstinence. About 70% reported tremors and taking a drink to ward off abstinence symptoms after drinking, but only 24.6% had progressed to the point of hallucinosis. The most prevalent social consequence was excessive spending for alcohol (85.1%), but less than half (44.7%) of the women acknowledged alcohol-related financial problems. Between 20% and

30% acknowledged that alcohol had interfered with their ability to care for their homes or themselves, to shop for food, or to cook, but no questions were asked about ability to care for children. There are strong associations in the literature between child abuse and substance abuse. Thus, specific probes for care and welfare of children appear warranted for women, as well as men, who abuse substances.

Antisocial Personality Disorder and Psychoactive Substance Use

In male patients with substance use disorders, comorbidity with antisocial personality disorder may be as high as 50% (Gerstley et al. 1990). In women, however, the prevalence of antisocial personality disorder is lower, and comorbidity with substance dependence by DSM-III-R criteria is lower (Blazer et al. 1985; Robins et al. 1984). In DSM-IV, antisocial personality disorder requires diagnosis of conduct disorder during childhood or adolescence. Conduct disorder has 15 criteria that reflect persistent violations of the rights of others or rule breaking, with about 6 criteria typically (but not exclusively) more characteristic of males than females (e.g., stealing with force, fighting with weapons, cruelty to animals, forced sexual activity, vandalism, fire setting). Highest estimated community setting rates for young males (16%) are about twice those for young females (9%). Antisocial personality disorder is applicable to people older than age 18 years and has 7 criteria. Three or more criteria are necessary for a diagnosis. Each criterion reflects violations of the rights of others, but they are broadly worded and less gender specific, including illegal behaviors, deceit, impulsivity, irritability and aggressiveness, reckless disregard for safety of self or others, failure to work or honor financial obligations, and lack of remorse. This disorder is said to be more common in males (3%) than in females (1%), but rates are higher among persons with concurrent substance use disorders.

It is possible that comorbidity of substance abuse and antisocial personality disorder is lower in women than in men because women have a lower rate of childhood conduct disorder, a precondition of antisocial personality disorder. Robins and Price (1991) suggested that numbers of childhood conduct disorder behaviors needed for a diagnosis of antisocial personality disorder be two or more for men and one or more for women. Some researchers assert that emphasis on behaviors may not be as telling as the apparent inability to form close relationships with others (Gerstley et al. 1990), an indicator that may be less gender specific.

Many studies of antisocial personality disorder and substance abuse have focused on men. However, in recent years, the behaviors of female substance abusers have drawn attention to possible associations between adult antisocial behaviors and antisocial personality disorder concurrent with substance use. In one study of 228 men and 118 women, 53% of the men and 29% of the women were found to have antisocial personality disorder (Felch et al. 1991). Women with antisocial personality disorder had rates of criminality and aggressiveness comparable to those reported by men who did *not* meet antisocial personality disorder criteria. Antisocial behaviors also were prevalent in women who used drugs and who did not meet full criteria for antisocial personality disorder because they lacked childhood antecedents. Typical adult behaviors included violence, weapon use, commission of felonies, and arrests for felonies. Men and women with antisocial personality disorder committed similar numbers of misdemeanors and had comparable social functioning.

Recently, we evaluated the temporal relationship between antisocial personality disorder and alcoholism in a selected population of female alcohol and drug users (Lex et al. 1994). For women, the temporal relationship between antisocial personality disorder and alcoholism is unclear. Driving while intoxicated is both a symptom of antisocial personality disorder and the alcohol-related problem most typically reported by women (Wilsnack et al. 1986). Accordingly, a period prevalence sample of 33 women incarcerated for drunk driving offenses was assessed with the Structured Clinical Interview for DSM-III-R (SCID; Spitzer et al. 1992) to determine whether the women had other symptoms of antisocial personality disorder. Excluding behaviors that only occurred while drinking, only 1 of the 33 women met DSM-III-R criteria for antisocial personality disorder. When behaviors while drinking were included, 18.2% of this sample met full criteria for antisocial personality disorder, and an additional 57.6% of the sample met criteria for adult antisocial personality disorder without a history of childhood conduct disorder. This pattern suggests that antisocial personality disorder was a consequence of substance abuse, rather than an antecedent, with childhood conduct disorder acting only as a limited predictor of antisocial personality disorder in adulthood. Relationships among gender, prodromal behaviors, and substance abuse appear more complex than anticipated and indicate the need to recognize "adult onset" antisocial personality disorder associated with substance abuse as a legitimate diagnosis that is manifested differently by women and men.

Recognition of Gender Differences

Alcohol Problems

Until the last two decades, alcohol problems in women received little systematic attention. It is now apparent that age, drinking patterns, and symptoms of alcohol dependence are different for women and men (Bohman et al. 1981; Clayton et al. 1986; Cloninger et al. 1986; Hesselbrock et al. 1984; Lex 1985; Mello 1980; Schuckit 1984). Alcohol dependence in women is associated with accelerated development of cardiovascular, gastrointestinal, and liver diseases (Blume 1986; Halliday et al. 1986; Lex 1985; Norton et al. 1987; Wilsnack et al. 1984), a process frequently referred to as *telescoping*. Several other gender differences have been observed. Onset of drinking problems in women occurs 4–8 years later than in men (Beckman 1976; Lisansky 1957). Alcohol-dependent women also drink less frequently and consume less alcohol than men (Schuckit 1984). Women report having fewer binges and less continuous drinking (Schuckit 1984) and recall fewer blackouts, less morning drinking, and fewer delirium tremens episodes (Tamerin et al. 1976). Women also report that before coming to treatment, they had shorter drinking histories (Crawford and Ryder 1986; Orford and Keddie 1985). Numerous reports associate alcohol abuse in women with serious reproductive dysfunctions (Gavaler 1988; Mello 1980, 1988; Van Thiel and Gavaler 1988; Wilsnack and Wilsnack 1991; Wilsnack et al. 1991), and it is well known that alcohol can seriously affect the developing fetus (Fisher and Karl 1988; Mello et al. 1989). Women who have alcohol problems also are at risk for polysubstance use, especially psychotropic prescription medications, marijuana, and cocaine (Clayton et al. 1986; Kreek 1987; Lex 1985; Lex et al. 1988, 1989; Wilsnack and Wilsnack 1991; Wilsnack et al. 1991).

Cutoff Levels and Women's Alcohol Use

Accumulating evidence underscores the need to reevaluate parameters of women's alcohol consumption levels and redefine excessive use by women (Wilsnack and Wilsnack 1991). Because of the telescoping phenomenon, cutoff levels for hazardous drinking by women should be lowered. For example, when consumption categories use the same definitions of heavy alcohol consumption (five or more drinks once per week) for women and men, rates are 22% for men and 6% for women (Caetano 1989; Herd 1989).

In contrast, a survey that examined alcohol consumption patterns of more than 22,000 Canadian men and women ages 15–29 years (Whitehead and Layne 1987) defined heavy drinking for men as about six drinks per episode, but heavy drinking for women was defined as four and a half drinks per episode. Using these gender-adjusted definitions, heavy consumption rates in this Canadian sample were similar for men and women when age, employment, and marital status were controlled. In addition, Mercer and Khavari (1990) surveyed 1,701 American college students in 1977 and reinterviewed 1,045 (61%) of them in 1985. Corrections for differences between men and women in amount of body fluid indicated both convergence in the amount of beer consumption and similar alcohol intake volume for each gender. Thus, some findings indicate a secular trend toward convergence in heavy alcohol use when the criterion for "heavy" drinking is adjusted for women.

In summary, a cutoff point somewhere between four and four and a half drinks per occasion appears to be a reasonable threshold for heavy drinking in women. This adjustment seems appropriate if findings about gender differences in "first-pass metabolism" in the gastric mucosa (Frezza et al. 1990) are substantiated. As noted, some confirmation of gender differences in alcohol metabolism is provided by women's higher risk for liver cirrhosis, which occurs with lower absolute alcohol intake (Zetterman 1992). Adequate attention must be devoted to this issue in future studies of women's drinking patterns.

Current Epidemiology of Alcohol and Illicit Drug Use

The latest cross-sectional household survey of alcohol and drug use ($N = 28,832$) was conducted during 1992 by the National Institute on Drug Abuse (1993). With regard to alcohol, a majority of all American women (60.2%) reported using alcohol during the previous year (versus 69.5% for men) and less than half (40.4%) during the previous month (versus 55.9% for men). In the younger age groups (18–34), rates reported for lifetime use were approximately 90% (about 90% for men and 88% for women). About 42% of boys and 37% of girls (ages 12–17) had ever tried alcohol, and about 15% of both had used alcohol in the past month (Table 14–1). Approximately 15% of women and 33% of men (ages 18–34) reported using alcohol at least once per week (Table 14–2).

More than 60% of all young adults ages 26–34 recalled use of some illicit drug in their lifetimes (Table 14–3). Reported rates were slightly lower among 18- to 25-year-old persons (53.3% of men and 50.0% of women) and were even lower for persons older than age 35 (34.1% of men and 22.8% of women). However, both men and women in the 18- to 25-year age group were more likely to continue illicit drug use during the past year (30.4% and 22.6%, respectively) and during the past month (16.7% and 9.5%, respectively).

In children ages 12–17, rates for ever having used an illicit drug were surprising insofar as girls had *higher* rates (16.6%) than boys (16.3%). This pattern persisted for illicit drug use within the past year (12.5% versus 11.0%, respectively) and for illicit drug use within the past month (6.5% versus 5.7%, respectively); this pattern is reflected in specific rates for cocaine use. Small sample size in these categories may contribute to unstable statistics, but it is also true that girls typically date older boys and that dating is a vector of drug use between males and females.

Access to marijuana and cocaine is still relatively common. For both men and women in the age categories reporting highest use (ages

Table 14-1. Prevalence estimates for alcohol: ever, past year, and past month (1992) by age and sex groups for total population

Age (years)	Sex	Ever used (%)	Used in past year (%)	Used in past month (%)
12–17	Combined	39.3	32.6	15.7
	Male	41.6	33.7	16.9
	Female	37.0	31.4	14.5
18–25	Combined	86.3	77.7	59.2
	Male	87.7	79.8	65.6
	Female	85.0	75.6	53.0
26–34	Combined	91.7	79.0	61.2
	Male	93.4	83.6	70.0
	Female	90.0	74.5	52.8
35+	Combined	87.0	62.6	46.5
	Male	93.8	69.0	56.1
	Female	81.0	57.0	38.0
Total	Combined	83.0	64.7	47.8
	Male	87.3	69.5	55.9
	Female	79.0	60.2	40.4

Note. United States population estimate: 205,713,288 persons.
Source. Adapted from National Institute on Drug Abuse 1993.

18–25 and 26–34) in 1992, about half had ever used marijuana, and between 16% and 30% had ever used cocaine (Tables 14–4 and 14–5). For persons using marijuana at least once per week (Table 14–6), the highest rate (8.8%) was reported by men ages 18–25 (versus 3.9% of women). In the 12- to 17-year-old group, use at least once per week reported by males (2.3%) was only negligibly greater than for females (2.0%) (Table 14–6).

Cocaine use was highest in the 18- to 25-year and 26- to 34-year age groups during the previous year and previous month. Men ages 18–25 had consistently higher rates of cocaine use than women—about 8.5% versus 4.2% for use in the previous year and 2.9% versus 0.8% for use in the previous month (Table 14–5). Men and women ages 18–25 had an identical rate (0.9%) for cocaine use of at least once per week (Table 14–7). Men ages 26–34 had higher rates of cocaine use than women (6.3% versus 3.5%, respectively)

Table 14–2. Prevalence estimates for alcohol: frequency of use within past year (1992) by age and sex groups for total population

Age (years)	Sex	At least once (%)	12 or more times (%)	Once a week or more (%)
12–17	Combined	32.6	11.2	4.1
	Male	33.7	12.1	5.0
	Female	31.4	10.3	3.3
18–25	Combined	77.7	50.0	24.1
	Male	79.8	59.1	32.4
	Female	75.6	41.2	16.0
26–34	Combined	79.0	50.3	25.1
	Male	83.6	63.1	36.1
	Female	74.5	37.9	14.5
35+	Combined	62.6	35.0	20.6
	Male	69.0	48.0	31.6
	Female	57.0	23.5	10.9
Total	Combined	64.7	37.5	20.3
	Male	69.5	48.6	29.7
	Female	60.2	27.2	11.5

Note. United States population estimate: 205,713,288 persons.
Source. Adapted from National Institute on Drug Abuse 1993.

during the previous year, the previous month (1.7% versus 1.1%, respectively), and at least once per week (1.0% versus 0.3%, respectively) (Tables 14–5 and 14–7). For use in the past year, males ages 12–17 reported a slightly lower rate (1.0%) than that reported by females (1.2%).

Until recently, heroin use was considered relatively rare and practiced by an aging group whose tendency to remain hidden made use and related factors difficult to measure (Kozel 1990). In the household survey of 1992, about 1.2% of men and 0.6% of women had ever used heroin, and most lifetime users were between ages 26 and 34 (1.6%). Use during the past year was greatest in the 18- to 25-year age group (0.5%), and there were twice as many male users (0.2%) versus female users (0.1%) (National Institute on Drug Abuse 1993).

Drug use is associated with crime in women and men. Of all female inmates in state prisons in 1986, 34% said they were under the influence of a drug at the time of their offense, 39% had used drugs daily

Table 14–3. Prevalence estimates for any illicit use: ever, past year, and past month (1992) by age and sex groups for total population

Age (years)	Sex	Ever used (%)	Used in past year (%)	Used in past month (%)
12–17	Combined	16.5	11.7	6.1
	Male	16.3	11.0	5.7
	Female	16.6	12.5	6.5
18–25	Combined	51.7	26.4	13.0
	Male	53.3	30.4	16.7
	Female	50.0	22.6	9.5
26–34	Combined	60.8	18.3	10.1
	Male	66.1	22.3	12.6
	Female	55.5	14.4	7.6
35+	Combined	28.0	5.1	2.2
	Male	34.1	6.7	3.2
	Female	22.78	3.7	1.4
Total	Combined	36.2	11.1	5.5
	Male	41.0	13.4	7.1
	Female	31.7	9.0	4.1

Note. United States population estimate: 205,713,288 persons.
Source. Adapted from National Institute on Drug Abuse 1993.

in the month before committing that offense, and 24% had used a "major" drug daily during that month (cocaine, heroin, methadone, lysergic acid [LSD], or phencyclidine [PCP]) (Bureau of Justice Statistics National Update 1991). Recent data from New York State (Canestrini 1991) indicate that female inmates have either a high prevalence of self-reported drug use during the 6 months before their incarceration or Michigan Alcoholism Screening Test (MAST; Selzer 1971) scores of nine or higher, or both.

In England and Wales (Maden et al. 1990), the number of women sentenced to prison between 1979 and 1988 increased by one-third, but drug-related offenses of incarcerated women grew 400%. When queried about drug use in the 6-month interval before their arrest, almost one-fourth were found to be drug dependent. Use of opiates alone, or in combination with other drugs, accounted for almost all drug use in females in British prisons.

Table 14–4. Prevalence estimates for marijuana: ever, past year, and past month (1992) by age and sex groups for total population

Age (years)	Sex	Ever used (%)	Used in past year (%)	Used in past month (%)
12–17	Combined	10.6	8.1	4.0
	Male	11.6	8.7	4.6
	Female	9.6	7.5	3.5
18–25	Combined	48.1	22.7	11.0
	Male	49.7	27.1	14.5
	Female	46.6	18.4	7.5
26–34	Combined	58.6	14.3	8.2
	Male	64.3	18.9	11.0
	Female	52.9	9.9	5.5
35+	Combined	24.8	3.3	1.6
	Male	31.2	4.5	2.3
	Female	19.2	2.2	1.0
Total	Combined	32.8	8.5	4.4
	Male	38.0	10.8	5.9
	Female	28.0	6.3	2.9

Note. United States population estimate: 205,713,288 persons.
Source. Adapted from National Institute on Drug Abuse 1993.

Polysubstance Use

In the United States, the use of alcohol concurrently with other substances is an established clinical reality in both sexes. Women with alcohol problems usually are at further risk for polydrug use, including cocaine, marijuana, opiates, and psychotropic prescription medications (Clayton et al. 1986).

A comprehensive study by Robbins (1989) examined gender differences in psychosocial problems associated with alcohol and other drug use by testing three hypotheses that could explain differential behaviors of women and men. Data were drawn from the 1985 National Household Survey on Drug Abuse. The first hypothesis was that differential psychosocial consequences of substance use for women derive in part from biological factors, especially alcohol metabolism (Robbins 1989). Because more women use psychoactive pre-

Table 14–5. Prevalence estimates for cocaine: ever, past year, and past
month (1992) by age and sex groups for total population

Age (years)	Sex	Ever used (%)	Used in past year (%)	Used in past month (%)
12–17	Combined	1.7	1.1	0.3
	Male	1.6	1.0	0.2
	Female	1.8	1.2	0.3
18–25	Combined	15.8	6.3	1.8
	Male	18.8	8.5	2.9
	Female	12.9	4.2	0.8
26–34	Combined	25.2	4.9	1.4
	Male	29.8	6.3	1.7
	Female	20.8	3.5	1.1
35+	Combined	6.9	0.9	0.2
	Male	8.8	1.3	0.3
	Female	5.2	0.6	0.1
Total	Combined	11.0	2.4	0.6
	Male	13.4	3.2	0.9
	Female	8.7	1.7	0.4

Note. United States population estimate: 205,713,288 persons.
Source. Adapted from National Institute on Drug Abuse 1993.

scription drugs, some of which are cross-tolerant with alcohol, vulnerability to alcohol-drug interactions may stem from liver clearance
rates. The second hypothesis was that substance use is popularly believed to be more stigmatizing for women. Similar observations have
been noted historically and cross-culturally (Lex 1985); thus, some
investigators have argued that potential compromise of women's sexual chastity or nurturing responsibilities underlies the greater stigma
directed toward women who use substances. The third hypothesis
was that men and women have different deviant behavior styles. Male
deviance is said to be antisocial and directed toward others, whereas
female deviance is thought to be channeled into internalized distress
and manifested as emotional upset. It is reasoned that women who
use substances at the behest of or in the company of a male partner
make stronger efforts to hide substance use, to curtail alcohol and
drug use except when caretaking expectations are in abeyance, and

Table 14-6.   Prevalence estimates for marijuana: frequency of use within past year (1992) by age and sex groups for total population

Age (years)	Sex	At least once (%)	12 or more times (%)	Once a week or more (%)
12–17	Combined	8.1	4.8	2.2
	Male	8.7	5.6	2.3
	Female	7.5	4.1	2.0
18–25	Combined	22.7	11.8	6.3
	Male	27.1	15.4	8.8
	Female	18.4	8.4	3.9
26–34	Combined	14.3	7.1	4.7
	Male	18.9	10.3	6.8
	Female	9.9	4.0	2.7
35+	Combined	3.3	2.0	1.0
	Male	4.5	2.9	1.3
	Female	2.2	1.2	0.6
Total	Combined	8.5	4.2	2.5
	Male	10.8	5.7	3.5
	Female	6.3	2.8	1.6

Note.   United States population estimate: 205,713,288 persons.
Source.   Adapted from National Institute on Drug Abuse 1993.

to strive to behave in "feminine" social roles despite drug or alcohol effects (Robbins 1989). Accordingly, women who use alcohol and other drugs report greater depression, anxiety, and guilt, whereas more men report alcohol- and drug-related belligerence, employment problems, and legal problems. Typically, the legal, financial, or job problems among men result in a greater likelihood of referral for treatment; thus, fewer women are referred for treatment (see "Gender and Treatment" later in this chapter).

Robbins found gender differences in the frequency distributions for 12 of 17 reported symptoms and consequences of substance abuse. Although not all differences were statistically significant, the results generally supported the "styles of pathology" hypothesis.

Note that the 1985 cross-sectional survey of persons residing in households, on which Robbins based her conclusions, underrepresented effects of marijuana and cocaine on individuals not living in conventional domestic settings. Studies of incarcerated or hospital-

Table 14–7. Prevalence estimates for cocaine: frequency of use within past year (1992) by age and sex groups for total population

Age (years)	Sex	At least once (%)	12 or more times (%)	Once a week or more (%)
12–17	Combined	1.1	0.3	0.1
	Male	1.0	0.3	0.1
	Female	1.2	0.3	0.1
18–25	Combined	6.3	2.1	0.9
	Male	8.5	2.3	0.9
	Female	4.2	1.8	0.9
26–34	Combined	4.9	1.8	0.7
	Male	6.3	2.2	1.0
	Female	3.5	1.4	0.3
35+	Combined	0.9	0.2	0.1
	Male	1.3	0.2	0.1
	Female	0.6	0.1	0.1
Total	Combined	2.4	0.7	0.3
	Male	3.2	0.9	0.4
	Female	1.7	0.6	0.3

Note. United States population estimate: 205,713,288 persons.
Source. Adapted from National Institute on Drug Abuse 1993.

ized populations of men and women might have yielded different results. Thus, the sociological interpretation may be correct, insofar as conclusions were drawn from observations of a less deviant or less severely impaired population. Robbins (1989) also questioned whether women's relatively increased vulnerability to disputes with their family and friends reflected a gender difference in expected behavior or reflected greater stigma and social disapproval directed toward women who abuse substances. Another explanation could be that women who abuse alcohol and other drugs are more likely to have families with other members who abuse substances (Lex 1991; Lex et al. 1990), thus generating greater family conflict and dysfunction. Women are also more likely to use substances in the company of spouses or mates who abuse substances (Kandel 1984; Kandel et al. 1986; Robbins 1989). This may also contribute to domestic discord.

Gomberg (1989a) interviewed 301 alcoholic women (ages 20–50), after detoxification in 21 Michigan treatment facilities, about their drug use and compared their responses with those of a matched control group of nonalcoholic women. Polydrug use was more common among alcoholic women. Compared with their nonalcoholic age peers, all alcoholic women reported more experience with cocaine, heroin, and marijuana. Younger alcoholic women typically reported using combinations of alcohol and other drugs, whereas older alcoholic women were significantly more likely to use medications, mainly minor tranquilizers, prescribed by a physician.

One study of treated prevalence rates of intercurrent psychiatric disorders investigated 260 male and 241 female patients with alcohol and drug problems (Ross et al. 1988). Diagnoses were made using the National Institute of Mental Health Diagnostic Interview Schedule (DIS; Robins et al. 1981). Individuals with polysubstance dependence had higher rates of intercurrent psychiatric disorders. Overall rates for cognitive impairment, schizophrenia, or affective disorders did not differ between women and men. Women had higher rates of anxiety and bulimia, which were not surprising, but also of psychosexual disorders—an unexpected finding. In all likelihood, these findings reflect use of the DIS, which has probes for recently delineated disorders, such as bulimia, recognized only within the past decade.

Another view is that consumption patterns are converging for women and men. This hypothesis has been controversial for more than a decade (Ferrence 1980; Ferrence and Whitehead 1980) and is related to an ideological debate (Lex 1985). Epidemiological data for alcohol and other drug consumption patterns in recent years yield little support for the idea that consumption behavior is similar for all women and men. However, younger age groups exhibit less gender difference in consumption patterns.

Marijuana

Kandel (1984) and Kandel and co-workers (1986) conducted longitudinal studies of substance users who were first identified in high school. Eighty-three percent of the original 1,651 adolescents were reinterviewed at ages 24–25. The majority of respondents, 78% of young men and 69% of young women, had used marijuana, but one-third of men and one-fifth of women also used other drugs. A correlation of 0.995 between increasing marijuana use and increasing use of other illicit drugs was found. Consequently, it is difficult to disentangle marijuana effects from effects of other substance use.

Job instability was associated with marijuana and other illicit drug use in both men and women. The amount of marijuana use reported in the initial survey predicted an increased number of unemployed intervals at follow-up. Illicit drug use also affected execution of adult family roles. Marijuana use predicted lower rates of marriage for women and was positively correlated with divorce or separation among both women and men and with abortions among women.

Marijuana users were heavily involved in social relationships in which marijuana use was common. Of women who had used marijuana four or more times per week during the past year, 96% reported that most or all of their friends used marijuana (Kandel 1984). Among women living with a spouse or partner, a male spouse's or partner's use had a strong effect on women's marijuana use (the "husband effect"). This influence was greater than peers' use and the individual's use of other illicit drugs.

Constriction of relationships to substance-using partners appears to increase women's exposure to both drugs and violence. Kantor and Strauss (1989) studied marijuana use by spouses of battered women. The investigators found a sixfold increase in marijuana use in the previous year among battered victims seen in an emergency room compared with nonvictims. Comparable findings for violence toward pregnant women by partners who used marijuana, cocaine, and alcohol were reported by Amaro and colleagues (1990).

Patterns of marijuana use in the community may be partially illustrated by laboratory studies. Two series of studies with similar protocols investigated marijuana self-administration in young men (Babor et al. 1975) and women (Babor et al. 1984). Based on drug-use histories and self-report questionnaires, subjects were classified as "moderate" or "heavy" users. Moderate smokers had used marijuana more than five times per month during the previous year, whereas heavy smokers had used marijuana five or more times per week during the previous year.

Subjects were studied on a research unit for 35 days in groups of three or four that included both moderate and heavy smokers. Study protocols included three phases: a 7-day drug-free baseline phase, a

21-day drug acquisition period during which marijuana cigarettes could be purchased on a free-choice basis, and a 7-day postdrug phase. During all study phases, subjects could work for points at a simple operant task that earned $0.50 per one-half hour of effort. During the 21-day acquisition period, points earned could either be exchanged directly for marijuana ($0.50 per cigarette) or accumulated until the conclusion of the study, added to points earned during the baseline period, and exchanged for money. Subjects who had sufficient points for purchase had no limit on the amount of marijuana they could smoke.

Male heavy smokers consumed about four cigarettes per day at the beginning of the 21-day marijuana acquisition period, and their use increased by one-half to about six and a half cigarettes per day by day 20. Male moderate smokers consumed about two cigarettes per day at the beginning and increased by one-half to about three cigarettes per day (Babor et al. 1975). In sharp contrast, marijuana use by female heavy smokers averaged three and a half cigarettes per day, and female moderate smokers consumed 1.4 cigarettes per day throughout the study period (Babor et al. 1984). No significant linear increases in marijuana smoking occurred for women.

Thus, distinct factors may influence marijuana use for men and women. Men's marijuana smoking appears influenced by availability. Women's marijuana smoking patterns, however, may reflect social influences, such as the temporal pattern of weekday versus weekend smoking (Lex et al. 1986) or influence of male partners (Kandel 1984; Kandel et al. 1986). However, fluctuations also could be related to the greater amount of female lipid tissue, which can store and gradually release tetrahydrocannabinol (Δ^9-THC). Furthermore, female moderate smokers increased their smoking on days when they reported heightened unpleasant moods, such as anger (Babor et al. 1984), which suggests that marijuana smoking was related to negative affect.

Another study series used daily diaries to obtain concurrent reports of marijuana and alcohol consumption by female marijuana smokers and alcohol and marijuana consumption by female social drinkers for three consecutive menstrual cycles (Lex et al. 1986, 1988). Subjects recorded the quantities and times of their alcohol and marijuana use, episodes of sexual activity, and occurrence of unusual life events (a definition of "stress") (Lex et al. 1986). Temporal variables were significantly associated with increased marijuana and alcohol consumption.

A prospective study of female social drinkers (Lex et al. 1988) used similar methods to examine alcohol and marijuana consumption patterns and mood states for roughly 90 days per subject (98+% completion rate). Heavy drinkers (mean $\geq$ 1.80 drinks per day) were significantly more likely to smoke marijuana than moderate drinkers (mean $\leq$ 1.75 drinks per day), and heavy drinkers also smoked significantly more amounts of marijuana.

Multiple regression analysis examined interaction of eight mood states with effects of six variables: heavy marijuana use, consumption of both marijuana and alcohol, occurrence of unusual events, sexual activity, menses, and weekdays versus weekends (Lex et al. 1989). Heavy marijuana smoking was the strongest predictor of mood states. Heavy marijuana smokers had lower scores on friendliness, elation, and vigor and higher scores on tension, anger, fatigue, and confusion than light smokers. Heavy marijuana smoking influenced *all* mood ratings except depression. Concurrent marijuana smoking and alcohol use was associated with increased scores for friendliness and vigor and decreased scores for tension and fatigue.

Low elation scores reported by female heavy marijuana smokers may indicate that marijuana smoking becomes associated with lessened euphoria among women who smoke heavily (Lex et al. 1989). Similar findings for young men have been reported by Mirin and associates (1971). Absence of changes in depression scores for female heavy marijuana users was an unanticipated finding that was different from increased depression reported by male heavy marijuana users (Mirin et al. 1971). Unusual events were significantly associated with increased tension, depression, anger, and confusion but unrelated to positive moods (Lex et al. 1989).

Opioids

One series of reports examined gender differences in the addiction careers of 546 male and female patients in methadone maintenance programs in southern California (Anglin et al. 1987a, 1987b; Hser et al. 1987a, 1987b). At admission, women were younger—age approximately 26 years versus 29 for men. Both women and men had an average of 10.5 years of education. Approximately 90% of men and women had been arrested, with first arrests at about age 16.5 and 18.5 years, respectively. About 80% of men and women were married, and about 85% had lived with a partner in a consensual union, with an average of 2.5 children. In this sample, approximately 60% of men also used marijuana, and 40% drank daily. White men were more likely to sell drugs than white women, but Hispanic women were more likely to be involved in drug dealing than Hispanic men. Overall, more men than women reported having been a gang member and having had school problems. Male addicts also had been arrested at younger ages and more frequently had been incarcerated for more than 30 days. They were also more likely to be on probation.

Note that about 15% of women, but no men, reported initiation into heroin use by their spouse or common-law partner. In contrast, men were more likely to initiate use in a group context, and no man reported living with an addicted woman before his initial heroin use. Women required less time to develop dependence, and many became dependent within 1 month. The mean number of total months from initiation into opiate use to opiate dependence was 14 months for women and 21 months for men. During the interval between initiation of use and physiological dependence, women also sharply curtailed nonopiate drug use and slightly decreased alcohol use. Women may replace use of other drugs with heroin, whereas men continue to experiment simultaneously with many drugs. Women and men seemed to follow similar opiate use patterns, but women's addiction careers seemed "compressed" into a shorter cycle (Hser et al. 1987b). This pattern of differential time to dependence for women is consistent with findings from other studies (Kosten et al. 1985) and is reminiscent of telescoping in alcohol dependence. Compared with male opioid users, women in this sample (Hser et al. 1987b) reported shorter durations of consistent daily use (23 months versus 32 months). About one-third of men and women reported that they had been able to abstain after becoming dependent, but women were abstinent for shorter intervals (approximately 3.5 months) than men (approximately 8 months). Female opiate users entered treatment after significantly less time—an average of about 5 years from first drug use to admission to a methadone maintenance program versus an average of 8 years for men.

Women were most likely to attribute their opiate use to social reasons, especially use by a partner (approximately 36%), but about 10% of men and women reported social use by friends as a major social reason for using opiates. For about 50% of men and 30% of women, "liking the high" and developing tolerance perpetuated use. Men also cited ready availability or cheaply priced heroin, but women were less likely to obtain their own heroin (Hser et al. 1987b). Influence of an opiate-using partner is a strong factor in opiate use by women, perhaps because opiate use becomes an adjunct to sexual activity (Lex 1990).

Kosten and colleagues (1985) studied 522 treated opiate addicts, including 126 women (24%). When rated on the Addiction Severity Index (McLellan et al. 1980), women had a severity rating of 4.0 for intercurrent psychological problems, whereas men averaged 3.3, although ratings were similar for other scales. Using Research Diagnostic Criteria (RDC; Spitzer et al. 1978), Kosten and colleagues (1985) found that intercurrent psychiatric diagnoses differed by gender, with more women having dysphoric and anxiety disorders (64% versus 49%) and more men having antisocial personality disorders (30% versus 17%). Women were twice as likely as men to have received their first psychiatric treatment by age 15 (10%).

Cocaine

There are comparatively few direct comparisons of male and female cocaine users in treatment. Wallace (1991) provided a brief literature review to preface discussion of the need for treatment of the pregnant crack addict and pointed out that cocaine-related deaths are declining, but arrests, admissions for treatment, and births of infants affected by cocaine are increasing. An article by Phibbs and colleagues (1991) documented the exorbitant costs of maternal cocaine use. A total of 355 cocaine-exposed infants were compared with a random sample of infants not exposed to cocaine ($n = 199$) delivered at Harlem Hospital in 1985 and 1986. Cocaine-exposed infants were more likely to be born to black mothers who were older, who had had more previous pregnancies, and who had not received prenatal care. Mothers of cocaine-exposed infants also were more likely to smoke tobacco cigarettes and to use alcohol. Infants exposed to cocaine had significantly lower birth weights (31.3% < 2,500 g and 3.7% < 1,500 g). At birth, cocaine-exposed infants also were an average of 1 week less than gestational age (38.1 weeks versus 39.2 weeks), and almost 20% had a gestational age less than 37 weeks. One-fourth (24.6%) were admitted to the neonatal intensive care unit. For babies exposed to multiple drugs, hospital costs were $8,450 versus $1,283 for babies exposed to cocaine alone, a more than fivefold increase, with lengths of stay averaging 10 days versus 2.7 days, respectively (Phibbs et al. 1991).

Many women who use crack exchange sex to obtain it. A recent study of prostitution in New York City assessed the impact of crack cocaine use (Maher and Curtis 1992). Unforeseen outcomes were deflated standard fees for sex acts and increased violence associated with these exchanges. As the cost of a cocaine "rock" dropped to about $2, ethnographic fieldwork disclosed that the conventional charges for sex acts also decreased, in some instances to $2–$3 per episode from $10 or higher.

Some studies suggest that increased numbers of women participating in more traditionally male criminal activities, such as assault or robbery, also reflect deflation of fees for sexual favors and the climate of violence in which these behaviors occur (Maher and Curtis 1992). Women's participation in the drug trade has been further marginalized, and movement into more violent activity can be seen as opportunistic rather than deliberate and calculated.

Women in treatment for cocaine-related problems appeared more likely to have an Axis I DSM-III-R diagnosis in addition to substance abuse, especially depression, whereas only men had antisocial personality disorder (Griffin et al. 1989). Women with a DSM-III-R diagnosis of depression had higher scores than men on the Hamilton Rating Scale for Depression (HRSD; Hamilton 1960) at admission, at 2 weeks after admission, and at 4 weeks after admission.

Women in this study gave four main reasons for their cocaine use: 1) depression, 2) feeling unsociable, 3) family and job pressures, and 4) health problems. Overall, men cited more intoxication effects from cocaine and were more likely to report that cocaine decreased libido (67% of men versus 38% of women reported the latter). Involvement or cohabitating with a drug-dependent partner may have contributed to the more rapid development of cocaine addiction in some women, an observation also found in female opioid addicts (Kosten et al. 1986) and in female alcoholic patients (Hesselbrock et al. 1985).

Morbidity and Mortality

Morbidity

The impact of excessive alcohol intake on women's physical health has been well documented. Development of hypertension, anemia, fatty liver, alcoholic hepatitis, and gastrointestinal complications occurs more rapidly in women than in men (Dunne 1988). Greater vulnerability to neurological damage in women also has been reported. A recent medical textbook (Zetterman 1992) reports that 10 years of daily exposure to 80 g of alcohol (about 6 ounces of 80-proof whiskey) can induce cirrhosis in women, in contrast to 160 g in men. Van Thiel and Gavaler (1988) cited more than 10 reports that indicate gender differences in onset and course of alcohol-related liver disease. Their conclusions are strengthened by the fact that these studies used different methodological designs, were conducted at different points in time, and examined subjects in five or more countries. An important finding is that alcohol-related liver damage in women appears to progress regardless of abstinence.

Frezza and co-workers (1990) reported that higher blood alcohol levels in women can be attributed to gender differences in first-pass or initial metabolism and oxidation by gastric tissue. In contrast to men, endoscopic gastric biopsies indicated less gastric alcohol dehydrogenase activity in female social drinkers and almost no activity in alcoholic women. This research has not specifically addressed the mechanisms underlying this difference, but it reinforces the notion that different consumption cutoffs apply to women and men.

Alcoholism in men has well-known associations with impotence, low testosterone levels, testicular atrophy, gynecomastia, and diminished sexual interest. Until very recently, however, relatively little research has focused on alcohol effects on reproductive function in women. Interpretation of data from women is complicated because most data are from studies of alcoholic women treated for liver disease, pancreatitis, or other intercurrent medical disorders. The adverse effects of chronic alcohol abuse on reproductive function via the hypothalamic-pituitary-gonadal axis may be caused by direct toxic effects of alcohol on the hypothalamus, pituitary gland, or ovaries or by a combination of these pathophysiological processes.

Use of drugs other than alcohol can exacerbate health problems and contribute to reproductive compromise. It is generally reported that one of every six couples experiences infertility, and women seeking help for obstetric and gynecologic problems have a higher rate of substance abuse problems. Busch and colleagues (1986) conducted a mail questionnaire study of two groups of women with a diagnosis of infertility problems or pelvic pain. Items in the questionnaire included type and amount of alcohol and drug consumption and patterns of use, the MAST (Selzer 1971), and a comparable inventory for drug dependence that included 21 questions. Subjects also identified the date of onset of use of various substances as well as dates of onsets of the pelvic pain or infertility problems. Of 74 women, 23 (31%) had either a potential or probable alcohol and/or drug use problem. Infertility was associated with alcohol problems in 23.2% of the women. Furthermore, 13 of 74 (18%) reported that use of alcohol and/or psychoactive substances increased after onset of pelvic pain or infertility.

These clinical findings corroborate results from a cross-sectional study (Wilsnack et al. 1984) in which 917 women were queried about dysmenorrhea, heavy menstrual flow, and premenstrual discomfort. Severity of menstrual distress symptoms increased linearly with amount of alcohol consumption.

Excessive alcohol intake in women also can result in amenorrhea, anovulation, luteal phase dysfunction, hyperprolactinemia, and spontaneous abortion. Opiate use may cause the same disorders in women. Marijuana smoking has been associated with amenorrhea, anovulation, luteal phase dysfunction, and spontaneous abortion, and cocaine use has been associated with amenorrhea, anovulation, hyperprolactinemia, and spontaneous abortion (Mello et al. 1989).

Mortality

Smith and colleagues (1983) examined predictors of mortality in alcoholic women in a prospective follow-up study. They used Feighner's criteria (Feighner et al. 1972) to ascertain alcoholism in 103 women who had been admitted to two psychiatric hospitals during 1967–1968. Follow-up data for 92 subjects reinterviewed in 1979 and 1980 found a 31% death rate. Compared with the overall female population in the city of St. Louis, excess mortality in alcoholic women yielded a ratio of 4.5:1. Approximately 75% of the original population was white. A higher mortality was observed for black women (42%) than white women (28%). Alcoholic women also were significantly younger at time of death (mean age, 51 years) than the general population of women in St. Louis (mean age, 66.5 years). The largest number of deaths were attributed to pancreatitis, hepatic cirrhosis, and other liver disorders (29%). Violence and accidents accounted for 26% of deaths at a mean age of 49.5 years (range, 28–70). Deaths in these categories were more than twice the overall rate for white women (ratio, 20:8) as for black women (ratio, 8:4). Only two deaths were identified as suicides by violent means; however, the deaths of two additional women who overdosed on combinations of alcohol and prescription medications also might have been suicides. Three deaths were accidental, attributed to fires related to smoking and drinking. The one homicide was a 54-year-old woman who was stabbed by a male drinking companion.

More global variables of duration and intensity of alcohol abuse were better predictors of mortality than highly specific alcohol-related symptoms. Only abstinence was associated with reduced mortality. Women who identified themselves as social drinkers had a higher than average proportion of deaths, and their death rate was comparable to those of sporadic/variable drinkers (20% versus 17%). The majority of deaths (54%) occurred in women who continued to drink steadily and in high volume.

One study compared suicidality in 301 alcoholic women with control women (Gomberg 1989b). Almost five times as many alcoholic women (40%) as control women (8.8%) acknowledged suicide attempts. Alcoholic women ranged in age from 20 to 50, with suicide attempts occurring more frequently in the younger alcoholic women.

No suicide attempts were reported by nonalcoholic control subjects. Younger alcoholic women also were more likely to use other psychoactive drugs than older alcoholic women.

Information from the Drug Abuse Warning Network (DAWN) discloses gender differences in drug-related emergency room episodes (National Institute on Drug Abuse 1992b). In 1991, 400,079 drug abuse episodes were treated in the 534 emergency rooms from which DAWN data were reported (National Institute on Drug Abuse 1992a). Of these episodes, 47.8% involved men and 51.9% involved women, for a male-to-female ratio of 1.0:1.09. About 1,200 patients died (0.3% of all episodes), with equal proportions among men and women. The motive for drug-induced and drug-related deaths was suicide in 43.8% of all cases, but women predominated (57.1% of women versus 29.6% of men), with a sex ratio of 1.0:1.93.

Data from drug-related medical examiner cases for which gender was recorded disclosed 4,733 male and 1,837 female deaths, with a sex ratio of 1.0:0.38 (National Institute on Drug Abuse 1992b). Of all drug deaths, 27% involved use of only one drug, whereas 73% involved multiple drugs. These distributions were similar for men and women (26.2% versus 28.7% and 73.8% versus 71.3%, respectively). Of 15,576 drugs mentioned in association with 6,601 deaths, narcotic analgesics (including heroin, methadone, codeine, and propoxyphene [Darvon]) accounted for 61.3%, cocaine accounted for 45.8%, and alcohol with combinations of other drugs accounted for 36.9% (National Institute on Drug Abuse 1992b). Rankings for these drugs were identical for each gender, but deaths associated with narcotic analgesics, with cocaine, and with alcohol in combination were proportionately greater among men (sex ratios of 1.0:0.84, 1.0:0.71, and 1.0:0.64, respectively). Women's deaths involved proportionately more antidepressant drugs (22.7% versus 8.6%, for a female-to-male ratio of 2.64:1.0) (National Institute on Drug Abuse 1992b).

Vital statistics for 1985 illustrate the role of alcohol in mortality rates (Rice et al. 1990). About 94,768 persons died from alcohol as a main cause; from alcohol-related malignant neoplasms, injuries, accidents, homicides, and suicides; or from alcohol-complicated respiratory tuberculosis, diabetes mellitus, pneumonia, influenza, and gastric diseases. Of these deaths, men accounted for 65,319 (69%), and women accounted for 29,448 (31%). Mortality caused by alcohol abuse in women increased with age—the highest percentage of deaths occurred in women age 65 and older (44.0%), but the highest percentage of deaths in men (29.8%) occurred at ages 45–64 years.

Available trend data for alcohol-related mortality in the United States based on ICD-9 (World Health Organization 1989) categories were used to calculate determinants of underlying causes of death in vital statistics compiled by the National Center for Health Statistics (Stinson and DeBakey 1992). Data collected between 1979 and 1988 indicate declining age-adjusted mortality rates for women and men for causes directly attributable to alcoholism. The new voluntary coding system for reporting alcohol involvement in accidents, diseases, and other effects in ICD-10 (World Health Organization 1992) is likely to increase precision in reporting alcohol-related mortality. Nonetheless, in 1988, about 5% of deaths were directly or indirectly related to alcohol use.

Gender and Treatment

The 1991 National Drug and Alcoholism Treatment Unit Survey (NDATUS; Substance Abuse and Mental Health Services Administration 1993) reported the demographic profile of patients receiving both public and private treatment for alcoholism and drug abuse on September 30, 1991. Women constituted 27.5% of all patients for whom gender was reported. Proportions of women ranged widely, from 33.1% of all patients in New York State to 14.4% in Louisiana. For a reporting base of 9,057 treatment units, 6,856 (75.7%) provided at least one type of specialized care, and 4,495 units (49.6%) offered specialized services to women.

An age-related cohort effect is obvious in the pattern of women's alcohol and other drug use. Analysis of data collected from 572 women who were admitted for inpatient alcohol and drug abuse treatment in 1986 and 1987 showed a clear difference between women older and younger than age 35 (Harrison 1989). Although the sample was predominantly white (79%), both age distinctions and effects of secular change were apparent. Likelihood of daily drinking was 2.5 times greater in women age 35 and older. As might be expected, women under age 35 also were regularly using marijuana, cocaine, other stimulants, opiates, and hallucinogens. Moreover, 56% of younger women began alcohol use before age 16, compared with 14% of women older than age 35. Polydrug use occurred by age 15 in almost half (47%) of women under age 35. In sharp contrast, only 3% of women older than 35 had tried drugs by age 15. Furthermore, younger women were more likely to use alcohol and drugs in public contexts (53%) rather than in isolation (21% of older women). It is of particular concern that initiation of alcohol use now occurs much earlier in the life cycle, before social roles crystallize. The impact of polydrug use is also clinically troublesome, especially because use of multiple drugs prevents the attribution of specific symptoms to specific drugs.

There are numerous studies of treatment for women with alcohol problems, although their quality and utility are uneven (Turnbull 1988). Prevalence rates may have been underestimated for women. Women may be less likely to use conventional alcoholism treatment facilities and more likely to seek help from private physicians. Some investigators also argue that women's drinking can remain more covert than that of men and that women are actively dissuaded by partners—often themselves heavy drinkers—from seeking treatment. Researchers have frequently alleged that available treatment facilities do not adequately accommodate problems presented by alcoholic women (Wilsnack 1991).

Vannicelli and Nash (1984) recalculated outcome data for 23 of 259 studies that had differentiated between alcoholic men and women. According to their analysis, no scientific evidence indicated that women respond poorly to treatment: 18 studies (78%) showed no differences in outcome, 4 studies (17%) showed better outcome for women, and no studies showed better outcome for men.

Vannicelli (1984) also identified three barriers to efficacious alcoholism treatment for women: 1) expectancies that women will not profit from treatment because they are more depressed, experience mood swings, and are self-centered; 2) traditionally stereotyped sex role expectancies that alcoholic women have limited potential for change; and 3) lack of information about prognosis for alcoholic women that has led to the assumption that treatment is ineffective. In addition, an expectancy effect or bias by male and female treatment

providers may exist. There is anecdotal evidence that providers in-
fantilize alcoholic women, thus undercutting growth and strength of
female patients. Furthermore, lack of research precludes development
of a scientific basis for designing treatment for women. Insufficient
data exist to evaluate the indications for individual therapy, group
therapy, and/or family therapy in women. Whether women need to
be treated separately or in mixed groups and the impact of female
versus male therapists are other issues that must be addressed.

Patterns of Compliance in
Men Versus Women

Duckert (1987) noted that alcoholic women are not likely to seek
treatment in conventional alcoholism services. Instead, they are
more likely to seek help for marital problems, family problems,
physical illnesses, or emotional problems. Clinicians believe that alcoholic women are difficult to engage in treatment, are highly ambivalent about treatment, and show poor motivation for treatment.
Attrition rates during the first month of treatment range from 28% to
80%. Moreover, patients who drop out have a poorer prognosis.

In Great Britain, self-referral constitutes the major intake route
for those who seek help for alcohol-related problems. British councils
on alcohol are said to be more successful in attracting women with
alcohol problems because the availability of female counselors may
reduce stigma, appointment schedules are flexible, and individual
counseling is emphasized.

Allan and Phil (1987) studied 112 men and women with alcohol
problems who were enrolled in a clinic by a community-based volunteer agency over a 6-month period. Only men (11% of original
referrals) attended the clinic for 6 months or more; all women dropped
out. Gender of counselors did not affect treatment retention because
78% of women were assigned to female counselors. However, referral
source was important. About one-half (49%) were self-referrals to the
agency, and the remainder were referred there by general practitioners, hospitals, and shelters. Individuals who had been referred remained in treatment longer; 14% of referred patients remained in
treatment for 6 months versus only 1.8% of self-referrals. Individuals

referred by shelters, employers, or courts had the highest rates of regular attendance. Because the vast majority of women were self-referrals or were referred by noncoercive sources, their high drop-out rate may be associated with lack of negative consequences for nonattendance and may reflect the nature of the referrals rather than indicate greater pathology.

A comprehensive study (Thom 1986) examined barriers to help seeking in 25 men and 25 women who were new admissions referred to an alcohol clinic. Women and men were similar in age (43.1 and 42.4, respectively) and did not differ significantly in marital status, in number living with children younger than age 16 years, in living situation, in employment, or in education level. Many women believed that their heavy alcohol consumption was a legitimate response to personal problems and did not perceive that alcohol use might further complicate their problems. They thought that drinking for the sake of drinking was the major reason that individuals should receive alcohol treatment; thus, they denied that the clinic was an appropriate place for them. A major obstacle for men was concern about having a problem that could not be solved without assistance. Men believed that they should be able to control their drinking on their own and found it difficult to ask for help. Some men reported that co-workers who learned that they attended an alcohol treatment clinic would view them as lacking masculinity. Women objected to being formally labeled as needing treatment from an alcohol clinic, but men worried that they would be labeled as needing psychiatric care.

Few patients (four women and no men) reported practical problems that made it difficult to attend the clinic. Child care was not a salient issue; instead, patients felt awkward about obtaining time off from work. An equal number of men and women ($n = 5$) were apprehensive about the hospital context; their fears included embarrassment about discussing personal problems, lack of knowledge about treatment requirements, being told never to drink again, and physicians as authority figures.

This study also examined reasons for referral (Thom 1987). Half of the men and women had first sought treatment within the year before the interview. Similar numbers of men ($n = 16$) and women ($n = 14$) were referred to the alcohol clinic by general practitioners.

However, almost double the number of women $(n = 9)$ versus men $(n = 5)$ were referred to the alcohol clinic from an emergency clinic, which suggests that women may delay treatment until health problems become urgent.

Only three men and six women failed to report a significant life event in the year before the interview. Major reasons for referral of women to alcohol abuse treatment included experience of physical violence, homelessness, and suicide attempts. Both men and women cited legal problems, death of a significant other, or marital dissolution. Job loss and health problems prompted men to seek treatment. Intriguingly, two men and three women reported that an encouraging life event prompted them to feel worthy and to have hope for the future, and influence of significant others also provided encouragement. More men $(n = 13)$ than women $(n = 4)$ attributed this influence to a spouse, whereas more women $(n = 6)$ than men $(n = 3)$ reported positive influence from their children.

Fifteen men and 14 women cited health problems, but only women $(n = 3)$ reported drug use as a health problem. Fourteen women versus 8 men reported depression, and 5 women versus 1 man reported generalized anxiety or panic attacks. Women were less likely to be in stable living arrangements and most frequently reported pressure from others and concern by others about their health as prompts to enter treatment. Men viewed encouragement from others as a positive factor, but women were more likely to perceive clinic attendance as a way to escape undesirable pressure from others, without expecting to make any concomitant changes in their lives.

Engagement in Treatment

A qualitative study of factors implicated in successful interventions for alcohol-dependent women involved 18 recovering alcoholic women who were identified through various community programs without use of systematic sampling (Robinson 1984). Findings indicated that humiliation and embarrassment rarely prompted women to seek treatment. Five women had been inpatients in psychiatric units; four had not received any help with their alcohol problem during these hospitalizations. Five women also reported seeing therapists who were either unapprised of the existence of an alcohol-dependence problem or who were unable to provide appropriate intervention. In addition, six women had physicians who provided no assistance. Furthermore, women who sought treatment from psychiatrists and other physicians reported receiving psychoactive medications that, in some instances, supplanted alcohol dependence as a substance of abuse.

Of these 18 women, 17 found Alcoholics Anonymous to be a good source of social support. Other social supports, however, appeared to be highly individual and included close friends, boyfriends or spouses, or parents. Perceived barriers to treatment also were highly individual, including desire for anonymity, lack of information, alcohol-dependent spouse, drug-dependent child, threat of divorce, need for monetary support from parents, fear of prosecution, refusal of spouse to pay medical expenses, and unpredictable work schedule.

Several investigators have compared differential treatment experiences of women and men. Beckman and associates (Beckman and Amaro 1986; Beckman and Kocel 1982) investigated the effects of three types of characteristics that might differentiate experiences of men and women in treatment settings. Sociodemographic, personal, social, and contextual characteristics were all associated with gender differences. Women's typically lower levels of disposable income and paucity of other economic resources were major potential obstacles to obtaining treatment.

A stepwise discriminant function analysis examined 12 independent variables, including health perceptions, health locus of control, drinking-related problems, negative effects of obtaining treatment, and negative effects of not obtaining treatment. Other variables included satisfaction with treatment, perceived success of treatment, and beliefs about family or genetic contributions to alcoholism. Findings generally supported the contention that women experience more difficulties in entering treatment but that family therapy and environmental intervention strategies counterbalanced obstacles. Women also may have had more difficulties than men in establishing trust in their alcohol counselor or therapist. A third important complicating factor for women was primary affective disorder, especially depression.

Accurate diagnosis is especially important because management and treatment of depression and of alcohol dependence require different strategies. A review by Turnbull (1988) reported that up to one-third of all women with alcohol problems may have a primary diagnosis of depression. Discrimination between the conditions that result in alcohol dependence is likely to reduce confounding in interpretation of women's need for treatment, and treatment can proceed most effectively only after identification of intercurrent disorders. High rates of major depression were identified among 572 female inpatients between 1986 and 1987 (Harrison 1989). This sample was divided into two groups—those older than age 35 and those younger than 35. Prevalence of depression was higher (71%) in younger women, although 62% of older women also reported a major depressive episode. Secular trends could be observed in the prevalence of anorexia nervosa and bulimia; about 25% of the younger women and 9% of the older women acknowledged an eating disorder. Antisocial behaviors in childhood also were more frequent in the younger age group.

As noted above, younger women are more likely to have histories of polydrug use. For disadvantaged women, often from minority backgrounds, multiple problems complicate treatment (Mondanaro 1989; Weiner et al. 1990). Women from these backgrounds need *habilitation* rather than rehabilitation. This means that the onset of drug abuse occurred so early in their adolescent development that their minimal occupational, child-rearing, and interpersonal skills, together with limited education, constitute serious disadvantages. Moreover, these women also are likely to have experienced abusive relationships with male partners who frequently use drugs themselves. This population is likely to depend on public assistance, yet public assistance programs are poorly equipped to contend with persons who have alcohol (or drug) problems (Schmidt 1990). Family backgrounds are likely to include alcohol or other drug use in family of origin and economic and emotional dependency on men who have introduced them to drug use (Weiner et al. 1990). Therefore, it is understandable that these women have low self-esteem and lack coping skills.

Some investigators have suggested that therapeutic communities or halfway houses are most appropriate for treating women from highly disadvantaged backgrounds (De Leon and Jainchill 1991; Huselid et al. 1991). It can be argued that the quality of social relationships may be a strong influence for women (Huselid et al. 1991). However, one study of 30 women completing a halfway-house program found that women who attributed their adverse life experiences to persistent and pervasive global influences were more successful. In contrast, women who minimized the importance of drug use effects across several dimensions of their lives and believed that they could control drug use were less likely to remain in treatment and achieve treatment goals. Huselid et al. interpreted these results as factors that could contribute to a "cautious abstinence." Halfway-house and therapeutic community models have been strongly influenced by Alcoholics Anonymous (Miller 1991). If abstinence is the primary goal for most treatment modalities for alcohol and drug abuse and dependence, then the effectiveness of Alcoholics Anonymous' principles (Emrick 1987) through participation in Alcoholics Anonymous or related 12-step programs appears appropriate for women and men.

Treatment Outcome

There appears to be little evidence indicating poorer prognosis for women than for men (Vannicelli 1984). Concerns about social conditions unique to women as mothers have promoted development of all-female treatment programs. Many of these programs provide child care or are targeted to pregnant women. Treatment outcomes for programs specifically targeted to women were reviewed by Duckert (1987). Results from those studies indicated that improvement rates ranged from 20% to almost 60%.

Herr and Pettinati (1984) presented outcome data for 48 homemakers and 24 employed women who had received 28-day inpatient alcoholism treatment in a psychiatric hospital. Outcome was assessed at the end of a 4-year interval. Average age at admission was 43 years. Adjustment was categorized as good, poor, or inconsistent. Approximately one-half of the homemakers and workers maintained a good adjustment over the 4-year interval, whereas 24% of homemakers versus 14% of employed women showed a poor adjustment.

At follow-up, 60% of homemakers still functioned as homemakers, and 59% of employed women were still in the labor force.

Improvements in adjustment and change of occupation were examined. Of 10 women who changed occupation, 9 improved at follow-up, compared with 7 of 13 who maintained the same occupation. A smaller number of women (3 homemakers and 3 employed women) did not change marital status at the time they changed occupations, suggesting that improvement in adjustment may have been related to change in occupation but independent of change in marital status. However, change in occupation cannot be considered as a single variable, because such a change might prompt a reallocation of leisure time or might be a consequence rather than a reason for improvement.

A series of reports by Haver (1987a, 1987b, 1987c) presented data from a follow-up study of 44 Norwegian women who had been treated for alcohol problems between 1970 and 1980. Follow-up interviews occurred approximately 6.5 years after first admission, when the mean age of the women was 32.2 years. A multiple regression analysis indicated that childhood violence experiences explained 11% of variance in outcome, but having a violent partner after treatment increased the explained variance to 25%.

The 44 women were evaluated for alcohol consumption during the year before follow-up interview (Haver 1987b). All of the women had consumed alcohol. Four women shifted from moderate to heavy drinking, and 4 women shifted from heavy to moderate drinking. Among the women who achieved total abstention after treatment, all relapsed one or more times subsequently.

Six women were long-term abstainers who changed their identities to nondrinkers by informing their drinking partners that they chose to abstain, by avoiding situations in which other people drank, by attending self-help groups, or through religious participation. Interestingly, even long-term abstainers relapsed into heavy drinking when prompted by a life crisis. Typical life crises were divorce or removal of children from the household, although these factors could be consequences and not predictors. Sixteen women (36%) were short-term abstainers who attempted to remain sober over time but could not maintain sobriety throughout the entire follow-up interval. These 16 women appeared to be able to respond to responsibilities such as holding a job or caring for children by reducing the frequency and consequences of their drinking. A shift to social drinking was reported by 17 women (39%), but a check of registry records indicated that only 8 of the women were providing accurate information. In these 8 individuals, abstinence occurred over months or years after treatment. Life situations changed for the better, with some separating from heavy drinkers and living with their children, with a new partner, or by themselves. Average consumption of social drinkers ranged from one or two glasses to four to six glasses of an alcoholic beverage per occasion. Among the long-term heavy drinkers, 4 women maintained heavy drinking after treatment, 2 retained jobs, and 2 had unstable employment.

Underhill (1986) identified many factors relevant to treatment programs for women. According to Underhill, the greater societal stigma attached to women with alcohol problems manifests itself in lower self-esteem, and this factor continues as women recover. For this reason, highly confrontational techniques were considered counterproductive. Underhill also emphasized that information about the concept of learned helplessness should be part of the education program for women involved in alcohol treatment. Similarly, concepts of assertiveness and recognition of negative affects, such as anger, were also considered important. Other relevant issues include prevalence of sexual abuse, including incest, physical abuse, and sexual assault. The prevalence rates of these events in the histories of women seeking treatment for substance abuse dependence are estimated to range from 40% to 74%. Some investigators have argued that women should receive treatment only in the context of same-sex groups, whereas others argue that the shared experience of substance abuse can be effectively handled in groups of men and women. Others have also suggested that men are more expressive about emotional problems in mixed groups and, accordingly, receive nurturing support from women, with the net result that men improve but women do not. This topic requires additional consideration.

In a recent review, Sullivan et al. (1992) asserted that improved functioning in family, work, and social adjustment is an important treatment goal. One promising strategy for ameliorating adjustment problems is case management. This approach addresses multiple needs through referrals to appropriate community resources. Case managers assess needs, develop pertinent plans, identify services, monitor positive changes, remain involved with patients, and evaluate efficacy of interventions.

Conclusion

It can be argued that the special needs of women—whether for enhancement of self-esteem, development of job skills, or training for parenthood—ideally can be met by case management. The concept and its practice are highly flexible, and sustained interaction between manager and patient can provide rapid responses as changes occur in social roles or status of drug use. Cause-and-effect sequences are readily identified so that evaluation of outcomes can be easily integrated into the case management process. Adaptability of case management to focus on all problematic life domains appears well suited for integration with "reality" or cognitive therapies.

References

Allan C, Phil M: Seeking help for drinking problems from a community-based voluntary agency: patterns of compliance amongst men and women. Br J Addict 82:1143–1147, 1987

Amaro H, Whitaker R, Coffman G, et al: Acculturation and marijuana and cocaine use: findings from HHANES 1982-1984. Am J Public Health 80:54–60, 1990

American Psychiatric Association: Diagnostic and Statistical Manual of Mental Disorders, 3rd Edition. Washington, DC, American Psychiatric Association, 1980

American Psychiatric Association: Diagnostic and Statistical Manual of Mental Disorders, 3rd Edition, Revised. Washington, DC, American Psychiatric Association, 1987

American Psychiatric Association: Diagnostic and Statistical Manual of Mental Disorders, 4th Edition. Washington, DC, American Psychiatric Association, 1994

Anglin MD, Hser YI, McGlothlin WH: Sex differences in addict careers, Vol 2: becoming addicted. Am J Drug Alcohol Abuse 13:59–71, 1987a

Anglin MD, Hser YI, Booth MW: Sex differences in addict careers, Vol 4: treatment. Am J Drug Alcohol Abuse 13:253–280, 1987b

Babor TF, Mendelson JH, Greenberg I, et al: Marihuana consumption and tolerance to physiological and subjective effects. Arch Gen Psychiatry 32:1548–1552, 1975

Babor TF, Lex BW, Mendelson JH, et al: Marijuana, effect and tolerance: a study of subchronic self-administration in women, in Problems of Drug Dependence 1984 (NIDA Res Monogr No 49). Edited by Harris LS. Rockville, MD, National Institute on Drug Abuse, 1984, pp 199–204

Beckman LJ: Alcoholism problems and women: an overview, in Alcoholism Problems in Women and Children. Edited by Greenblatt M, Schuckit MA. New York, Grune & Stratton, 1976, pp 65–96

Beckman LJ, Amaro H: Personal and social difficulties faced by women and men entering alcoholism treatment. J Stud Alcohol 47:135–145, 1986

Beckman LJ, Kocel KM: The treatment-delivery system and alcohol abuse in women: social policy implications. Journal of Social Issues 38:139–151, 1982

Blazer DG, George KL, Landerman R, et al: Psychiatric disorders: a rural/urban comparison. Arch Gen Psychiatry 42:239–242, 1985

Blume SB: Women and alcohol: a review. JAMA 256:1467–1470, 1986

Bohman M, Sigvardsson S, Cloninger CR: Maternal inheritance of alcohol abuse cross-fostering analysis of adopted women. Arch Gen Psychiatry 38:965–969, 1981

Bureau of Justice Statistics National Update: Nearly Half of the Women in State Prisons for a Violent Crime in 1986 Were Under Sentence for a Homicide. Washington, DC, U.S. Government Printing Office, 1991

Busch D, McBride AB, Benaventura LM: Chemical dependency in women: the link to ob/gyn problems. J Psychosoc Nurs Ment Health Serv 24:26–30, 1986

Caetano R: Concepts of alcoholism among whites, blacks and Hispanics in the United States. J Stud Alcohol 50:580–582, 1989

Canestrini K: Identified Substance Abusers, New York State Department of Correctional Services, April 1991. Albany, NY, New York State Department of Correctional Services, Division of Program Planning, Research and Evaluation, 1991

Clayton RL, Voss HL, Robbins C, et al: Gender differences in drug use: an epidemiological perspective, in Women and Drugs: A New Era for Research (NIDA Res Monogr No 65). Edited by Ray BA, Braude MC. Rockville, MD, National Institute on Drug Abuse, 1986, pp 80–99

Cloninger CR, Sigvardsson S, Reich T, et al: Inheritance of risk to develop alcoholism, in Genetic and Biological Markers in Drug Abuse and Alcoholism (NIDA Res Monogr No 66). Edited by Braude MC, Chao HM. Rockville, MD, National Institute on Drug Abuse, 1986, pp 86–96

Corrigan EM, Butler S: Irish alcoholic women in treatment: early findings. Int J Addict 26:281–292, 1991

Crawford S, Ryder D: A study of sex differences in cognitive impairment in alcoholics using traditional and computer-based tests. Drug Alcohol Depend 18:369–375, 1986

De Leon G, Jainchill N: Residential therapeutic communities for female substance abusers. Bull N Y Acad Med 67:277–290, 1991

Duckert F: Recruitment into treatment and effects of treatment for female problem drinkers. Addict Behav 12:137–150, 1987

Dunne F: Are women more easily damaged by alcohol than men? Br J Addict 83:1135–1136, 1988

Edwards G: The alcohol dependence syndrome: usefulness of an idea, in Alcoholism: New Knowledge and New Responses. Edited by Bultman I. Baltimore, MD, University Park Press, 1977, pp 136–156

Edwards G, Gross MM: Alcohol dependence: provisional description of a clinical syndrome. BMJ 1:1058–1061, 1976

Emrick CD: Alcoholics anonymous: affiliation processes and effectiveness as treatment. Alcohol Clin Exp Res 11:416–423, 1987

Feighner JP, Robins E, Guze SB, et al: Diagnostic criteria for use in psychiatric research. Arch Gen Psychiatry 26:57–63, 1972

Felch LJ, Brooner RK, Bigelow GE: Gender differences in the antisocial behavior of intravenous drug abusers (abstract), in Problems of Drug Dependence 1991: Proceedings of the 53rd Annual Scientific Meeting (NIDA Res Monogr No 119). Edited by Harris LS. Rockville, MD, National Institute on Drug Abuse, 1991, p 446

Ferrence RG: Sex differences in the prevalence of problem drinking, in Research Advances and Drug Problems, Vol 5: Alcohol and Drug Problems in Women. Edited by Kalant OJ. New York, Plenum, 1980, pp 69–124

Ferrence RG, Whitehead PC: Sex differences in psychoactive drug use: recent epidemiology, in Research Advances in Alcohol and Drug Problems, Vol 5: Alcohol and Drug Problems in Women. Edited by Kalant OJ. New York, Plenum, 1980, pp 125–201

Fisher SE, Karl PI: Maternal ethanol use and selective fetal malnutrition, in Recent Developments in Alcoholism. Edited by Galanter M. New York, Plenum, 1988, pp 277–289

Frezza M, di Padova C, Pozzato G, et al: High blood alcohol levels in women: the role of decreased gastric alcohol dehydrogenase activity and first-pass metabolism. N Engl J Med 322:95–99, 1990

Gavaler JS: Effects of moderate consumption of alcoholic beverages on endocrine function in post-menopausal women: bases for hypotheses, in Recent Developments in Alcoholism. Edited by Galanter M. New York, Plenum, 1988, pp 229–251

Gerstley LJ, Alterman AI, McLellan AT, et al: Antisocial personality disorder in patients with substance abuse disorders: a problematic diagnosis? Am J Psychiatry 142:173–178, 1990

Gomberg ESL: Alcoholism in women: use of other drugs. Alcohol Clin Exp Res 13:338, 1989a

Gomberg ESL: Suicide risk among women with alcohol problems. Am J Public Health 79:1363–1365, 1989b

Griffin ML, Weiss RD, Mirin SM, et al: A comparison of male and female cocaine abusers. Arch Gen Psychiatry 46:122–126, 1989

Halliday A, Booker B, Cleary P, et al: Alcohol abuse in women seeking gynecologic care. Obstet Gynecol 68:322–326, 1986

Hamilton M: A rating scale for depression. J Neurol Neurosurg Psychiatry 23:56–62, 1960

Harrison PA: Women in treatment: changing over time. Int J Addict 24:655–673, 1989

Haver B: Female alcoholics, III: patterns of consumption 3–10 years after treatment. Acta Psychiatr Scand 75:397–404, 1987a

Haver B: Female alcoholics, IV: the relationship between family violence and outcome 3–10 years after treatment. Acta Psychiatr Scand 75:449–455, 1987b

Haver B: Female alcoholics, V: the relationship between family history of alcoholism and outcome 3–10 years after treatment. Acta Psychiatr Scand 76:21–27, 1987c

Herd D: The epidemiology of drinking patterns and alcohol-related problems among U.S. blacks, in Alcohol Use Among U.S. Ethnic Minorities (NIDA Res Monogr No 18). Edited by Spiegler D, Tate D, Aitken S, et al. Rockville, MD, National Institute on Drug Abuse, 1989, pp 3–50

Herr BM, Pettinati HM: Long term outcome in working and homemaking alcoholic women. Alcohol Clin Exp Res 8:576–579, 1984

Hesselbrock MN, Hesselbrock VM, Babor TF, et al: Antisocial behavior, psychopathology and problem drinking in the natural history of alcoholism, in Longitudinal Research in Alcoholism. Edited by Goodwin DW, Dusen KTV, Mednick SA. Boston, MA, Kluwer-Nijhoff, 1984, pp 197–214

Hesselbrock MN, Meyer RE, Keener JJ: Psychopathology in hospitalized alcoholics. Arch Gen Psychiatry 42:1050–1055, 1985

Hser YI, Anglin MD, Booth MW: Sex differences in addict careers: addiction. Am J Drug Alcohol Abuse 13:231–251, 1987a

Hser YI, Anglin MD, McGlothlin W: Sex differences in addict careers: initiation of use. Am J Drug Alcohol Abuse 13:33–57, 1987b

Huselid RF, Self EA, Gutierres SE: Predictors of successful completion of a halfway-house program for chemically dependent women. Am J Drug Alcohol Abuse 17:89–101, 1991

Kandel DB: Marijuana users in young adulthood. Arch Gen Psychiatry 41:200–209, 1984

Kandel DB, Davies M, Karus D, et al: The consequences in young adulthood of adolescent drug involvement. Arch Gen Psychiatry 43:746–754, 1986

Kantor GK, Strauss MA: Substance abuse as a precipitant of wife abuse victimizations. Am J Drug Alcohol Abuse 15:173–189, 1989

Kosten TR, Rounsaville BJ, Kleber HD: Parental alcoholism in opioid addicts. J Nerv Ment Dis 173:461–469, 1985

Kosten TR, Rounsaville BJ, Kleber HD: Ethnic and gender differences among opiate addicts. Int J Addict 20:1143–1162, 1986

Kozel NJ: Epidemiology of drug abuse in the United States: a summary of methods and findings. Bull Pan Am Health Organ 24:53–62, 1990

Kreek MJ: Multiple drug abuse patterns and medical consequences, in Psychopharmacology: The Third Generation of Progress. Edited by Meltzer HY. New York, Raven, 1987, pp 1597–1604

Lex BW: Alcohol problems in special populations, in The Diagnosis and Treatment of Alcoholism, 2nd Edition. Edited by Mendelson JH, Mello NK. New York, McGraw-Hill, 1985, pp 89–187

Lex BW: Review of alcohol problems in ethnic minority groups. J Consult Clin Psychol 55:293–300, 1987

Lex BW: Male heroin addicts and their female mates: impact on disorder and recovery. J Subst Abuse 2:147–175, 1990

Lex BW: Gender differences and substance abuse, in Advances in Substance Abuse, Vol 4. Edited by Mello NK. London, Jessica Kingsley Publishers, 1991, pp 225–296

Lex BW, Griffin ML, Mello NK, et al: Concordant alcohol and marihuana use in women. Alcohol 3:193–200, 1986

Lex BW, Palmieri SL, Mello NK, et al: Alcohol use, marijuana smoking, and sexual activity in women. Alcohol 5:21–25, 1988

Lex BW, Griffin ML, Mello NK, et al: Alcohol, marijuana, and mood states in young women. Int J Addict 24:405–424, 1989

Lex BW, Teoh SK, Lagomasino I, et al: Characteristics of women receiving mandated treatment for alcohol or polysubstance dependence in Massachusetts. Drug Alcohol Depend 25:13–20, 1990

Lex BW, Goldberg ME, Mendelson JH, et al: Components of antisocial personality disorder among women convicted for drunken driving. Ann N Y Acad Sci 708:49–58, 1994

Lisansky ES: Alcoholism in women: social and psychological concomitants. Quarterly Journal of Studies on Alcohol 18:588–623, 1957

Maden A, Swinton M, Gunn J: Women in prison and use of illicit drugs before arrest. BMJ 301:1133, 1990

Maher L, Curtis R: Women on the edge of crime: crack cocaine and the changing contexts of street level sex work in New York City. Crime, Law and Social Change 18:221–258, 1992

McLellan AT, Luborsky L, Woody GE, et al: An improved diagnostic evaluation instrument for substance abuse patients: the Addiction Severity Index. J Nerv Ment Dis 168:26–33, 1980

Mello NK: Some behavioral and biological aspects of alcohol problems in women, in Alcohol and Drug Problems in Women. Edited by Kalant OJ. New York, Plenum, 1980, pp 263–312

Mello NK: Effects of alcohol abuse on reproductive function in women, in Recent Developments in Alcoholism. Edited by Galanter M. New York, Plenum, 1988, pp 253–276

Mello NK, Mendelson JH, Teoh SK: Neuroendocrine consequences of alcohol abuse in women. Ann N Y Acad Sci 562:211–240, 1989

Mercer PW, Khavari KA: Are women drinking more like men? An empirical examination of the convergence hypothesis. Alcohol Clin Exp Res 14:461–466, 1990

Miller CE: Women in a drug treatment therapeutic community, in Preventions and Treatments of Alcohol and Drug Abuse: A Socio-Epidemiological Sourcebook. Edited by Forster B, Salloway JC. Lewiston, NY, Edwin Mellen Press, 1991, pp 361–392

Mirin S, Shapiro L, Meyer R, et al: Casual versus heavy use of marijuana: a redefinition of the marijuana problem. Am J Psychiatry 127:1134–1140, 1971

Mondanaro J: Chemically Dependent Women: Assessment and Treatment. Lexington, MA, D.C. Heath and Company, 1989

National Institute on Drug Abuse: Annual emergency room data 1991 (Series 1, No 11-A, DHHS Publ No ADM-92-1955). Washington, DC, U.S. Government Printing Office, 1992a

National Institute on Drug Abuse: Annual medical examiner data 1991 (Series 1, No 11-B, DHHS Publ No ADM-92-1955). Washington, DC, U.S. Government Printing Office, 1992b

National Institute on Drug Abuse: National household survey on drug abuse: population estimates 1992 (DHHS Publ No SMA-93-2053). Washington, DC, U.S. Government Printing Office, 1993

Norton R, Batey R, Dwyer T, et al: Alcohol consumption and the risk of alcohol related cirrhosis in women. BMJ 295:80–82, 1987

Orford J, Keddie A: Gender differences in the functions and effects of moderate and excessive drinking. Br J Clin Psychol 24:265–279, 1985

Phibbs CS, Bateman DA, Schwartz RM: The neonatal costs of maternal cocaine use. JAMA 266:1521–1526, 1991

Rice DP, Kelman SK, Miller LS, et al: The economic costs of alcohol and drug abuse and mental illness 1985 (DHHS Publ No ADM-90-1694). Washington, DC, U.S. Government Printing Office, 1990

Robbins C: Sex differences in psychosocial consequences of alcohol and drug abuse. J Health Soc Behav 30:117–130, 1989

Robins LN, Price RK: Adult disorders predicted by childhood conduct problems: results from the NIMH epidemiologic catchment area project. Psychiatry 54:116–132, 1991

Robins LN, Helzer JE, Croughan J, et al: National Institute of Mental Health Diagnostic Interview Schedule. Arch Gen Psychiatry 38:381–389, 1981

Robins LN, Helzer JE, Weissman MM, et al: Lifetime prevalence of specific psychiatric disorders in three sites. Arch Gen Psychiatry 41:949–958, 1984

Robinson SD: Women and alcohol abuse-factors involved in successful interventions. Int J Addict 19:601–611, 1984

Ross HE, Glaser FB, Stiasny S: Sex differences in the prevalence of psychiatric disorders in patients with alcohol and drug problems. Br J Addict 83:1179–1192, 1988

Rounsaville BJ, Kranzler HR: The DSM-III-R diagnosis of alcoholism, in American Psychiatric Press Review of Psychiatry, Vol 8. Edited by Tasman A, Hales RE, Frances AJ. Washington, DC, American Psychiatric Press, 1989, pp 323–340

Rounsaville BJ, Spitzer RL, Williams JBW: Proposed changes in DSM-III substance use disorders: description and rationale. Am J Psychiatry 143:463–468, 1986

Schmidt LA: Problem drinkers and the welfare bureaucracy. Social Services Research 37:390–406, 1990

Schuckit MA: Subjective responses to alcohol in sons of alcoholics and control subjects. Arch Gen Psychiatry 42:879–884, 1984

Selzer ML: The Michigan Alcoholism Screening Test: the quest for a new diagnostic instrument. Am J Psychiatry 127:1653–1658, 1971

Smith EM, Cloninger CR, Bradford S: Predictors of mortality in alcoholic women: a prospective follow-up study. Alcohol Clin Exp Res 7:237–243, 1983

Spitzer RL, Endicott J, Robins E: Research Diagnostic Criteria: rationale and reliability. Arch Gen Psychiatry 35:773–782, 1978

Spitzer RL, Williams JBW, Gibbon M, et al: The Structured Clinical Interview for DSM-III-R (SCID), I: history, rationale, and description. Arch Gen Psychiatry 49:624–629, 1992

Stinson FS, DeBakey SF: Alcohol-related mortality in the United States, 1979-1988. Br J Addict 87:777–783, 1992

Substance Abuse and Mental Health Services Administration: National drug and alcoholism treatment unit survey (NDATUS): 1991 main findings report (DHHS Publ No SMA-93-2007). Washington, DC, U.S. Government Printing Office, 1993

Sullivan PS, Wolk JL, Hartmann DJ: Case management in alcohol and drug treatment: improving client outcomes. Families in Society: Journal of Contemporary Human Services 73:195–203, 1992

Tamerin JS, Tolor A, Harrington B: Sex differences in alcoholics: a comparison of male and female alcoholics, self and spouse perceptions. Am J Drug Alcohol Abuse 3:457–472, 1976

Thom B: Sex differences in help-seeking for alcohol problems, I: the barriers to help-seeking. Br J Addict 81:777–786, 1986

Thom B: Sex differences in help-seeking for alcohol problems, II: entry into treatment. Br J Addict 82:989–997, 1987

Turnbull JE: Primary and secondary alcoholic women. Social Casework 69:290–297, 1988

Underhill BL: Issues relevant to aftercare programs for women. Alcohol Health and Research World 11:46–47, 1986

Vannicelli M: Barriers to treatment of alcoholic women. Substance and Alcohol Actions/Misuses 5:29–37, 1984

Vannicelli M, Nash L: Effect of sex bias on women's studies on alcoholism. Alcohol Clin Exp Res 8:334–336, 1984

Van Thiel DH, Gavaler JS: Ethanol metabolism and hepatotoxicity: does sex make a difference?, in Recent Developments in Alcoholism. Edited by Galanter M. New York, Plenum, 1988, pp 291–304

Wallace B: Chemical dependency treatment for the pregnant crack addict: beyond the criminal-sanctions perspective. Psychology of Addictive Behaviors 5:23–35, 1991

Weiner HD, Wallen MC, Zankowski GL: Culture and social class as intervening variables in relapse prevention with chemically dependent women. J Psychoactive Drugs 22:239–248, 1990

Westermeyer J: Methodological issues in the epidemiological study of alcohol-drug problems: sources of confusion and misunderstanding. Am J Drug Alcohol Abuse 16:47–55, 1990

Whitehead PC, Layne N: Young female Canadian drinkers: employment, marital status and heavy drinking. Br J Addict 82:169–174, 1987

Wilsnack SC: Barriers to treatment for alcoholic women. Addiction Recovery 11:10–12, 1991

Wilsnack SC, Wilsnack RW: Epidemiology of women's drinking. J Subst Abuse 3:133–157, 1991

Wilsnack SC, Wilsnack RW, Klassen AD: Drinking and drinking problems among women in a U.S. national survey. Alcohol Health and Research World 9:3–13, 1984

Wilsnack SC, Wilsnack RW, Klassen AD: Epidemiological research on women's drinking, 1978-1984, in Women and Alcohol: Health-Related Issues. Washington, DC, U.S. Government Printing Office, 1986, pp 1–68

Wilsnack SC, Klassen AD, Schur BE, et al: Predicting onset and chronicity of women's problem drinking: a five-year longitudinal analysis. Am J Public Health 81:305–318, 1991

World Health Organization: International Classification of Diseases, 9th Revision. Geneva, World Health Organization, 1989

World Health Organization: The ICD-10 Classification of Mental and Behavioural Disorders. Geneva, World Health Organization, 1992

Zetterman RK: Cirrhosis of the liver, in Diseases of the Liver and Biliary Tract. Edited by Gitnick G, LaBrecque DR, Moody FG. St. Louis, MO, Mosby–Year Book, 1992, pp 447–466

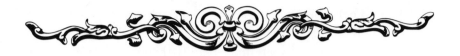

CHAPTER 15

Health Care Provision for Men and Women

Edith S. Lisansky Gomberg, Ph.D.

W omen report more medical use of psychoactive drugs than men do (Robbins and Clayton 1989). In order to understand the use and abuse of psychoactive drugs, in this review, I survey gender differences in health behaviors, psychiatric diagnoses, and patterns of use of benzodiazepines and other sedatives. I describe several explanatory hypotheses about the observed gender differences. Finally, I briefly review relevant information about special populations—that is, alcoholic women, older people, and minorities.

Gender Differences in Response to Illness

Data from the National Ambulatory Medical Care Survey (Verbrugge 1980) support the idea that men delay seeking medical diagnosis longer than women and are more reticent to admit they have symptoms during a physician visit. Little evidence suggests that men and women vary in the perception, interpretation, or description of their symptoms. Likewise, little evidence indicates sex differences in the accuracy of symptom description. Sex differences seem to exist in health-related *behaviors* more than in subjective awareness of symptoms.

Self-report surveys designed to examine gender issues in response to illness have all found sex differences (Kessler 1986). Men and women with serious health problems have similar rates of seeking professional help, but women with less serious health problems are more likely than men to seek help. Several studies have shown that women seek psychiatric help more readily than men at comparable levels of self-reported distress (Kessler et al. 1981).

Utilization of Medical Resources

The number and percentage of office visits to physicians by sex and by age can be calculated from Vital and Health Statistics of the National Center for Health Statistics (DeLozier and Gagnon 1991). Women make more office visits than men (60% versus 40%, respectively). It is interesting to note differences occurring during the life span. When males and females younger than age 15 years are compared, boys have a slightly higher number of physician visits than girls (per capita averages are 2.6 and 2.5 visits per year, respectively). After this age, women utilize the resources of physician visits more than men do; the difference peaks in the age group of 25–44, presumably because these are the childbearing years. During these years, women average 3.2 visits per year versus 1.6 visits for men. For the oldest group—75 years and older—the average number of physician visits is near parity: 5.9 for women and 5.8 for men.

When hospitalization and outpatient treatment are compared for both women and men, women up to their late 40s are hospitalized slightly more often than men, even when obstetric hospitalizations are omitted. After age 50, men have much higher hospitalization rates and at all ages (except 65 and older), and men have longer hospital stays than women. This is linked to the more serious nature of medical conditions in men age 50 years and older (Verbrugge 1982).

Physicians' Responses to Women and Men

Does a symptom receive the same response from a physician regardless of the sex of the patient? The evidence is contradictory and confusing. Armitage and colleagues (1979) compared male physicians' responses to five medical complaints presented by male and female patients in their 40s: back pain, headache, dizziness, chest pain, and fatigue. Although the number of physician visits was equal, men received more extensive work-ups than women in all five of the complaints. The investigators suggest that physicians were responding to current stereotypes in which the male is typically stoic and the female is typically hypochondriacal. (Of course, it is not clear whether the extensive work-up results in better medical care.) In another study (McCranie et al. 1978), 117 physicians completed an evaluation in a case booklet. The questions included tentative diagnosis, further diagnostic procedures, treatments, and medications. Male and female patients with identical symptoms were described in the case booklet. The male general practitioners who were the respondents were *not* more inclined to diagnose the females' symptoms as psychological or to prescribe more psychotropic medication for the female patients. Furthermore, both Mitchell et al. (1986) and Rowland et al. (1987) reported no effect of patient gender on physicians' attention to problem drinking among medical patients. However, these latter studies highlight the problem of inadequate attention to alcohol abuse in both sexes rather than demonstrating gender differences.

One viewpoint is that many competent and responsible physicians overlook organic disease in women and consider their symptoms to be due to stress, " ... that time of life," or to psychosexual problems. The author speculates that, perhaps for reasons of his own, the male physician needs to perceive the woman patient as " ... weak, vulnerable and emotional" (Brozovic 1989, p. 689).

The evidence for this viewpoint is ambiguous. However, some data do suggest that physicians are more perfunctory with female patients. Evidence supports a gender difference in the amount of time and attention devoted to women's problems both in medical treatment and medical research. A study of procedures prescribed for patients hospitalized with coronary heart disease (Ayanian and Epstein 1991) reports that women undergo fewer diagnostic and therapeutic procedures than male patients.

Incidence and Prevalence of Mental Disorder in Men and Women

The National Institute of Mental Health's multisite Epidemiologic Catchment Area (ECA) study has recently summarized its findings, including prevalence of psychiatric disorder among men and women in the general population (Robins and Regier 1991). The ECA study reversed the findings of earlier studies and established that *more men than women have had a psychiatric disorder during their lifetimes*—36% versus 30%. No gender difference was found in the percentage with active disorder in the past year (20% for both sexes). The discrepancy with earlier studies (e.g., during the 1960s) can be explained by the inclusion, in the early studies, of illnesses then considered to be psychosomatic and their relative omission of substance abuse and antisocial personality diagnoses (Leighton et al. 1963; Srole et al. 1962).

Men manifest certain types of disorders more than women do, and women manifest other types of disorders in greater proportion. Men had higher rates of alcohol abuse and antisocial personality; women had substantially higher lifetime rates of somatization disorder, obsessive-compulsive disorder, and major depressive episode. It would appear that the findings of Dohrenwend and Dohrenwend (1976) are accurate: generally, women have higher rates of neuroses and depression, and men have higher rates of antisocial personality disorder and alcohol abuse. If gender distribution of mental disorder is related to prescription of psychoactive drugs, note that, at present, alcohol abuse and antisocial personality disorder are not as likely to elicit psychoactive medication prescription as are the neuroses and depression (Shader and Greenblatt 1993).

Rate of Prescriptions in Women and Men

Women receive prescriptions more often than men (Verbrugge and Steiner 1985). Vital and Health Statistics of the National Center for Health Statistics (DeLozier and Gagnon 1991) do not contain a breakdown of "drug visits and drug mention" in terms of gender, but it is relevant that almost 70% of such drug visits embrace four medical specialties: family practice, internal medicine, pediatrics, and obstetrics/gynecology.

Verbrugge and Steiner (1985) examined how often physicians prescribe therapeutic drugs to men and women with the same medical complaint or who receive the same diagnosis. For most common complaints and diagnoses, women receive prescriptions more often than men; the differences were moderate (women's medical contacts were 1%–18% more likely to result in prescriptions), but the differences were consistent across a wide variety of health problems. When medically relevant factors such as patient status, seriousness of the diagnosis, presence of injury, prior visit status, and acute versus chronic medical problems are controlled, the sex difference persists. Sex differences in prescriptions are statistically significant for the following conditions: weight gain, skin wounds, upper and lower extremity pain, and fatigue symptoms and for the following diagnoses: cystitis, obesity, hypertension, and neuroses. The authors concluded that "psychosocial factors" probably explain the sex difference in prescriptions. These factors include patient behavior, such as requests for medication, and physician behavior, such as "sex-biased prescribing."

Although the following comment is more than two decades old, it still appears to be valid (Sims 1974, p. 156): " . . . A fairly liberal use of medically prescribed drugs is not generally considered deviant behavior for women."

On a historical note, it is relevant that the typical opiate user in the 1880s in the United States was a 30- to 50-year-old white woman who functioned reasonably well (Ray and Ksir 1990). She could have ordered her medication through the mail from Sears Roebuck; two ounces of laudanum cost 18 cents.

In addition to receiving more prescriptions, women may be more likely than men to take their prescribed drugs and, perhaps, to have more adverse drug reactions even when number of drugs prescribed and their dosages are controlled (Hamilton and Parry 1983).

Gender Differences in Prescription Rate and Utilization Rate

Women are prescribed psychoactive drugs more often than men, and women use psychoactive drugs more frequently than men. Data collected by different investigators during the last decades have clearly indicated that women are more likely to use tranquilizers, sedatives, and other psychoactive drugs (Mellinger and Balter 1983; Parry et al. 1973). Not only does the disproportionate use of psychoactive drugs by women appear repeatedly in epidemiological studies in the United States, but the same gender ratio appears in studies from many different countries: Canada (Cooperstock 1978), the United Kingdom (Taylor 1987), Denmark (Hansen 1989), and France (Pariente et al. 1992). Previous cross-national studies have shown the same patterns of male and female differences in prescribed psychoactive drug use (Balter et al. 1974).

Analysis of gender differences in psychoactive drug use, as reported in a 1982 National Household Survey on Drug Abuse (NHSDA) (Robbins and Clayton 1989), shows some interesting patterns of gender and age differences. Women generally reported more frequent use of prescribed psychoactive drugs within the past year than did men, and female use peaked in the 45- to 64-year age group. However, it is significant that in the 65 and older age group, Robbins and Clayton (1989) reported that men were more likely than women to report use in the past year of sedatives, tranquilizers, and stimulants. Note that these reports focus on *prescribed* drug use. Men reported more frequent use of sedatives, tranquilizers, stimulants, and analgesics obtained in ways other than by prescription.

The gender ratio among older people and their use of prescribed psychoactive drugs is unclear. Glantz and Backenheimer (1988) asserted that the data show "considerably" greater drug use among elderly women than among elderly men, and one study (Cafferata et al. 1983) suggested a 2:1 female-to-male ratio. However, a report on psychoactive drug use, stress, and coping in an older adult sample (Huffine et al. 1989) indicated that when income, marital status, and education are controlled, gender differences in psychoactive drug use (and in alcohol use) disappear. Contradictory findings about psychoactive drug use in the elderly therefore include more male use than female use (Robbins and Clayton 1989), more female use (Glantz and Backenheimer 1988), or no gender difference (Huffine et al. 1989).

However, several sources of information suggest that psychoactive drug use is more problematic for elderly women than for elderly men. It is true that elderly men are more likely to seek the services of a physician than they did at earlier ages and are more likely to receive a psychoactive drug prescription. However, older women are more likely than older men to be long-term users (Mellinger et al. 1984). Data from the Drug Abuse Warning Network (DAWN Annual

Data 1989) include tables of different drugs involved in emergency room visits. Elderly persons, age 60 and older, are most likely to have difficulty with nonbarbiturate sedatives, tranquilizers, barbiturate sedatives, and antidepressants. For all of these drug emergencies, a higher percentage of women appear in emergency rooms than men. For tranquilizers in general, the total DAWN system percentages are 37.9% for men and 61.1% for women; for antidepressant-related emergencies, the DAWN percentages are 35.1% for men and 64.1% for women (note that these percentages represent all age groups).

Lest we think of all psychotropic drug use as being a "problem," there is a caveat. The use of anxiolytic drugs and sedatives is *not* per se problematic, and such drugs may be beneficial in relieving discomfort. For instance, sensible use of medications " . . . to relieve disabling symptoms" often facilitates "productive psychotherapy" (Mogul 1985, p. 1080).

Kleber (1990) noted that patients often ask physicians who prescribe benzodiazepines whether the drugs are "addicting" or have potential for abuse. The answer is complex, and a half-century of World Health Organization (WHO) committees seeking to clarify definitions of dependence, tolerance, habituation, and so forth have not lessened the confusion. One WHO Expert Committee recommended that the term *abuse* be abolished and be replaced by unsanctioned use, hazardous use, dysfunctional use, and harmful use (Kleber 1990). To compound the confusion, it is difficult to distinguish between physical and psychological dependence. Kleber's (1990) classification of benzodiazepine dependency could be useful: therapeutic dosage dependency, primary high-dose dependency, and secondary dependency (i.e., in the context of multiple drug use). It is admittedly an assumption, but most people, young or old, male or female, probably use the drugs at "usual therapeutic doses." The use of sedatives and tranquilizers, usually with alcohol, for "a high," or regular use at high doses, constitutes the problem behaviors and characterizes those who appear in emergency rooms and/or other clinical facilities (Cole and Chiarello 1990; Woods et al. 1988, 1992).

The use of psychotropic drugs by women has become a political issue in which male physicians treating female patients are seen as manifesting " . . . a double standard of health care," based on sex bias in diagnosis (Nellis 1980, p. 92). An image of a neurotic, dependent female patient and an uncaring male physician often colors such description. It must be noted again that, in general, women utilize medical services more than men, and they receive more prescriptions of all types than male patients. Even when considering that women have more contact with medical care, women still receive a disproportionate share of tranquilizer prescriptions. We must assume that physicians see female patients as more anxious, more neurotic, and more emotional than male patients and thus prescribe more psychotropic drugs for women.

The consequences of the gender difference in prescription of sedatives and tranquilizers are not trivial. These drugs have a high abuse potential, and the patient is at some risk of becoming dependent on the substance. Most of the psychoactive drugs prescribed are potentiated by alcohol, and the use of tricyclic antidepressants plus alcohol for suicide attempts occurs frequently. Some of the best known and most widely used drugs have negative side effects in some patients. The undoubted benefits of the controlled use of sedatives and tranquilizers must be balanced against the risks of drug abuse, misuse, and dependence.

Further research must examine the different patterns and effects of psychoactive drug use at different points in the life span of women. The disproportionate number of women who use psychoactive drugs exists in most populations, including college-age women (Golding and Cornish 1987; McLaney and Del Boca 1991), young and middle-aged adults in general population surveys (e.g., Mellinger and Balter 1983), and older women (Glantz and Backenheimer 1988). Most women comply with controlled use of prescription drugs. Problems exist among two groups: 1) those who abuse medication and whose primary drugs of abuse are the psychoactive drugs themselves, and 2) those who abuse other drugs (e.g., alcohol or cocaine) and who use psychoactive drugs in addition to their primary drug of abuse.

Women Who Abuse Psychotropic Drugs

Pihl and colleagues (1986) compared a nonclinical sample of women in Montreal who used psychotropic drugs alone, alcohol alone, both psychotropic drugs and alcohol, and neither alcohol nor psycho-tropic drugs. The average age of the women who used psychotropic drugs was 47.4, somewhat older than the other groups. Pihl and col-leagues concur with the most commonly reported finding that women who use psychotropic drugs have a relatively larger number of physical and psychological problems. The authors concluded that women who use alcohol and those who use psychotropic drugs rep-resent different populations, with "psychotrope users . . . subjectively more anxious, tense, depressed, ill, and under greater stress than al-cohol users" (p. 998).

In addition, and not surprising, women who use psychotropic drugs are more likely to seek professional help for emotional difficulties.

Many attempts have been made to account for differences be-tween psychoactive drug prescription and use in men and women. Explanations include health issues, sex bias in prescribing, subjective stress, and coping.

Health issues. The use of anxiolytic drugs is associated with com-plaints of poor physical and psychological health (Ashton 1991). Women experience unique problems involving pregnancy, lactation, premenstrual states, and menopause—these may be "natural" events but are often accompanied by problems. Although the pathways to psychoactive drug use are not altogether clear, Cafferata and Meyers (1990) demonstrated that data from the U.S. National Medical Care Expenditure Survey show that gender differences were accounted for by the greater likelihood of women to seek help for medical illness. Several studies by a Quebec research group reported that vague and ill-defined health problems seen by the prescribing physician may be economical, social, or psychological rather than medical (Marinier et al. 1982). In Massachusetts, Hemminki and co-workers (1989) stud-ied a large sample of women between ages 45 and 55 and found that the same women used several different types of drugs. The major distinction between users and nonusers was that the users were in poorer health.

Psychiatric disorder. Although the results of the ECA study (Rob-ins and Regier 1991) indicated a higher lifetime prevalence rate of psychiatric disorders in men than in women, they are based on the high male-to-female ratio of alcohol abuse and sociopathic personality disorder. Women have considerably higher lifetime rates than men for depression, anxiety, and other nonpsychotic disorders. Anxiolytics and antidepressants are widely used to treat those disorders in which women prevail. Investigators generally believe that women are more likely than men to express psychological complaints to their doctors and that more women have diagnosable psychiatric disorders (Ashton 1991).

Women's gender role.   This is a vague concept that usually refers to women's role as nurturer, wife, mother, and general caretaker in the family. Ogur (1986) reviewed the standard explanatory models of addiction—for example, behavioral theories and biochemical theories—and offered an adaptive model of addiction that explains female prescription drug addiction as an attempt to cope with sex-role stereotyping and women's low status in society. Marcus and Seeman (1981) offer a more specific definition of sex role. Gender differences in morbidity (i.e., higher rates among women) are hypothesized to be related to fixed role obligations, and data from a Los Angeles Health Survey were utilized to test the hypothesis. When investigators controlled for role obligations, particularly employment status, sex differences in reporting disability days were attenuated, but self-reports of chronic conditions continued to show significant differences between men and women, independent of these roles.

Related to the idea of gender roles is an explanation in terms of fewer outlets (Ashton 1991). Women have fewer opportunities than men do for controlling symptoms by activities outside the home. Cooperstock and Lennard (1979) believe that women use more psychoactive drugs because societal norms permit them to express feelings such as anxiety, to perceive emotional problems in themselves, and to use medical care for emotional problems. Ashton (1991) adds to this that men are permitted to seek outlets (e.g., the use of alcohol) to cope with stress.

Stress and coping skills.   Interview studies of women in Quebec (Marinier et al. 1985) showed those who use psychotropic drugs to be older, in poorer health, and less educated than abstainers. Women also showed a higher prevalence of nervousness, anxiety, depression, and restlessness. It is significant that psychoactive drug use was associated with anxiety, depression, and nervous tension, whereas alcohol use was not (Pihl et al. 1986). Psychoactive drug users are described as being under greater stress than alcohol users, and Pihl and colleagues (1986) speculate that a "lack of skill at coping" results in a greater degree of subjective stress. The drug users had more deficits in problem-solving skills than the abstainers and were more likely to seek professional help for emotional disturbance than the abstainers.

Gender bias in medical diagnosis. Ogur (1986) rejects most theoretical explanations of female prescription drug abuse and posits an adaptive model that includes the theme of sex-role stereotyping, low status in the society, and the power dynamic of the male physician–female patient interaction. Ashton (1991) states more moderately that there may be a gender bias in medical diagnosis and choice of medication. Brozovic (1989) believes that the medical profession is guilty of a special kind of discrimination against women patients, based on a view of women as weak and emotionally unstable. The evidence that men and women with the same symptom or illness receive different responses from physicians was reviewed earlier in this chapter, and the conclusion remains that the evidence is equivocal and ambiguous. Cafferata and Meyers (1990) clearly believe that gender differences in prescriptions for psychoactive drugs are not a result of physician-patient interaction or of gender-determined treatment norms by physicians.

An integrated explanatory model. Perhaps all the models described contribute to the gender disparities in prescription and use of psychoactive medications. Women utilize health care resources more than men do, and women make more complaints about health status. Gender differences in morbidity do exist. Women more often seek help for psychiatric disorders that are likely to receive pharmacological intervention. These differences do not exclude the idea of sex stereotyping and gender bias in physician diagnosis and prescription. It may be as important to examine female sex role, male versus female stressors, and outlets for symptom control as to examine morbidity tables and health care utilization statistics. Historically, evidence reveals that women in the nineteenth century were the major users of "tonics" (often laced with alcohol, cocaine, etc.). A case can be made that gender and the use of drugs for medicinal/therapeutic purposes are inextricably linked (Gomberg 1982; Smith 1991). Female sex role assigns women as the primary nurturer within the family; we may hypothesize that a prescription or medication is a form of socially sanctioned nurturance for women. That hypothesis would be difficult to test although some epidemiologists claim that psychosocial factors such as these will help explain gender differences in prescriptions (Verbrugge and Steiner 1985). Many authors have noted the importance of patient-caretaker interaction (Brozovic 1989; Cafferata and Meyers 1990; Ogur 1986; Verbrugge and Steiner 1985). Some gerontologists have noted that older persons often have a special attachment to their medication.

Subgroups of Women

Minority Women

Few data exist for minority women's use of psychotropic drugs, but Robbins and Clayton (1989) have analyzed gender-related differences in psychoactive drug use by black, white, and Hispanic men and women, based on data from the NHSDA conducted in 1982. Regardless of ethnic group or race, men reported more nonmedical use of sedatives, tranquilizers, stimulants, and analgesics than did women, but when the sexes were compared for medical (i.e., prescribed) use, black, white, and Hispanic women all reported more use during the preceding year. The sole exception was use of sedatives in Hispanic women, which peaked for women ages 35–44 and for men older than age 65. It is interesting that use of sedatives peaked for black women between ages 45 and 64 but for white women at ages 65 and older. For tranquilizer use within the last year, black, white, and Hispanic women all reported peaks in the 45- to 64-year age group. Analgesic use peaked for both black and Hispanic women in the 45- to 64-year age group but for white women between ages 18 and 25 (Robbins and Clayton 1989).

A recent national study of drug abuse again shows greater use of sedatives among Hispanic and black women than men, greater use of tranquilizers among white women, and greater use of analgesics among white and black women (National Institute on Drug Abuse 1993).

Older Women

Older persons have higher rates of use of sedatives and tranquilizers than younger persons (Gomberg 1992; Levenson 1981). National surveys that include the 95% of elderly people living in the community showed elevated use of psychoactive medications. Robbins and Clayton (1989) studied the medical use of psychoactive drugs in patients ages 65 and older and reported increased use in men versus women, at least for sedatives, tranquilizers, and stimulants. Older women reported greater use of analgesics. There is no ready explanation for this shift among older persons, although several hypotheses have been offered (e.g., that older men are more likely to use medical care facilities than younger men). It may also be that depression and anxiety appear more frequently among older men than older women, who, it is theorized, adapt better to aging. Older women reported greater use of analgesics (Robbins and Clayton 1989) and greater use of multiple analgesics (Chrischilles et al. 1990). Whereas male multiple analgesic use is linked to the experience of pain, female use appears to be linked to pain, a history of ulcers, limited physical functioning, and more depression symptoms.

It is of interest that older women are viewed as being at risk for self-perpetrated abuse of psychoactive drugs (Glantz and Backenheimer 1988). These investigators believe that elderly women are at greater risk for iatrogenic drug abuse involving psychoactive drugs than any other age-by-gender group. A study of the prevalence and correlates of long-term regular use of anxiolytics (Mellinger et al. 1984) reports regular users to be older persons, predominantly women, with high levels of emotional distress and chronic somatic health problems. In a recent study (Gomberg 1993a), I compared use of drugs such as sedatives and tranquilizers between older alcoholic women and men and found that the women reported more drug dependence, more tolerance, and more withdrawal effects. When the reported widespread use of anxiolytics and other psychoactive drugs in nursing homes, which have primarily female residents, is incorporated into these data, the discrepancy looms even larger (Cooper 1988).

Women Who Abuse Substances

As Chan (1991) has noted, the prevailing trend is for substance abusers to have a primary drug of preference but also to use a variety of other drugs. Among substance abusers, like the general population, it is the young people who tend to use banned substances, "street drugs," and legal drugs obtained nonmedically. Among the middle-aged and elderly population, both substance abusers and nonsubstance abusers are likely to misuse, abuse, and develop dependency on legal psychoactive substances (Gomberg 1993a).

The fact that alcoholic women more frequently use prescribed psychoactive drugs than alcoholic men has been noted by many researchers, most recently by Ross (1989) and Ross et al. (1988). A study of alcoholic women, compared with nonalcoholic women, matched for age and social class, showed significantly more psychoactive (and other) drug use among the alcoholic women for both lifetime and past year use (Gomberg 1990, 1993b). When alcoholic women from this sample were compared by age group, those in their 20s had a significantly higher proportion of stimulant and sedative use. They were more likely to have obtained psychoactive drugs through nonmedical channels, and they were significantly more likely to combine sedatives, stimulants, tranquilizers, and analgesics with alcohol than alcoholic women in their 30s and 40s (Gomberg 1990). The younger the alcoholic woman, the more likely she was to be a multiple drug abuser, although all age groups of women—20s, 30s, and 40s—displayed little difference in their use of tranquilizers.

The Drug Problem

When the media and the public show concern about "the drug problem," it is usually for banned substances and their illegal sale and use.

Men use street drugs more frequently than do women. This is also true for alcohol and its abuse (see Chapter 14). The reverse is true for prescribed psychotropic drugs; women constitute the majority of users. Although such use may not normally be considered to constitute a psychiatric addiction for which explanations must be adduced and interventions formulated, it is clear that the understanding of gender differences will contribute to the comprehension of this widespread and potentially serious phenomenon. Changes in patterns of health care provision can prevent and remediate the problem.

References

Armitage KJ, Schneiderman IJ, Bass RA: Response of physicians to medical complaints in men and women. JAMA 241:2186–2187, 1979

Ashton H: Psychotropic-drug prescribing for women. Br J Psychiatry 158 (suppl 10):30–35, 1991

Ayanian JZ, Epstein AM: Differences in the use of procedures between men and women hospitalized for coronary heart disease. N Engl J Med 325:221–225, 1991

Balter MB, Levine J, Manheimer DI: Cross-national study of the extent of antianxiety/sedative drug use. N Engl J Med 290:769–774, 1974

Brozovic M: With women in mind. BMJ 299:689, 1989

Cafferata GL, Meyers SM: Pathways to psychotropic drugs: understanding the basis of gender differences. Med Care 28:285–300, 1990

Cafferata GL, Kasper J, Bernstein A: Family roles, structure, and stressors in relation to sex differences in obtaining psychotropic drugs. J Health Soc Behav 24:132–143, 1983

Chan AWK: Multiple drug use in drug and alcohol addiction, in Comprehensive Handbook of Drug and Alcohol Addiction. Edited by Miller NS. New York, Marcel Dekker, 1991, pp 87–113

Chrischilles EA, Lemke JH, Wallace RB, et al: Prevalence and characteristics of multiple analgesic drug use in an elderly study group. J Am Geriatr Soc 38:979–984, 1990

Cole JO, Chiarello RJ: The benzodiazepines as drugs of abuse. J Psychiatr Res 24:135–144, 1990

Cooper JW: Medication misuse in nursing homes. Generations 12:56–57, 1988

Cooperstock R: Sex differences in psychotropic drug use. Soc Sci Med 12B:179–186, 1978

Cooperstock R, Lennard HL: Some social meanings of tranquilliser use. Sociology Health Illness 1:331–347, 1979

DeLozier JE, Gagnon RO: Summary: National Ambulatory Medical Care Survey: Advance Data From Vital and Health Statistics, No 203. Hyattsville, MD, National Center for Health Statistics, 1991

Dohrenwend BP, Dohrenwend BS: Sex differences and psychiatric disorders. American Sociological Review 81:1447–1454, 1976

Drug Abuse Warning Network Annual Data. Rockville, MD, National Institute on Drug Abuse, 1989

Glantz MD, Backenheimer MS: Substance abuse among elderly women. Clinical Gerontologist 8:3–25, 1988

Golding JF, Cornish AM: Personality and life-style in medical students: psychopharmacological aspects. Psychology and Health 1:287–301, 1987

Gomberg ESL: Historical and political perspective: women and drug use. Journal of Social Issues 38:9–24, 1982

Gomberg ESL: Drugs, alcohol and aging, in Research Advances in Alcohol and Drug Problems, Vol 10. Edited by Kozlowski LT, Annis HM, Cappell HD, et al. New York, Plenum, 1990, pp 171–213

Gomberg ESL: Medication problems and drug abuse, in Mental Health and the Elderly. Edited by Turner FJ. New York, Free Press, 1992, pp 355–374

Gomberg ESL: Gender issues, in Recent Developments in Alcoholism, Vol 11: Ten Years of Progress. Edited by Galanter M. New York, Plenum, 1993a, pp 95–107

Gomberg ESL: Women and alcohol: use and abuse. J Nerv Ment Dis 181:211–219, 1993b

Hamilton JA, Parry B: Sex-related differences in clinical drug response: implications for women's health. J Am Med Wom Assoc 18:126–132, 1983

Hansen EH: Sex differences in the use of psychotropic drugs: an annotated review of Danish studies, in Women, Alcohol and Drugs in the Nordic Countries (NAD Publ No 16). Edited by Haavio-Mannila E. Helsinki, Nordic Council for Alcohol and Drug Research, 1989, pp 97–132

Hemminki E, Ferdock MJ, Rahkonen O, et al: Clustering and consistency of use of medicines among middle-aged women. Med Care 27:859–868, 1989

Huffine CL, Folkman S, Lazarus RS: Psychoactive drugs, alcohol, and stress and coping processes in older adults. Am J Drug Alcohol Abuse 15:101–113, 1989

Kessler RC: Sex differences in the use of health services, in Illness Behavior: Multidisciplinary Perspectives. Edited by McHugh S. New York, Plenum, 1986, pp 135–148

Kessler RC, Brown RL, Broman CL: Sex differences in psychiatric help seeking: evidence from four large-scale surveys. J Health Soc Behav 22:49–64, 1981

Kleber HD: The nosology of abuse and dependence. J Psychiatr Res 24 (suppl 2):57–64, 1990

Leighton DC, Harding JS, Macklin DB, et al: The Character of Danger: Psychiatric Symptoms in Selected Communities. New York, Basic Books, 1963

Levenson AJ: Psychotropic drug use in the elderly: an overview (editorial). Am Fam Physician 24:194, 1981

Marcus AC, Seeman TE: Sex differences in reports of illness and disability: a preliminary test of the "fixed role obligations" hypothesis. J Health Soc Behav 22:174–182, 1981

Marinier R, Pihl RO, Wilford C, et al: Psychotropic drug usage in Quebec urban women: pharmacological aspects. Drug Intelligence and Clinical Pharmacy 16:556–562, 1982

Marinier R, Pihl RO, Wilford C, et al: Psychotropic drug use by women: demographic, lifestyle and personality correlates. Drug Intelligence and Clinical Pharmacy 19:40–45, 1985

McCranie EW, Horowitz AJ, Martin RM: Alleged sex-role stereotyping in the assessment of women's physical complaints: a study of general practitioners. Soc Sci Med 12:111–116, 1978

McLaney MA, Del Boca FK: Students' motivations for using alcohol and other drugs (abstract). Alcohol Clin Exp Res 15:354, 1991

Mellinger GD, Balter MB: Psychotherapeutic drugs: a current assessment of prevalence and patterns of use, in Social Medication: Conflicting Signals for Prescribers and Patients. Edited by Morgan JP, Kagan DV. Lexington, MA, Lexington Books, 1983, pp 137–154

Mellinger GD, Balter MB, Uhlenhuth EH: Prevalence and correlates of the long-term regular use of anxiolytics. JAMA 251:375–379, 1984

Mitchell WD, Thompson TL, Craig SR: Under consultation and lack of follow-up for alcohol abusers in a university hospital. Psychosomatics 27:431–433, 1986

Mogul KM: Psychological considerations in the use of psychotropic drugs with women patients. Hosp Community Psychiatry 36:1080–1085, 1985

National Institute on Drug Abuse: National household survey on drug abuse: population estimates 1992 (DHHS Publ No SMA-93-2053). Washington, DC, U.S. Government Printing Office, 1993

Nellis M: The Female Fix. New York, Houghton Mifflin, 1980

Ogur B: Long days' journey into night: women and prescription drug abuse. Women Health 11:99–115, 1986

Pariente P, Lepine JP, Lellouch J: Self-reported psychotropic drug use and associated factors in a French community sample. Psychol Med 22:181–190, 1992

Parry HJ, Balter MB, Mellinger GD, et al: National patterns of psychotherapeutic drug use. Arch Gen Psychiatry 28:769–784, 1973

Pihl RO, Murdocuh D, Lapp JE, et al: Psychotrope and alcohol use by women: one or two populations. J Clin Psychol 42:991–999, 1986

Ray O, Ksir C: Drugs, Society and Human Behavior, 5th Edition. St. Louis, MO, Mosby, 1990

Robbins C, Clayton RR: Gender-related differences in psychoactive drug use among older adults. Journal of Drug Issues 19:207–219, 1989

Robins LN, Regier DA (eds): Psychiatric Disorders in America. The Epidemiologic Catchment Area Study. New York, Free Press, 1991

Ross HE: Alcohol and drug abuse in treated alcoholics: a comparison of men and women. Alcohol Clin Exp Res 13:810–816, 1989

Ross HE, Glaser FB, Stiasny S: Sex differences in the prevalence of psychiatric disorders in patients with alcohol and drug problems. Br J Addict 83:1179–1192, 1988

Rowland N, Maynard A, Beveridge A, et al: Doctors have no time for alcohol screening. BMJ 295:95–96, 1987

Shader RI, Greenblatt DJ: Use of benzodiazepines in anxiety disorders. N Engl J Med 328:1398–1405, 1993

Sims MA: Sex and age difference in suicide rates in a Canadian province. Life-Threatening Behavior 4:139–159, 1974

Smith MC: A Social History of the Minor Tranquilizers: The Quest for Small Comfort in the Age of Anxiety. New York, Haworth, 1991

Srole L, Langner TS, Michael ST, et al: Mental Health in the Metropolis: The Midtown Manhattan Study. New York, McGraw-Hill, 1962

Taylor D: Current use of benzodiazepines in Britain, in The Benzodiazepines in Current Clinical Practice. Edited by Freeman H, Rue Y. London, Royal Society of Medicine Services, 1987, pp 13–18

Verbrugge LM: Sex differences in complaints and diagnoses. J Behav Med 3:327–355, 1980

Verbrugge LM: Sex differentials in health. Public Health Rep 97:417–437, 1982

Verbrugge LM, Steiner RP: Prescribing drugs to men and women. Health Psychol 4:79–98, 1985

Woods JH, Katz JL, Winger G: Use and abuse of benzodiazepines: issues relevant to prescribing. JAMA 260:3476–3480, 1988

Woods JH, Katz JL, Winger G: Benzodiazepines: use, abuse, and consequences. Pharmacol Rev 44:151–347, 1992

CHAPTER 16

Conclusion

Mary V. Seeman, M.D., C.M., F.R.C.P.C.

Men and women are differentiated from each other in all cultures and have been throughout history from virtually all perspectives. But are men and women essentially different? In this book, we take an essentialist position on the issue of women, men, and psychiatric illness. We conclude that real, essential gender differences do exist in the expression of psychopathology. Some may consider it reductionistic to divide human beings in a binary way, male or female, and to view psychopathology along this somewhat arbitrary dimension. It has been argued that maleness and femaleness are overlapping constructs (Harding 1986), that they do not depend on biological sex (Bleier 1991), and that bisexual or intersexual organisms exist in nature (Fausto-Sterling 1993) and are, perhaps, the rule in the human species. In humans, the initial polarization imposed by genetic sex can be readily reversed by environmental events, such as hormones, surgery, name and role assignment, didactic teaching, identification with role models, social expectation, and experiential shaping. It is currently fashionable to deconstruct the duality of man versus woman in the same way that twentieth-century moral philosophers questioned the opposition of traditional bipolar constructs such as good and bad, truth and falsehood, and selfishness and altruism. Current political events proclaim the transiency of once rigid class distinctions and of contrasting and once identifiable ideologies such as left versus right. Modern art forms illustrate the illusory quality of the dividing line that once existed between artist and patron; dramatist and audience; and author, protagonist, and reader (Foucault 1977).

Fluidity and fusion in many streams of intellectual life are not, however, currently reflected in Western psychiatric theory. Here, the trend is in the opposite direction, toward categorization, precision, and demarcation of ever more specific psychopathological syndromes. Psychiatry is experiencing a structuralist phase. The motive force behind this movement is a complex amalgam of attitudinal shifts and economic pressures that has influenced medical decision making. The scientific motive is the hope that more precise taxonomy will effect greater correspondence between a specific set of symptoms and a specific evolution of pathophysiological processes on one hand and a personal history of individual pathopsychological development on the other. The current ideal in psychiatric research is to delimit unambiguous symptom and sign sets so finely and accurately that vulnerability to their expression can be matched to unique sequencing errors in the genetic code. The further hope is that such findings could sequentially lead to understanding specific gene products, their exact cellular function, and, eventually, their regulatory mechanisms—genetic, environmental, and experiential. The ultimate hope is that such knowledge will permit effective therapeutic intervention at all levels, from the molecular to the individual, interpersonal, and societal.

This strategy, matching syndromes to gene defects, is beginning to bear fruit in the expanded understanding of many medical diseases, although it is too early to establish whether it holds promise for complex disease, especially for psychiatric disease. One may even argue with the concept that the psychopathology discussed in this book—depression, substance abuse, eating disorders, sleep disorders, somatoform disorders, and dissociative identity disorders—is related to genetically influenced disease. The antidisease argument is currently less frequently advanced for schizophrenia, although it could be, has been, and, undoubtedly, will be advanced again as medical science progresses and as changing research technology and methodology shed light on diverse aspects of causality.

While reifying the male/female dichotomy and embracing essentialism, this book deconstructs or puts aside the disease/nondisease distinction. In other words, the authors of these chapters generally espouse the view that the two sexes differ in essential ways—essential enough to influence the frequency or severity with which they express various psychiatric illnesses—but they collectively affirm a poststructuralist stance, advancing the unity of medical/social, biological/psychological, and nature/nurture perspectives on psychiatric distress. The authors are from disparate academic backgrounds: psychology, sociology, epidemiology, history, psychiatry, and psychoanalysis. A truly comprehensive view on this complex subject—gender and psychopathology—would have required contributions from anthropologists, molecular geneticists, embryologists, primatologists, endocrinologists, neuroscientists, educators, artists, pediatricians, linguists, philosophers, theologians, economists, political scientists, and many others.

We assert that psychiatric diseases are inherently multidetermined but that biological sex (genetics, anatomy, hormones) and psychosocial gender (assigned and adopted roles within family, political, and economic structures) taken together are two powerful determinants.

The facets of psychiatric disease that appear to differ between the two sexes are

- The prevalence of certain syndromes (some found more commonly in men, others in women)
- The age at onset of certain syndromes (some begin earlier in one sex than in the other)
- The character and diversity of symptoms (sometimes identical in both sexes, sometimes not)
- The course and severity of illness (sometimes more progressive and more lethal in one sex than in the other)
- The response to existing interventions (sometimes particular to one sex or the other)
- The known risk factors (often distinct in women and men)

These seeming differences must be understood so that more can be learned about each illness in order to provide more effective treatment for individuals with psychiatric disease.

One central puzzle that emerges in this book is the role of puberty.

Why, for instance, do so many psychiatric syndromes begin postpu-
bertally, and why, at puberty, do the two sexes begin to travel such
a markedly bifurcated route? For example, women develop depressions, eating disorders, somatoform disorders, and personality disorders such as dissociative identity disorder, and men progress to
schizophrenia and substance use disorders.

These observations are consistent with the theory that gender-
specific modes of responding to adversity affect the types of disorders
that emerge in reaction to various nonspecific stresses of adulthood
(Dohrenwend et al. 1992).

Gender specificity is perhaps best illustrated by the phenomenon
of depression. To qualify for a diagnosis of depression, an individual
must impart a set of subjective feelings to a diagnostician or, in the
case of epidemiological surveys, transpose those feelings into endorse-
ments of questionnaire items. In other words, symptoms must first be
acknowledged, then shared. It is well known that, regardless of how
questions are worded, women, as a group, consistently evaluate their
general physical health as poor compared with men (Verbrugge 1985).
This continues in the face of morbidity and mortality statistics that
show these subjective evaluations to be the opposite of the objective
evidence. In that context, it is not surprising that diagnostic entities
that rely on subjective symptom endorsement, such as depression,
appear to be more prevalent among women. Paradoxically, but perhaps understandably, suicide, a result of depression, occurs much
more frequently in men.

In general, behavioral manifestations of disorder, as opposed to
subjective distress, are more frequently observed in men. Diagnostic
entities that rely, in large measure, on behavioral manifestations of
disease rather than on the verbal communication of distress tend to
be more prevalent in men. This view can be best applied to substance
use disorders.

The prevalence of schizophrenia is thought to be approximately
equal in men and women but, nevertheless, manifests an age at onset
difference. Men reportedly become ill 4–6 years earlier than women.
Can this discrepancy at least be partially accounted for by the fact
that subjective appreciation of distress is impaired in this illness and
that behavioral manifestations may be necessary before a diagnosis
is made?

Women seek help for medical problems more readily than men, even when their symptoms are subjectively less severe than that of a male comparison group (Verbrugge 1985). This behavior may help to explain the apparently greater prevalence in women of somatoform disorders such as irritable bowel syndrome, chronic fatigue, and fibromyalgia. It may also shed some light on the tendency for women to receive more prescriptions for sedative medication and also on the gender ratio reported in subjectively distressing disorders such as dissociative states.

The gender ratio in eating disorders is not, however, explicable by women's greater tendency to acknowledge distress and to seek help for it. Patients with anorexia and bulimia characteristically deny discomfort and do not seek help voluntarily. Eating disorder diagnostic entities are among those based, in large part, on objective rather than on subjective criteria. Explanations grounded in developmental issues such as conflictual identification with the mothering person, the influence of gender-specific sexual abuse, and social expectations that create an unrealistic body image ideal may play a greater role.

Whatever the explanatory chain, it presupposes a gender-specific line of development beginning in early childhood. Nonetheless, before puberty, boys report greater health problems and seek more health services than girls do (Verbrugge 1985). This is also true for psychiatric health; boys have more childhood psychiatric disorders than girls do (Earls 1987). Does something happen at puberty to change disturbed boys into stoic men and well-adjusted girls into self-conscious women? The abrupt change may be more apparent than real. It may mean, simply, that mothers and female teachers bring boys to medical attention because of the boys' hard-to-manage behavior and the ensuing subjective distress experienced by their female caretakers. Girls may be distressed at young ages, but their distress may not affect their demeanor, and they may only be able to express their unhappiness to diagnosticians after they become mature enough to articulate it in medically meaningful terms.

Sex-specific vulnerabilities to specific symptoms, behaviors, and etiologically distinct illnesses, however, probably also exist. Risk factors for some psychiatric illnesses may be linked to genes on the X chromosome (Mandel et al. 1992) or to autosomal genes turned on or off under the influence of sex hormones. Contributory factors to some illnesses may be infective agents against which men and women have different immune reactions at discrete times and reproductive stages. Hypo- or hyperimmune responses to such agents may result in dimorphic symptom pictures—that is, acute respiratory illness in men versus chronic illness (fibromyalgia, chronic fatigue, insomnia) in women. This is, of course, speculation.

Depending on culture and socioeconomic status, men and women are exposed to differential physical risks (e.g., head injury) secondary to differences in lifestyle and occupation. At various ages and stages, men and women are probably also exposed to disproportionate levels of psychological stress and socioeconomic pressure and are restricted in specific ways with respect to the range and diversity of available coping strategies. Crying, screaming, engaging in sex, clinging to parental figures, swearing, drinking, seeking solitude, demanding attention, kicking a ball, spending money, lifting weights, eating to excess, avenging, confiding, confessing, and so on are all possible responses to adversity that are each sanctioned in one sex more than in the other. Subcultures place further sex-specific restrictions on permissible expressions of frustration or help seeking.

As a result of development, certain characteristics are thought to be more prevalent in one sex than in the other. Many consider empathy or the ability "to put oneself in another's shoes" to derive principally from the female experience (Jordan et al. 1991). The enhanced development of this capacity is thought to result from a process of mutual identification between mothers and daughters, each aware of and quick to validate the other's subjective state. Although this characteristic is usually considered to confer a relational advantage to women, it may act as an obstacle to successful coping in some situations. Women may be inhibited from expressing legitimate anger or exasperation because they do not want to burden another person, to disappoint or hurt another person, or to threaten the harmony of a relationship. One aspect of this phenomenon is the paradox that large social networks buffer men from stress-related disorder but aggravate the situation for women. The troubles of their friends become their troubles, so that relatively isolated women appear to cope better than those with large friendship circles. By the same token, marriage is protective of mental health for men but not for women. This may be less related to power relations within marriage and more related to the confidante role that women play. They buffer stress for their husbands and families but are consequently burdened by the confidences they elicit.

Men's jobs—more highly paid, more visible, and more competitive—are usually considered to be more stressful than women's, although this view can be challenged. Women's relative lack of authority in work situations as well as the tedium they experience in repetitive tasks and the perceived inequity of the remuneration they receive may contribute to a level of occupational stress that is equal to or greater than men's. Role conflict with respect to career and child rearing is an additional stress factor affecting women more than men. The feminine capacity for empathy and feeling the other person's pain makes women, more than men, experience guilt about leaving children or aging parents with caretakers while they devote their energy to careers.

Psychopathological differences between men and women do, and logically should, differ over the course of a lifetime. An individual's relative susceptibility to react with symptoms to a life event fluctuates over time and depends, in part, on initial endowment, on past personal experience, and on the timing of an adverse event. A destabilizing event may be borne with greater equanimity at some stages of life than at others. The large monthly hormonal fluxes that define women's experience may (although this is debatable) create a physiological central nervous system (CNS) environment that is more vulnerable to symptom formation than the more stable hormonal environment of the male CNS. Once a set of symptoms has been expressed, neural circuits used in the initial formation of these symptomatic pathways take on a life of their own and may, henceforth, be triggered by barely perceptible changes in homeostasis. This sensitization process could account for the "repetition compulsion" of symptoms, behaviors, and attitudes acknowledged to be maladaptive. The periodicity of hormonal cycles in women compared with the daily, but smaller, fluctuations in men may account for sex differences in symptomatic expression such as episodic aggression, mood variability, and impulsive acts (Halbreich et al. 1988). Although aging initiates many sexually dichotomous processes, especially with respect to physical well-being and socioeconomics, it normalizes the hormonal environment and makes certain gender contrasts less prominent than in youth.

Because so much of what happens in the course of life reverberates what occurred before and shapes not only future behavior but recollections of the past, it is impossible to know how much, if any, of the sex difference observed in psychopathology is attributable to basic differences in male and female brains. Early in fetal life, hypothalamic circuitry becomes sex specific and thereafter governs reproductive behavior. The limbic system, the seat of emotions, is demonstrably sexually dimorphic in humans, and brain pathways mediating cognition and pain sensitivity may also be dimorphic. Individual catecholaminergic neuronal loops, implicated in many psychiatric disorders, appear to be morphologically and functionally sex specific at birth (Pilgrim and Riesert 1992). This means that boys and girls begin postnatal life with subtle differences in their brains that influence their perception of the world and their responses to it. The overlapping but, as a group, sufficiently distinct responses, in turn, evoke differences in feedback from caretakers. This process progressively entrains sexually divergent behaviors and, over time, reinforces sexually divergent neuronal pathways. Each new experience is registered in the developing brain via electrical activity and neurochemical signaling. Thus, experience modifies the structure and functioning of nerve cells and can even alter the expression of genes. The distinction between biological and psychological factors is artificial because both exert their effects through the substrate of neuronal firing that leads to altered behavior and, sometimes, to psychopathology (McEwen 1991).

In conclusion, I would like to draw readers' attention to two books that cover topics similar to those in this book. One was published in 1979 and was coedited by one of the authors of this volume (Gomberg and Franks 1979); the other appeared in 1982 (Al-Issa 1982). Over the years, emphases have changed, and data gathering has become more scientific. Statistical analyses have become more complex but also more accurate. New imaging techniques have evolved and psychiatric genetics loom ever larger. Power imbalances between the sexes have come into sharper focus. In the past, sexual abuse of females was almost never mentioned as an explanation for gender differences in psychopathology. Male and female developmental tracks have received more serious attention. More psychiatric drugs are in common use, and their interactions with neurotransmitter receptors and with hormone receptors are becoming clearer. There is greater fidelity to diagnostic categories. Forgotten syndromes (chronic fatigue syndrome, dissociative states) have reemerged. Reading from a historical perspective expands our horizons and evokes our humility. The older texts constitute an excellent background from which to evaluate whatever progress has been made. In summary, there are a few new answers, but the old questions remain.

References

Al-Issa I (ed): Gender and Psychopathology. New York, Academic Press, 1982

Bleier R: Gender ideology and the brain: sex differences research, in Women and Men, New Perspectives on Gender Differences. Edited by Notman MT, Nadelson CC. Washington, DC, American Psychiatric Press, 1991, pp 63–74

Dohrenwend B, Levav I, Shrout P, et al: Socioeconomic status and psychiatric disorders: the causation-selection issue. Science 255:946–952, 1992

Earls F: Sex differences in psychiatric disorders: origins and developmental influences. Psychiatric Developments 1:1–23, 1987

Fausto-Sterling A: The five sexes. The Sciences, March/April 1993, pp 20–25

Foucault M: Language, Counter-Memory, Practice. Translated by Bouchard DF, Simon S. Edited by Bouchard DF. Ithaca, NY, Cornell University Press, 1977

Gomberg ES, Franks V (eds): Gender and Disordered Behavior: Sex Differences in Psychopathology. New York, Brunner/Mazel, 1979

Halbreich V, Holtz Alt I, Paul L: Premenstrual changes: impaired hormonal homeostasis. Endocrinol Metab Clin North Am 17:173–194, 1988

Harding S: The Science Question in Feminism. Ithaca, NY, Cornell University Press, 1986

Jordan JV, Kaplan AG, Baker Miller J, et al: Women's Growth in Connection. New York, Guilford, 1991

Mandel J-L, Monaco AP, Nelson DL, et al: Genome analysis and the human X chromosome. Science 258:103–109, 1992

McEwen BS: Sex differences in the brain: what they are and how they arise, in Women and Men, New Perspectives on Gender Differences. Edited by Notman MT, Nadelson CC. Washington, DC, American Psychiatric Press, 1991, pp 35–42

Pilgrim C, Riesert I: Differences between male and female brains—developmental mechanisms and implications. Horm Metab Res 24:353–359, 1992

Verbrugge LM: Gender and health: an update on hypotheses and evidence. J Health Soc Behav 26:156–182, 1985

Index

Page numbers printed in **boldface** *type refer to tables or figures.*